YOUR C
WEIC

HELPING WITHOUT HARMING

BIRTH THROUGH
ADOLESCENCE

ELLYN SATTER
MS RD LCSW BCD

kelcy press

MADISON, WISCONSIN

Your Child's Weight: Helping Without Harming
(Birth Through Adolescence)
Copyright © 2005 by Ellyn Satter

Kelcy Press
4226 Mandan Crescent, Suite 57
Madison, WI 53711-3062
(877)844-0857

ISBN 0-9671189-1-3

Satter, Ellyn
Your child's weight; helping without harming birth
through adolescence/Ellyn Satter
p.cm.
Includes bibliographic references and index
ISBN 0-9671189-1-3
1. Pediatrics. Nutrition and feeding of infants and children. 2. The family.
Children. Child development 3. The family. Youth. Adolescents I. Title

Printed in the U.S.

Production manager: Clio Bushland
Copyeditor: Mary Ray Worley
Layout and Cover Art: Karen Foget
Typesetting: Sherpe Advertising Art
10 9 8 7 6 5 4 3 2

Kelcy Press books are available at special discounts for bulk purchases.
For more information, please contact Kelcy press at (877)844-0857 or
see www.KelcyPress.com

Your Child's Weight is distributed to the trade by:
Publishers Group West
1700 Fourth Street
Berkeley, CA 94710
(800)788-3123
orders@pgw.com

DEDICATED
to all who parent, in the *finest* sense.
And to *all* our children.

ALSO BY ELLYN SATTER

CHILD OF MINE:
Feeding with Love and Good Sense

SECRETS OF FEEDING A HEALTHY FAMILY

HOW TO GET YOUR KID TO EAT...
BUT NOT TOO MUCH

ELLYN SATTER'S FEEDING IN PRIMARY CARE
PREGNANCY THROUGH PRESCHOOL:
Easy-to-Read Reproducible Masters

ELLYN SATTER'S NUTRITION AND FEEDING FOR
INFANTS AND CHILDREN:
Handout Masters

ELLYN SATTER'S FEEDING WITH
LOVE AND GOOD SENSE:
Video and Teacher's Guide

Ellyn Satter's
Montana FEEDING RELATIONSHIP
Training Package

CONTENTS

   Emphasize *providing*, not *depriving*. Trying to get children to
   eat less or move more in the name of weight control backfires. It makes them preoccupied with food, inclined to move
   less when they get the chance, and prone to gain too much
   weight.

   Follow Ellyn Satter's Division of Responsibility in Feeding.
   Feed well, parent well, and accept your child's natural size
   and shape. Your child needs to be able to trust you to *provide;*

you need to trust him to *eat* and *grow*.

9. **Teach Your Child: Be All You Can Be** 291
Love your child the way she is and teach her to be capable,
including loving her body. Stowing your agenda about your
child's size and shape opens the door to your parenting her
well and feeling good about her.

10. **Understand Your Child's Growth** 323
Growth charts provide a snapshot of your child's physical,
nutritional, emotional, and developmental health. Most of
your child's growth depends on genetics. To protect against
interference, understand growth charts.

Appendixes 383
  A. Position Statement: Eating Management to Prevent and
     Treat Child Overweight
  B. Satter Feeding Dynamics Approach: Child Weight
     Management
  C. Children and Food Regulation: The Research
  D. Cooking in a Hurry
  E. Assessment of Feeding/Growth Problems
  F. Treatment of Feeding/Growth Problems
  G. Feeding and Parenting in the School Setting
  H. Development of Physical Self-Esteem: Birth Through
     Adolescence
  I. Health Risks of Child Overweight
  J. Dairy Products, Bone Health, and Weight Management
  K. Books and Resources by Ellyn Satter
  L. Order blank

FIGURES

STORIES ABOUT CHILDREN

PREFACE

 I see the problem from both
ends. I train other health professionals to teach and support
positive feeding and parenting. They tell me how much trouble
parents today have feeding their children and feeding themselves. I also treat the casualties—children and adults whose
eating and weight struggles are so pressing that they become
engulfing and life-limiting. One informs the other. Defining
optimum feeding and parenting illuminates what has gone
wrong for those who struggle. Treating those who struggle
emphasizes how desperately important it is to do things right
in the first place.

Your Child's Weight: Helping Without Harming is about doing
things right in the first place. It is about good parenting—about
doing an excellent job with respect to feeding and physical
activity and letting your child grow up to get the body that is
right for her. Doing your job means your child does not have to
worry about eating and weight. The two little girls on the cover

capture what I want for your child—they are happy and having fun, they know they will be provided for, and weight could not be further from their minds. That is as it should be.

Your Child's Weight: Helping Without Harming is about *providing,* not about *depriving*. If your goal is to have a slim child and you are looking for the magic diet and ready to do whatever it takes to achieve that, this is *not* the book for you. On the other hand, if you are willing to stow your agenda about your child's size and shape, shoulder your responsibilities with respect to feeding and parenting, and raise your child to get the body that is right for her, read on. If, in fact, like a lot of parents you were reluctant to pick this book up because you dread even entertaining the *thought* that your child might have a weight problem, with all the misery that entails, then this *is* the book for you.

Your instincts are good. It's amazing you still have them, because the pressure on today's parents to deprive children of food and try to force their weight down is simply enormous. Current attitudes and approaches blame children and parents for a child's fatness and promise cures that we can't deliver. Such approaches lead parents to believe that children are fat because they eat too much and exercise too little and that children can become slim if they eat less and exercise more. In taking these approaches, we set parents and children up for disappointment and unnecessary self-blame.

We health professionals have done the same to ourselves. In encouraging parents and children to try for weight loss, we administer programs we don't believe in and accept outcomes that leave us feeling discouraged and dishonest.

The truth of the matter is that you can do everything just "right" and your child may still grow up to be relatively fat. However, you must reassure yourself—and him—that his size and shape are normal for him. Moreover, he will be thinner than had you struggled with him about his weight. Being thin is not the most important thing for your child. Most important is knowing you love him and accept him for being just who he is—thin or fat, tall or short. To give him that, you simply *can't* get caught in the pursuit of thinness.

However, not restricting your child's food intake doesn't

mean you do nothing at all. In *Your Child's Weight* I will teach you Ellyn Satter's Division of Responsibility in Feeding: The parent is responsible for *what, when,* and *where;* the child for *how much* and *whether.* Following the division of responsibility in feeding throughout your child's growing-up years means that you will have roughly 18 years, *per child,* of good parenting with respect to food. That's a *lot,* and it won't be easy.

The division of responsibility in feeding is not for sissies. Doing an excellent job of feeding your child will put you decidedly out of step with what goes on around you. As a society, we are abominable about feeding ourselves, only marginally better about feeding our children, and obsessed with weight. Whether we know it or not, in being so offhand about eating, we *scare* ourselves and we scare our children. To feed well, you must make an absolute priority of providing food for yourself and your family. Family meals are key to that providing—and to parenting. To maintain that priority, you have to discard the norms: being casual and ad-lib about eating, grazing, feeding children rather than eating with them, eating on the run. And you have to do it over the long haul.

It won't be easy for you to do your part with respect to feeding, and it won't be easy to trust your child to do her part with *eating.* To accept her eating and weight, you will have to resist your own misgivings as well as the interference from the many who will urge you to *do something* about your relatively large (or even average) or enthusiastically eating child. You could hardly ask for a more destructive backdrop for raising your child to be competent with respect to eating and growth.

This book teaches you to go beyond that destructive backdrop and do an excellent job of feeding and parenting. The theme is *helping without harming.* While my message is fundamentally different from what you ordinarily hear, it is sound. It is based on my long clinical practice and is tested by the research evidence. You will learn about both throughout.

A minor theme in *Your Child's Weight: Helping Without Harming* is doing treatment. You and your child will need treatment if his weight veers abruptly up or down, if you worry a lot about his weight, or if you have repeated struggles that you just can't resolve on your own. The treatment segments show you—and show readers who are health professionals—what treatment based on feeding dynamics looks like.

There are many who helped develop and refine the Satter Feeding Dynamics-Based Approach to Child Overweight. I am thinking of my colleagues who are committed to the model, of the parents who resist societal norms and the conventional wisdom to act on behalf of their children, of the researchers who ask the right questions and tell the truth about their results, and of the program planners and policy makers who predicate their thinking on accepting children and helping them make the most of what nature has provided them. You will hear about many of those people as we go along in *Your Child's Weight: Helping Without Harming*.

I would particularly like to thank the Ellyn Satter Institute Consultants Ines Anchondo, R.D., L.D., C.S.P., M.P.H.; Edie Applegate, M.S., R.D., L.D., C.D.E.; Clio Bushland, M.S.; Pam Estes, M.S., R.D., C.D.; Elizabeth Jackson, M.S., R.D.; Lisa Modesti, R.D., C.D.E.; and Patty Nell Morse, R.D., C.D.E. These creative, committed, and caring women think and present and challenge and reach out to parents and professionals in every way they can think of. I am most grateful to the content readers, who criticized, suggested, questioned, and reorganized: Paul Bushland; Harsha Bhagtani, M.D.; Nancy Crassweller, M.S.; Forence Deza, M.D.; Barbara Lohse, Ph.D., R.D.; James G. McGuire M.D., F.A.A.P.; Ann Merritt, M.S., R.D., L.D.; Jennifer Motl, R.D.; Sallie Rixey, M.D., Me.D.; Lora Stratton, R.N., B.Sc.N.; and Carol Walsh, M.S., R.D., C.D., L.D.E.

I celebrate my book-production team: Clio Bushland, ingenious production manager; Karen Foget, designer extraordinaire; Howard Sherpe, stalwart and resourceful typesetter; and Mary Ray Worley, acute and committed copyeditor.

The alert reader will note that Clio Bushland's name appears on most all the lists. Clio is my very-important-right-hand-woman who does it all: sounding board, reader, production manager, computer maven—the list goes on. I depend on her more than I can say.

Not the least, I thank my children and grandchildren, who live fully, and my friends who do the same. They make life rich.

EATING...
is more than deciding
what and how much to eat.
FEEDING...
is more than choosing food
and getting it into a child.
EATING AND FEEDING...
reflect people's histories,
their relationships with themselves
and with others.
Feeding a child
is about the connection
between parent and child,
about trusting or controlling,
about providing or neglecting,
about accepting or rejecting.
Eating
is about the connection
with our bodies
and with life itself.
Eating can be joyful,
full of zest and vitality.
Or it can be fearful,
bound by control and avoidance.
My mission
is to help children and adults
be joyful and capable
with eating.

-Ellyn Satter

CHAPTER
1
HELP WITHOUT
HARMING

The mother was getting more and more impatient with me, and I didn't blame her. Her disgusted expression told me all too clearly that the hour she and her 9-year-old son had spent in my clinical dietitian's office had been anything but helpful. The doctor had sent them to see me with the vague notation "weight problem." The boy, I will call him Sean*, was chubby, and he looked *miserable*. He slumped in his chair, staring at the floor and occasionally casting sidelong and wary glances at his mother.

I was trying my best to address the issue at hand without doing any *more* damage to that unhappy little boy. So I talked about the Basic Four Food Plan. This was 30 years ago, *long*

---

* Mrs. Thompson's and Sean's names, and possibly their genders, have been changed to protect their privacy. With the exception of stories about my own children, the other children and their parents whose stories are told in *Your Child's Weight* have been disguised as well.

before the Food Guide Pyramid was ever created. And I talked about meal planning and about having fruits and vegetables and about portion sizes and about nutritious snacks. All the while, I watched Sean out of the corner of my eye, hoping he would perk up at something I said. Truth be told, I didn't know *what* I was driving at, but I *did* know that nothing good would come of sending that little boy out of my office feeling so worthless.

I thought I was being tactful and indirect. I very carefully avoided *any* euphemism or double-talk that would say to him, "You are too fat—don't eat so much." I didn't say a *word* about food restriction or following a diet. I stayed strictly on the topics of choosing healthy food and planning nutritious meals. I was only fooling myself. Mrs. Thompson decoded my message, and it made her angry: "He is too fat. Don't feed him so much." Sean decoded it as well, and it made him feel ashamed: "You are too fat, don't eat so much."

Finally, Mrs. Thompson had had enough of my nutritional guidelines. "I am already doing all that!" she snapped. "And look at him! He is still fat! I have another one at home who is too thin, and I am trying to make *him* eat *more*. How am I supposed to make one eat *less* and the other one eat *more*?"

Silence. After what seemed like a *long* time, I gathered my wits together and blurted (some of my best answers have been blurted), "It's not your job to control how much they eat! *Your* job is to put meals and snacks on the table. *Their* job is to decide how much to eat!"

Mrs. Thompson looked even more furious. Sean straightened up, heaved a big sigh that I took to be relief, sat back in his chair, and looked at me for the first time all day. "Good grief," I thought. "What was that? What *did* I just say? Is that really *true*?" But it was better than anything else I had said that day, so I let it stand. I have since discovered that it *is* true, but I wish I had *also* reassured that frustrated mother: "You don't have to make it your job to determine how their bodies turn out. That is up to nature, and to them."

Mrs. Thompson had every right to be angry with me. I was being critical. Based on Sean's appearance, I was making the judgment that she wasn't doing a good job of feeding him. Not only that, I was asking her to do the impossible—to get Sean thin.

I *could* have given her a diet, but I wasn't willing to do that. I had started raising my own children, and they taught me about the importance of the feeding relationship. Their joyful response to food, their intuitive capabilities with eating, and my own satisfaction in feeding them was so rewarding and *right*. My youngest was chubby and *loved* to eat, and I loved feeding him. I often reflected, "I am so glad I don't feel the need to restrict him. It would spoil this."

I was fifteen years into my career by then and had been down a *lot* of blind alleys. I had tried all the direct and indirect ways of restricting children's food intake that are still in vogue today: limiting portion sizes, emphasizing low-calorie foods like fruits and vegetables, cutting fat and sugar down to the minimum. I even learned behavioral modification and taught that to parents as an indirect way of limiting calories. Nothing worked. I thought for a long time that my approaches were flawed, but I know now that for the pediatric population, as for the adult population, significant and sustained weight loss is virtually nonexistent.[1]

To my credit, I did follow up, and I learned from my mistakes. I found that no matter what form it took, restricting a child's food intake was destructive to the feeding relationship and to parent-child relationships overall. Parents became police officers, the "overweight" child became an irritable food bandit, and siblings became spying tattle-tales. Worst of all, telling a child, directly or indirectly, "You are too fat, and you must eat less" made him feel bad all over. The process made parents feel bad as well. No loving parent deliberately hurts a child by saying to him, "You are not all right the way you are." But buying into the perception that their child was too fat and making efforts to slim him down did just that.

It began to dawn on me that the children I worked with got *fatter*, not *thinner*. The food-preoccupied child was prone to overeat when he got the chance and therefore was likely to gain excessive weight.

I didn't do follow-up with the Thompsons—I didn't feel I had taught them anything that was *worth* following up on. I was in clinical limbo. I was finding out what *not* to do, but I wasn't yet entirely clear on what *to* do.

WHAT TO DO INSTEAD

Figuring out what *to* do took a long time. It sent me back to graduate school to become a family therapist. I read *stacks* of research articles and discovered researchers who were thinking along the same lines I was. I studied child development and clarified what needs to happen at each stage of a child's life in order to support the child's normal growth and development-with eating and in all other ways. I practiced family therapy, and psychotherapy, looking for a bridge between the child's emotional functioning and his eating and weight.

Sean and Mrs. Thompson stayed in the back of my mind as I worked in detail with many other families. As the complexity of the problem became ever more apparent, I learned not to give *answers*, as I had so high-handedly attempted with the Thompsons, but to ask *questions*. Through it all, these were my guiding principles:

- *The answers lie in the child.*
- *Whatever I do, it must not hurt the child.*

About 10 years after that unhappy pair left my befuddled presence, I had figured out what to do. In a nutshell, my solution was this:

- *Feed well.*
- *Trust the child to eat as much as he or she needs.*
- *Let the child have the body that nature intended.*

I have written about this solution before—in journal articles,[2-5] in both the original and revised versions of *Child of Mine: Feeding with Love and Good Sense*, and in *How to Get Your Kid to Eat . . . But Not Too Much*. I have taught my principles and this solution in many workshops and have trained many professionals. The principles are in appendix A, "Position Statement: Eating Management to Prevent and Treat Child Overweight," and the solution is in appendix B, "Satter Feeding Dynamics Approach: Child Weight Management."

For a while, it seemed that the child care world was ready to focus on feeding well, trusting children to eat well, and letting children have bodies that reflected their genetic endowments. However, the current concern about child overweight has made that practical and wellness-based approach seem inadequate. Today's parents and clinicians are too upset and confused about the topic of child overweight to consider feeding and parenting well and supporting normal growth and development to be an adequate solution. They feel that children can no longer be trusted to eat as much as they need.

If that is indeed the case—that children can't be trusted to eat and grow well—it has more to do with lack of *support* than lack of *capability*. The norms of appropriate *feeding* have eroded. The dedication to family meals that Mrs. Thompson and her age-mates took for granted is no longer a given. Lacking the family meal as a focal point, child feeding at all ages and stages has become distorted. The norm has become casual feeding on the one hand and, on the other, food restriction and avoidance in the name of health and weight control. As I commented in the preface, "As a society, we are abominable about feeding ourselves, only marginally better about feeding our children, and obsessed with weight."

If raising children today seems hard, it is because it *is* hard. To a greater extent than parents 30 years ago, today's parents struggle to provide for themselves and for their children. Money is tighter, parents work longer hours, extended families are even more dispersed, the overstressed health care system falls even shorter of guiding and teaching good parenting and feeding, and social supports for families have eroded more and more. Today's parents raise children in a world they didn't grow up in, with opportunities and dangers far different from those of even a generation ago. Those changes leave parents uncertain about how to take an effective leadership role with their children. Values have changed as well. Today's parents have difficulty making children their priority. Jobs, money, social advancement, the trappings of wealth and power—all compete in importance with raising children. Society and culture come into this as well, because parents are *not* encouraged to make better choices on behalf of their children.

Little wonder that today's children are anxious. In fact, research shows that the average American child in the 1980s exhibited more anxiety than child psychiatric patients in the 1950s.[6]

The emphasis in the media and health care world on the "epidemic" of child overweight contributes to parents' dilemmas. As I did with Mrs. Thompson, however indirectly, health professionals are telling parents today, "Your child is too fat—don't feed him so much." Such a judgment makes parents hesitant to provide and undermines to an even greater extent their confidence in feeding their children. In the flutter of solutions to the "epidemic," I see clinicians, policy makers, program planners, researchers, and even legislators making the same mistakes and doing the same harm that I did 30 years ago. Moreover, they are doing it in a far more public and far-reaching way, with far less opportunity to do damage control. Those "solutions" put even more pressure on today's parents and distort feeding to an even greater extent.

All of this leads me to my conclusion:

• Today's crisis is *not* one of child overweight.
• It is a crisis of *parenting* and *feeding*.

ADDRESS FEEDING AND PARENTING

How do we address the issue of children and weight and at the same time make a contribution to resolving that larger crisis of *parenting* and *feeding*? By doing an excellent job with feeding. *Your Child's Weight: Helping Without Harming* is as much about *parenting* as it is about *feeding*. Feeding embodies your entire relationship with your child. In this book you will learn to maintain the division of responsibility in feeding, which will support you in keeping your priorities straight, define your role with your child, help you understand him, and guide you in doing good parenting from the time he is born until he leaves home. Differentiating your job of *feeding* from your child's job of *eating* provides a concrete example of sorting out control issues in other areas as well. Knowing when to take leadership and when to let go is the essence of good parenting.

Sean and Mrs. Thompson Do-Over

To illustrate, let's turn back to Sean and his mother. If they were to appear in my office today, what would I do differently? To begin, I would find out for sure whether there actually *was* a problem. I would review Sean's growth records before I met with him and his mother. In that earlier session, I hadn't seen the clinical record. It had missed the shuttle from the satellite clinic, and I did not have the information I needed to help them. All I could do was look at Sean—yes, he *was* chubby. I could try to decipher the physician's cryptic referral: *weight problem*. But that deciphering would have been unlikely to have done any good, because the doctor was likely as unclear—and as reluctant to do harm—as I was. I could take my cue from what I *thought* was the mother's conviction: *Sean was too fat.*

On the other hand, examining Sean's growth chart—a graphic representation of his body weight over time*—would tell me whether his chubbiness was normal or abnormal *for him.* If he had grown along a consistent percentile on his growth chart, *even if that percentile was high,* there *was* no weight problem. His weight was normal *for him.* He was just a large and rather chubby-looking child. One task would still need to be done, however. That task would be to support his *continued* normal growth and development. I would explain the growth chart to Sean and his mother and point out that he was growing consistently and well—he was just a relatively large boy.

In contrast to that earlier session, I would emphasize feeding dynamics, *not* food selection. I *would* discuss food selection briefly, but it would be for the purpose of providing a backdrop and support for the feeding relationship. I would find out how

---

* Growth charts graph children's weights or heights against their age and classify them by percentiles. I will explain a little more in chapter 2, "Feed and Parent in the Best Way," and a lot more in chapter 10, "Understand Your Child's Growth."

Sean was fed—whether the family had regular meals, if Sean was allowed to have snacks, if he was allowed to graze. I would find out what food the family ate, but the purpose would be to allow me to *support,* not *criticize.* I would bend over backward to avoid saying *anything* that would undermine Mrs. Thompson's ability to get meals on the table.

Then I would turn to the feeding relationship. Based on Sean's consistent growth, I would congratulate his mother on doing a good job of feeding. I would congratulate *Sean* on doing a good job of eating and growing. I would teach them the division of responsibility in feeding:

- Parents are responsible for the *what, when,* and *where* of *feeding.*
- Children are responsible for the *how much* and *whether* of *eating.*

Then I would work with them to distinguish Mrs. Thompson's *feeding* jobs from Sean's *eating* jobs. As she so indignantly pointed out to me, Sean's mother *was* doing a good job of feeding. However, growing out of her own concerns about Sean's weight and interference from people like me, she was likely intruding on Sean's prerogatives of *what* and *how much* to eat. She had done all she could, and she needed to stop interfering. Instead, Sean needed her trust—trust that he would eat the amount he needed to grow in the way nature intended for him to grow.

Then I would emphasize to both Mrs. Thompson and Sean that they needed to protect themselves from *interference.* There are many people who would look at Sean's chubby appearance, criticize his weight, and expect them both to do *something* to make him thinner. They both needed to ignore that interference and trust that Sean would eat the right amount to continue to grow in the commendable way that he was. Ironically, I would try to immunize them both against the very thing I had done to them in that original session.

Distinguish Between Consistent and Accelerating Weight
I would have taken a different approach if, on the other hand,

Sean's weight was *inconsistent*—if it was accelerating and crossing percentiles on his growth chart. However, even when a child is relatively heavy, or gaining weight rapidly, I do *not* ask, "How do I get this child to lose weight?" Instead, I ask, "What is happening in this child's life to distort his ability to grow predictably?" That question is based on an absolutely fundamental principle: *It is normal for each child to eat and move in a way that allows him to grow predictably in accordance with his genetic endowment.* If he does not, then *something is the matter.* My job as a clinician is to find out what is the matter.

Answering that question requires time and investigation. I would offer to collaborate in that investigation with Mrs. Thompson. If she didn't want to investigate further, we would be back to the principles I just described: Feed well, trust Sean to eat as much as he needs, let him have the body that nature intended, avoid interference. The growth chart would likely show evidence to support that approach. In reviewing lots of growth charts, my colleagues and I have found that a child's weight often starts to accelerate right after the imposition of food restriction and attempts at weight loss.

Establishing and maintaining the division of responsibility in feeding is a powerful intervention, one that will stabilize the child's weight. That is, it will stop his weight from accelerating and let it go back to moving consistently along his normal growth curve. However, I have found that some parents and their health professionals have difficulty settling for such a straightforward and unglamourous approach. Surely, they feel, there is more to it than that. In their skepticism, they don't quite bring it off. They might be able to do their jobs of *feeding,* but they can't quite trust their child to do his job of *eating.* Often unconsciously, they continue to interfere—emphasize "healthy" food, hold back on portions, push fruits and vegetables, cut out treats, give a child a *look* if he seems to eat too much. The child knows it is all code for "You are too fat—don't eat so much." Even if he tries to restrict *himself,* the child can't help but periodically overeat. His weight continues to accelerate, and the intervention "fails."

What does it take for parents to buy in to the division of

responsibility in feeding and to *truly* trust the child to do his part with eating? They must have a satisfactory answer to a single *key* question. *What is undermining this child's ability to grow in a way that is right for him?* Until that question is answered to their satisfaction, parents continue to see the child as a chronic overeater with a strong tendency to gain too much weight. Consciously or unconsciously, they continue to try to compensate for their child's seeming inability to regulate his eating by directly or indirectly restricting his food intake. The child consequently loses his ability to regulate, gets fatter and fatter, and grows up seeing himself as a glutton.

IDENTIFY DISTORTIONS

This is the critical question: What is undermining this child's ability to grow in a way that is right for her?* It is a question about *feeding dynamics,* not about *food selection.* Embedded in the question is a fundamental principle: It is normal for children to grow normally. Based on their internal regulators of hunger, appetite, and fullness, children are excellent at eating the amount they need. Based on their natural energy levels and inclination to be active, children have a strong drive to move in a way that is right for them. Children are such good regulators that they intuitively eat more or less depending on their growth rate, activity, and the amount of calories in their food. They even make up for errors in regulation. If they overeat for whatever reason—they are offered exceptionally tasty food, or they are overly hungry—they compensate for that overeating by not getting hungry as soon or by eating less the next time.

Based on their natural levels of eating and activity, children have a powerful and resilient tendency to grow consistently and predictably, in the way nature intended them to grow. It takes a *lot* to disrupt that regulatory ability to the extent that it

---

* You will have noted a switch from *he* to *she.* When I'm not referring to a specific individual child, I have addressed the ever-awkward *he-she* pronoun dilemma by using both *he* and *she* intermittently in this chapter and in chapter 7, "Optimize Feeding: Your Adolescent." The other chapters use only one pronoun or the other.

distorts growth. Moreover, those disruptive factors have to be *powerful* and *continuous*. Being offered too much fat or too few fruits and vegetables won't do it. Being offered too-large portion sizes won't do it. Going to fast-food restaurants won't do it. What will do it? Distortions in the feeding relationship.

From that careful framing of the question grows a clear course of action for *one child at time:* to identify the disruptions that are making *this child* gain too much weight. Throughout the course of my career, with many families, I have done the careful sleuthing to answer that question. The answer is different for each child and each family. I have found that generally a child's weight accelerates because of one or a combination of typical disruptive factors such as these:

- Misinterpretation of normal growth
- Restrained feeding
- Poor feeding practices
- Stress

Misinterpretation of Normal Growth

Often the child is naturally large. Her growth charts show that she has been growing at a consistently high level from infancy. The weight dilemma grew out of an overzealous diagnosis of overweight. That diagnosis labeled as *abnormal* the child's *normal* growth, precipitated the recommendation to lose weight, and initiated interference with her eating. In other words, her "weight problem" was in the eyes of the diagnostician. That faulty diagnosis, in turn, created the weight problem.

There is a word for this incorrect labeling: *iatrogenic*. According to Merriam-Webster, an *iatrogenic condition* is a malady "induced by a physician—used chiefly of ailments induced in a patient by autosuggestion [self-suggestion] based on a physician's words or actions during examination." The physician said the child is too fat, and therefore she was perceived— by herself and others—as being too fat.

Physicians aren't the only ones who apply the overweight label and set off the train of events that disrupt the child's normal growth. Other professionals do it as well. So do parents, extended families, neighbors, and society in general. Sometimes the child isn't even large but is simply the child of heavy parents and therefore is perceived as being "at risk" of becoming overweight.

Restrained Feeding

If indeed there has been weight acceleration, I most often find the cause to be restrained feeding. The child's food intake has been restricted, she has been pressured about her eating and, in consequence, her weight gain has accelerated. The growth chart tells the story—weight gain accelerates shortly after the onset of restrained feeding. Prior to food restriction, her growth was likely to have been consistent—she demonstrated her ability to regulate food intake. She may have grown at a constitutionally high level from birth, but sometimes her weight was even at or near average. Overzealous health professionals or parents restrict for the misguided purpose of heading off obesity. An average child of heavy parents might have become the target of this interference.

Food restriction is only one of the circumstances that make children afraid of going hungry. Erratic and unpredictable feeding—being casual about providing family meals and structured snacks—mimic restrained feeding. It makes children gain too much weight for the same reasons. The child doesn't know for sure that she will get fed, and as a consequence, she becomes food-preoccupied and prone to overeat when she gets the chance. Sometimes there is plenty of money and no one taking time to provide food. Other times, there simply isn't enough money to buy food.

The research literature lends clear support for my clinical observations. Parents who worry about their children's weight and try to get or keep them thinner tend to raise fatter children.[7,8] Preschoolers in a group setting whose parents overcontrolled their eating were poor at stopping eating when they were full.[9] Five-year-old girls who qualified for the "at-risk for overweight" designation showed significantly higher levels of restraint, disinhibition, weight concern, body dissatisfaction, and greater weight acceleration by age 9 years than girls whose weight was lower.[10] When parents severely restricted access to "forbidden" foods, their school-age daughters were more likely to eat in the absence of hunger and be fatter as well as to feel ashamed of themselves for eating.[11] Girls who dieted during high school were fatter by graduation than those who did not diet.[12]

Poor Feeding Practices

Of course, restrained feeding is a poor feeding practice. However, in this section, I am focusing on additional inappropriate feeding practices. Often, as a result of inaccurate advice or their concern about their child, parents make errors in feeding. If those errors persist, the child's weight gain accelerates because the distortions in feeding undermine her ability to eat the amount she needs to grow consistently. The problems create stress around feeding, and that stress undermines the child's natural ability to eat the amount she needs to grow well.

For instance, parents of a relatively large—or small—infant may try to get her to eat less—or more—food than she wants, and so feeding becomes nerve-racking and unsatisfying for everyone. Parents may start solid foods too early or too forcefully, and parents and child consequently become embroiled in extreme and prolonged struggles around eating. Other parents may misinterpret the toddler's erratic and unpredictable eating behavior as food refusal and get pushy, or they may cater to the child, who then learns to use eating to manipulate her parents. Parents may overestimate the self-reliance of the preschooler, school-age child, or teenager and stop providing the support of family meals. The children then become overwhelmed, not knowing how to feed themselves.

In many cases, health professionals contribute to those errors in feeding by making poor feeding recommendations. Often the errors are those of omission—health professionals do not teach parents recommended feeding practices. Professionals also often let moderate problems slide until they became *severe* problems—failing to ask questions that would identify and resolve problems early.

Again, there is support in the research for my clinical observations. A California study that followed almost 300 children from age 6 months to 16$^1/_2$ years found that children who later became fat were more likely to have had feeding problems and to have been fed in a less structured fashion when they were young. The problems were with poor feeding practices, not food selection. Children who later became fat ate no more calories, no more low-nutrient-density or sweet foods. They were no more likely to have been bottle-fed, were started no earlier on solid foods, and were no more likely to have been given high-fat milk than children who remained slim.[8] A Scottish follow-up study showed that children who had suffered from leukemia when they were young became fatter in later life.[13] While researchers looked for physiological explanations, I think of feeding dynamics. Growing out of their legitimate concern for their child, parents have likely tried to override the child's treatment-induced poor appetite and therefore gotten into struggles around feeding. Ongoing research at Children's Medical Center in Washington, D.C., clearly links feeding errors to children's difficulties in eating the right amount to grow well.[14]

Stress

Stress appears to make a child gain too much weight in a two-step process. First, restrained feeding or other poor feeding practices teach the child to eat for emotional reasons. Later on, the child experiences extreme stress and intuitively acts out by overeating and gaining weight.

A child learns to eat for emotional reasons when parents regularly and consistently use food to deal with feelings—to diffuse, soothe, or entertain. This error in learning generally takes place somewhere in the first 4 years and is most strongly put in place with the toddler. To learn to tolerate and express her anger, sadness, boredom, and other negative feelings, the toddler depends on parents to accept those feelings and apply appropriate solutions. The parent tolerates the child's anger, accepts her sadness, redirects her boredom. Regularly using food to soothe or distract the toddler teaches her to use food for emotional reasons. Then, if and when the child enters a period of unusual stress, she reacts by demanding food. Depending on the severity of the stress, her food demands can become so extreme that she gains too much weight.

What about the research? A study in Buffalo, New York, showed that children exposed to experimental stress who had been fed in a restrained fashion ate more; those who had not been restrained ate less.[15] A large Danish study showed that children who showed evidence of neglect tended to be fatter.[16] Lack of structure stresses children, and there is considerable evidence that structure around feeding is eroding. Parents wait for food requests before they feed their toddler, as well as short-order cooking for her.[17] Letting young children eat on the run is increasingly the trend,[18] and family meals are decreasing in frequency.[19]

PHYSICAL ACTIVITY

The same patterns and distortions I describe with respect to feeding apply to children and activity as well. Defining a child as being too fat makes her move less because it makes her feel her body is bad. Rather than being natural and spontaneous about moving and playing, the child holds back and becomes self-conscious. Pressure to be more active as a way of slimming a child down takes away her natural love of movement and makes activity into a *chore*. Defining a child as being too fat blunts the child's natural creativity, growth, and development with respect to physical movement by making her feel anxious. Stress affects activity as well. Depressed children often become indolent. Anxious children become guarded in all ways, including movement.

FEED AND PARENT WELL, THEN TRUST

From studying the distortions in feeding and parenting that make children gain too much weight, I have learned the critical importance of doing things right in the first place. In *Your Child's Weight: Helping Without Harming*, I will teach you to do an excellent job of feeding from the time your child is born until she leaves home. What it all boils down to is this: *Feed and parent well, accept your child's size and shape, and avoid interference.*

Maintain the Division of Responsibility in Feeding

Children *are* capable, and they *can* be trusted. If you parent well with respect to feeding and activity, even your large child will eat and grow in a way that is right for her. Even your large child is entitled to depend on you to do your feeding jobs and then to be trusted to do her eating—and growing—jobs. Even your large child is entitled to go to the table hungry, eat until she is satisfied, and then stop, knowing another meal or snack is coming and she can do it again. Even your large child is entitled to be unconscious and unconcerned about it all, free from worry about eating, moving, and weight.

Chapter 2, "Feed and Parent in the Best Way" outlines in detail the division of responsibility in feeding by defining your feeding tasks and your child's eating capabilities. Chapter 3, "Make Family Meals a Priority," expands on your task of providing consistent and reliable family meals. It lays out the importance of family meals for your child's social, emotional, intellectual, and nutritional development and gives strategies for orchestrating and maintaining family meals.

Avoid Food Restriction in *Any* Form
In chapter 4, "Help Without Harming: Food Selection," I do my level best to focus on food selection without taking the fun out of eating or sending you on guilt trip. It isn't easy. Restrained eating and deprivation are so deeply embedded in our societal attitudes toward food and eating that I often find that even my most benign messages take on a restrictive spin when others hear them. I have worked hard to be clear and positive with my advice regarding food selection. My take on food selection boils down to this: "Choose the foods you like; be knowledgeable and reliable about providing for your family."

However, what I *say* is less important that what you *hear*. If my recommendations make you feel guilty about including the foods you enjoy in your meals and snacks, modify the recommendations. I depend on *you* to decode my messages. To clarify your own understanding, consider *intent*. Are my food selection recommendations *intended* to make your child eat less and weigh less? I know they are *not*, but if you decode them that way, you need to modify my recommendations to fit *you*. Are your decisions about food selection *intended* to make your child eat less and weigh less? If the answer is *yes*, it is restrained feeding and you need to lighten up.

Also consider your child's eating behavior. If your decisions about food selection make her food-preoccupied and prone to overeat when she gets the chance, feeding is restrained.

Optimize Feeding: Birth Through Adolescence

The way you apply the division of responsibility in feeding for an infant is different from the way you do it for a teenager, although the principles remain the same. You do your jobs, on the one hand, and trust your child to do hers, on the other. Chapter 5, "Optimize Feeding: Birth Through Preschool," chapter 6, "Optimize Feeding: Your School-Age Child," and chapter 7, "Optimize Feeding: Your Adolescent," focus on child development as it applies to feeding throughout the growing-up years.

Maintain the Division of Responsibility with Respect to Physical Activity

Children are born loving their bodies, curious about them, inclined to move, and driven to be as physically competent as they can possibly be. Good parenting with respect to children's physical activity preserves those qualities throughout the growing-up years. Parents provide *structure, safety,* and *opportunities.* Children choose *how much* and *whether* to move and the *manner* of moving. Chapter 8, "Parent in the Best Way: Physical Activity," focuses on your child's development in the arena of physical activity, with the goal of preserving her positive attitudes about her body and her joy in moving. Joyful activity is sustainable.

Even your large child is entitled to like her body and must be trusted to find ways of moving it that are right for her. As with eating, falling prey to agendas will undermine your child's normal growth and development. Resist current attitudes that say, "Well, diet doesn't seem to work to slim children down, but surely activity will." Such attitudes will turn you into a personal trainer rather than a parent, encouraging, cheerleading, nagging, and even coercing your child to *move* in the name of weight control.

Consider Your *Whole* Child

Chapter 9, "Teach Your Child: Be All You Can Be," encourages you to accept your child the way she is and raise her to be capable. Most people see child overweight as a *physical* and *health* issue. You know better. Labeling your child as *overweight* and taking steps to control her weight, whether direct or indirect, make her feel flawed and inferior in *all* ways. You do *not* have to define your child as defective and try to change her natural body. Instead, put your efforts into parenting and feeding well and feeling good about her. Help your child develop in ways that *really* matter: good character, common sense, effective ways of responding to feelings, problem-solving skills, and the ability to get along with others. Children who are relatively fat, like children with other characteristics that make them distinct, need better-than-average social skills in order to succeed.

Distinguish Between Normal Fatness and Excess Weight Gain
Current health policy labels as many as one in seven children overweight or "at risk of overweight."[20] Accepting such a diagnosis for your large child puts pressure on you and pressure on your feeding relationship with your child. Chapter 10, "Understand Your Child's Growth," helps you protect you and your child from those pressures by illustrating the contradiction between health policy standards and the principles of normal growth and development. On the other hand, if your child's weight is *accelerating* and rapidly crossing growth percentile curves, her growth may be distorted. Understanding growth charts will help you to recognize that divergence early, promptly correct problems in feeding and parenting, and let your child go back to growing predictably.

DOES THE FEEDING DYNAMICS APPROACH *WORK*?
My audiences ask me, "Does the feeding dynamics approach *work*?" The answer depends on what they mean by "work." Does it *work* to support normal growth and development? Yes it does. I will be discussing lots of research and clinical observations that demonstrate that point.

Does the feeding dynamics approach *work* to correct disruptions in feeding and parenting and thereby set right your child's too-rapid weight gain? Yes it does, provided you can *truly* establish the positive feeding dynamics I teach in *Your Child's Weight*. Does the feeding dynamics approach *work* to keep your child's weight down to a certain level or get her to lose weight? No, it does not. Defined weight outcome is absolutely contradictory to my principles and approach. Keep in mind that even ambitious, multidisciplinary weight-management programs don't "work" to produce long-term weight loss either. They produce modest weight loss, and that loss is almost without exception regained on follow-up. Moreover, these conventional approaches undermine growth and development. They deprive parents of nurturing and children of *being* nurtured.

Striving for weight loss does harm. It hurts your child, and it hurts you. For your child, getting enough to eat is basic to getting her needs met. For you, giving your child enough to eat is fundamental to nurturing. You don't have to go there. Instead, do the best job of feeding and parenting that you possibly can, and accept your child, just the way she is.

NOTES

1. Epstein et al., "Treatment of Pediatric Obesity."
2. Satter, "Childhood Eating Disorders."
3. Satter, "The Feeding Relationship."
4. Satter, "Internal Regulation."
5. Satter, "Moderate View on Fat Restriction"
6. Twenge, "The Age of Anxiety?"
7. Birch and Fisher, "Mother's Child-Feeding Practices."
8. Crawford and Shapiro, "How Obesity Develops."
9. Johnson and Birch, "Parents' and Children's Adiposity."
10. Shunk and Birch, "Girls at Risk for Overweight."
11. Birch, Fisher, and Davison, "Learning to Overeat."
12. Stice et al., Naturalistic Weight-Reduction Efforts."
13. Reilly et al., "Premature Adiposity."
14. Chatoor, "Feeding Disorders."
15. Roemmich, Wright, and Epstein, "Dietary Restraint."
16. Lissau and Sorensen, "Parental Neglect."
17. Skinner et al., "Mealtime Communication Patterns."
18. Jahns, Siega-Riz, and Popkin, "Increasing Prevalence of Snacking."
19. Eisenberg et al., "Correlations Between Family Meals and Psychosocial."
20. Barlow and Dietz, "Obesity Evaluation and Treatment."

ELLYN SATTER'S DIVISION OF RESPONSIBILITY IN FEEDING

Parents provide *structure, support,* and *opportunities.* Children choose *how much* and *whether* to eat from what the parents provide.

The Division of Responsibility for Infants:
• The parent is responsible for *what*
• The child is responsible for *how much* (and everything else).

The parent helps the infant to be calm and organized and feeds smoothly, paying attention to information coming from the baby about timing, tempo, frequency, and amounts.

The Division of Responsibility for Toddlers Through Adolescents:
• The parent is responsible for *what, when, where*
• The child is responsible for *how much* and whether

The Parents' Feeding Jobs:
• Choose and prepare the food.
• Provide regular meals and snacks.
• Make eating times pleasant.
• Show children what they have to learn about food and meal-time behavior.
• Do not let children graze for food or beverages between meals and snack times.
• Let children grow up to get bodies that are right for them.

Fundamental to parents' jobs is trusting children to decide *how much* and *whether* to eat. If parents do their jobs with respect to *feeding,* children do their jobs with respect to *eating.*

Children's Eating Jobs:
• Children will eat.
• They will eat the amount they need.
• They will eat an increasing variety of food.
• They will grow predictably.
• They will learn to behave well at the table.

CHAPTER
2
FEED AND PARENT
IN THE BEST WAY

To raise your child to have the body that is right for him, make eating and feeding positive, rewarding, and important. *How* you feed is far more important than *what* you feed in terms of allowing your child to grow appropriately. While *what* you feed is certainly important for nutritional health, child weight problems are *behavioral* problems. You cannot solve behavioral problems by focusing on food selection.

Where your child's body weight is concerned, helping without harming requires good parenting and a positive relationship between you and your child. Restrictive feeding practices, supervising and controlling your child's eating and activity in the name of weight control, and making size and shape your central focus by their very nature are destructive. They involve negative parenting, damage the parent-child relationship, and hurt your child's feelings about himself and other people. In the long run, such approaches will make your child fatter, not thinner.

TWO CHILDREN WHOSE PARENTS MADE A DIFFERENCE

At age 17, Dan was well over six feet tall. He had slimmed down a *lot* from when he was younger. He was about normal weight and was pear-shaped and looked kind of soft. That is a typical body type for many men. Dan looked good, he was dressed nicely, and he seemed to feel good about himself. His mother told me that his eating and weight were not big concerns for him or the family.

It could easily have turned out otherwise. Dan had been chubby throughout his growing-up years. His parents worried about him, and his mother confided how hard it was to hold steady. "I take him for one of our very rare ice cream cones, and I know others are looking at us and saying, 'why is she giving that overweight child ice cream? No wonder he is so heavy!'" But Dan's parents thickened their skins. They were consistent about carrying out their feeding responsibilities and letting Dan be responsible for his eating. They also gave him opportunities to be active, and then they waited to see what happened with his size and shape. Their approach took real courage, but it paid off.

With Mary and her mother, however, it was another story. According to family legend, Mary's doctor warned her mother that if she allowed 6-month-old Mary to remain "obese" that Mary would "develop too many fat cells that would forever want to be filled up" and therefore she would be fat for life.* From that day forward, Mary's mother set out to slim Mary down. She was successful, if you can call underfeeding an infant "successful." Take a look at Mary's growth chart in figure 2.1, on page 25.

Between birth and 5 months, Mary grew predictably and well. She was weighed each time she went for a health check, and her weight was plotted against her age on a growth chart like the one pictured in figure 2.1. Her data points followed right along the top curve for growth, the one labeled 97. Her

---

* The doctor was talking about Hirsch's fat cell theory of obesity, popular in the late 1970s and periodically revived ever since. Hirsch may have been right about *fat cells,* but he was wrong about *people.* Fat babies are no more likely to become fat adults than are thin ones.

weight *tracked,* which was good and meant she was growing well. Plotting along that top curve meant Mary was a relatively big girl—she was heavier than 97 percent of other girls her age. I will explain growth charts in detail in chapter 10, "Understand Your Child's Growth."

However, Mary's doctor didn't understand that her consistently high weight data meant she was growing well. He thought her large size meant that she was too fat. As a conse-

FIGURE 2.1 MARY WEIGHT-FOR-AGE BIRTH TO 24 MONTHS

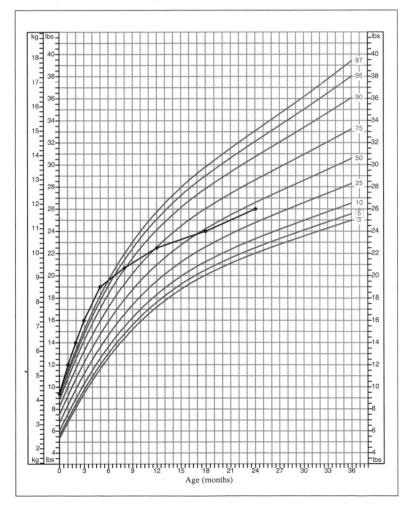

quence, he encouraged her parents to limit her food intake to get her weight down. Her parents did just that, and between age 6 and 18 months, Mary's weight fell off dramatically. Her relatively high weight fell to average—from above the 97th percentile to the 50th percentile. In other words, Mary's weight was about 20 percent lower than it would have been had she continued to grow in her own natural way. Think of it! Twenty percent is a *lot* of weight! Mary was growing *very* poorly.

Mary's parents continued their vigilance until Mary was 10 years old. As you can see in figure 2.2, during that time, Mary's weight went up a bit, but it continued to plot right along the 75th percentile. When Mary was 10 years old, a crisis erupted in the family. Her father left the family, and her mother was depressed and overwhelmed. At that point, Mary's mother not only stopped restricting her, but stopped *feeding* her as well. Those events were disastrous for Mary emotionally, and the place her distress showed the most was in her weight. After years of food restriction, Mary had long since lost track of her internal regulators of hunger, appetite, and satisfaction. When her mother's external controls were gone, Mary was left with no controls at all.

Mary ate until she could hold no more, and over the next two years she gained a considerable amount of weight. In her struggles to regain control, Mary went to Weight Watchers, lost a lot of weight, then immediately gained it back. As Mary put it, "The minute I hit bottom I started eating again." Then Mary turned to purging as a way of managing her overeating. I met her when she was 19 years old, and by that time she was bulimic.

Strikingly, after food restriction was lifted, when Mary was between 10 and 12 years old, her weight rose to the 97th percentile and leveled off. That was just where it had been between birth and age 6 months. It appeared that the 97th percentile may have been where her weight belonged all along. On the other hand, most relatively fat infants and toddlers slim down. Restricting Mary's food intake may have deprived her of that natural slimming process.

Disastrous as the eating and weight issues were for Mary, they were the least of her troubles. Worse by *far* was the impact on her emotional welfare. In depriving her of food and making her be slimmer, Mary's mother inadvertently deprived Mary of *nurturing* and taught her that she was flawed. That certainly wasn't her mother's intent—she was doing what she thought was best for Mary. In telling this story, I do not want to in any way point the finger at Mary's mother and say she was bad. She was acting on the best advice she had. But nurturing with

FIGURE 2.2 MARY WEIGHT-FOR-AGE 2 TO 19 YEARS

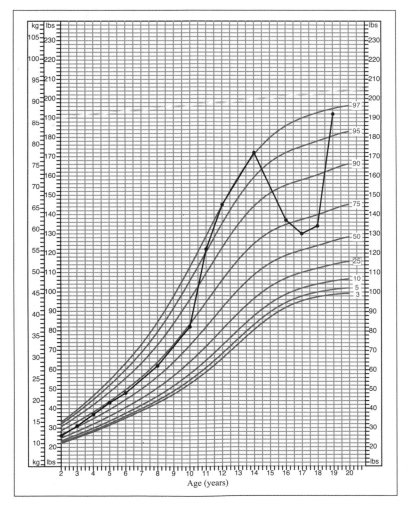

food is absolutely synonymous with nurturing overall. You can't withhold one without withholding the other. Moreover, children don't distinguish between flaws in *weight* and flaws in *themselves*. As far as Mary was concerned, her mother was dissatisfied with *her*.

It is generally recognized that overweight children score low not only on physical self-perception but on overall self-worth.[1] What is less well recognized, however, is that it isn't the child's weight per se that makes the overweight child feel bad about himself and causes him to be socially handicapped. The injury is in the parents' *attitude* toward the child and his weight.

Researchers at Pennsylvania State University found that 5-year-old girls whose weight was at the 85th percentile or above felt particularly bad about themselves if their parents were *concerned* about their being overweight. Their self-regard was even more impaired if parents restricted food intake. Compared with other 5-year-olds whose parents were concerned—*even those who weighed the same*—restricted girls didn't feel as good about their bodies, didn't think they were as smart, and didn't feel they had as much physical ability. Again, these results were independent of the girls' actual weight.[2]

The moral of the story? Children who are perceived as being too fat and whose food intake is restricted will suffer emotional harm and be subject to periods of overeating and weight gain throughout life.

Feeding: Helping Without Harming
In contrast to Mary's mother, Dan's parents kept their nerve and did a good job of feeding and parenting throughout his growing-up years. Dan grew up to be a competent eater and developed the body that was right for him. Mary's mother was too restrictive with feeding, and Mary grew up to be incompetent with her eating. Mary was afraid she wouldn't get enough to eat and had lost touch with her internal regulators.

Your child knows how much he needs to eat. He has powerful sensations of hunger and satisfaction. He has a powerful sense of appetite—he is tuned in to tastes, smells, and textures of food, and part of his sense of satisfaction is feeling pleasure from eating. To retain his eating abilities, he depends on you to do a good job of feeding. Your job is to find the middle ground with regard to feeding—to be supportive without being controlling; to give autonomy without being neglectful. As with all other issues in parenting, it is much harder to find the middle ground than to go to the extremes.

To find that middle ground, you must trust your child to grow in the way that nature intended for him to grow. Despite his current size and shape, he may grow up to be tall or short, fat or thin, big or little. Children generally slim down as they grow up. The fat infant, toddler, or preschooler is no more likely to grow up to be fat than is the thin one. In fact, it isn't until a child is 9 to 13 years old, depending on the study you read, that the likelihood of his remaining fat in later life pulls even with his likelihood of slimming down.[3] Despite the conviction that leaving childhood slim guarantees slimness for life, most overweight adults were not overweight as children.[4] In fact, only about 10 percent of obese men in a large study in England were obese at age 11.[5]

But your child can't do the job of growing up to be a competent eater and to have the body that is right for him all by himself. You have to help him. He can eat appropriately and grow in the way nature intended for him only if you do a good job of feeding throughout his growing-up years. That applies to you the parent as well as to the other grown-ups in your child's life. Notice I said *feeding*. As I have said before, feeding is *providing*. It is not *restricting*. Restricting hurts both emotionally and physically and in the long run will make your child fatter, not thinner.

FEEDING DEMANDS THE DIVISION OF RESPONSIBILITY
You do not have to restrict your child as Mary's mother did. Instead, do your jobs of feeding and parenting, let your child do his jobs of eating and growing, and support him by accepting the body that nature has given him.

In chapter 1, "Help Without Harming," I introduced you to Ellyn Satter's Division of Responsibility in Feeding. Here we will discuss the topic in more detail.

Feeding requires a division of responsibility between you

and your child. In infancy, the division of responsibility in feeding is simple:

- You are responsible for *what.*
- Your child is responsible for *how much* (and everything else).

At first, you get to decide only whether to breastfeed or bottle-feed and what goes into the bottle. Your job is to guide feeding based on information coming from your child: How often, how much, how fast, at what level of skill. Pay attention to your child's nonverbal messages about food, sleep, and comfort; follow his lead; and do your best to keep him comfortable and happy. This is far easier said than done, as I will explain in chapter 5, "Optimize Feeding: Birth Through Preschool."

However, don't try to keep your *toddler* comfortable and happy, or neither of you will get your needs met. He will become a tyrant, and you will become his slave. Give your toddler room to explore along with structure and limits. Work hard to find this balance, because the patterns you establish now will continue throughout your child's growing-up years.

For toddlers and older children, the division of responsibility in feeding becomes more detailed:

- You are responsible for *what, when,* and *where.*
- Your child is responsible for *how much* and *whether.**

You are responsible for *feeding;* your child is responsible for *eating.* Your job involves determining structure, location, and food selection. Rather than continuing to feed on demand, institute structured sit-down snacks to allow your toddler to come to meals hungry but not famished and ready to explore the food there. Then let your child—now and always—decide how much and whether to eat of the food you have made available. You must trust your child to do his jobs of eating once you have done yours of feeding.

---

* Or, as my colleague Edie Applegate puts it, *if at all.*

Beware of Counterfeits

Before we go on, a word about nutrition politics. For the first time, in *Your Child's Weight,* I am putting my name on the division of responsibility. I am labeling it Ellyn Satter's Division of Responsibility in Feeding. I don't like doing it—it feels self-important and doesn't roll off the tongue. I also realize it will be off-putting for some readers. But because protecting the basic integrity of the division of responsibility in feeding is so important, I am doing it anyway.

Many who base their work on the division of responsibility in feeding understand it thoroughly and apply it as I intended. Others straddle the fence—they try to have it both ways. They recite the division of responsibility on the one hand, and then interfere with the child's eating on the other. Rather than trusting the child to eat as much or as little as he wants from what the parent has provided, they emphasize "healthy" food, recommend portion sizes, push fruits and vegetables, and teach fat restriction.

Such contradictory messages destroy the power of the division of responsibility. As I said in chapter 1, parents know that such recommendations are code for "He is too fat—don't let him eat so much." Even if parents miss it, the child *certainly* knows that such recommendations mean "You are too fat—don't eat so much." Parents then restrict the child's eating, consciously or unconsciously. Even if he *tries* to hold himself back, the underfed child becomes food-preoccupied and overeats. His weight continues to accelerate, and the intervention "fails." Even more seriously, parents attempting to act on such contradictory messages trust sometimes and take away trust others. That inconsistency leaves the child not knowing *what* to expect and is worse for him than sticking with one or the other.

A child can be a capable eater only when his grown-ups do their jobs, and then *truly* trust him to know what and how much to eat. No cheating, no fingers crossed, and no sneaky, indirect ways of holding down food intake. To make the division of responsibility *work,* adults *have* to be conscientious both about doing their tasks with feeding and about *not interfering* with children's prerogatives.

Changing "choose and prepare food" to "choose and prepare *healthy* food," as some do, changes the intent. Given society's obsession with food restriction and body weight, the word *healthy* decodes as "don't eat so much, and don't eat what you like." I don't *want* to put in the word *healthy*. I don't *want* my message decoded in this way. I *intend* for you to choose food *you* like, prepared the way *you* like it, not food *I* like or food somebody else thinks you *should* be eating. I intend for you and your child to eat until you are satisfied. I can even live with your off days when meals turn out to be nutritionally worthless. As far as children are concerned—and the rest of us, for that matter—structure and reliability are most important. Even the most reprehensible family meal is better than no meal at all.

My point is to warn you to be alert when you read handouts or look for helpers. Don't be taken in by information and advice that takes away your trust in your child's ability to eat as much as he needs. Consider *intent*. If the *intent* is to make your child eat less and weigh less, it is restrained feeding. In the long run, restrained feeding will undermine your child's ability to eat the amount he needs to grow predictably and well. It is *definitely* not Ellyn Satter's Division of Responsibility in Feeding.

The Division of Responsibility Applies to the School-Age and Teenage Child
The division of responsibility in feeding still applies during the school-age and adolescent years. When he is older, your child still depends on you to take primary responsibility for the *what, when,* and *where* of feeding. School-age and teenage children do best in all ways when they have regular family meals. If you have fed well through the preschool years, your school-age and teenage child will be good at regulating his food intake and sneaking up on new food and learning to like it. He will still be capable of intuitively managing the *how much* and *whether* of eating.

Gradually, during his school-age and teenage years, your child will learn to manage the *what, when,* and *where* for himself. Your role is coach: You dole out tasks and responsibility as he is able to manage them. As a school-age child, he chooses his after-school snack from what you make available and sees to it that he eats it right after school so he doesn't spoil his dinner. He chooses his school lunch and decides what to eat at friends' houses and what to buy at the convenience store to serve as his afternoon snack. As an adolescent, he gains more and more skills with food selection, planning, shopping, and cooking. His food management will become fully independent after he learns to do for himself what you have done for him. That will be when he is grown and ready to leave home.

At all stages of development, the principles of parenting with respect to feeding are absolutely the same as the principles of parenting in general. You respect your child and trust that he wants to please you and grow up to be all he can be. You identify your jobs, are faithful about executing them, and distinguish your jobs from your child's jobs. You are clear about the tasks your child needs to master, and you give privileges and autonomy as he becomes skilled and responsible. You identify your own needs and are clear and firm about meeting them.

YOUR JOB OF FEEDING
What does your job of feeding involve? You must provide food, make eating times pleasant and predictable, and show your child what it means to grow up with respect to eating. Then you must trust him—to eat what he needs and as much as he needs and to grow in the way that is right for him.

Choose and Prepare Food
You are the one who knows the most about food, nutrition, and menu planning. Your child is growing up to be at *your* table and to learn to eat the food *you* eat. That's the way it works. Someday he will have his own table, and then he can decide. Your child will do best with eating when you take appropriate leadership with food management, set up the structure, and then give him choices within that structure.

Your child is taking over your job of choosing food if you ask what he wants for dinner, short-order cook for him, restrict the menu to foods he readily accepts, or get up from the table to make substitutes. Current product marketing teaches you to cater to your children. It promotes the idea that children need their own special foods, like expensive pre-packaged lunches or green ketchup, advertises kid-friendly foods that "your child will love," and plants the idea that pickiness and food refusal is normal behavior that you are obligated to work around. Not only that, but advertising promotes mutiny in your offspring by teaching them to pester you for particular foods and particular brands. Ignore it all.

Provided that you do your jobs with respect to feeding—*including and particularly maintaining structure*—your child will do an adequate job of eating the amount he needs to grow appropriately. You can easily learn meal- and snack-planning principles. When applying the principles, don't try for perfect. Your child does not need the perfect diet in order to keep from becoming overweight. Conventional wisdom says otherwise— it assumes that we are fat because we eat the wrong food and that if we eat the right food we will be slim. You know what we are supposed to do—eat less fat and sugar, eat more fruits and vegetables, avoid the "toxic foods" we all know and love, avoid the "evil" fast-food franchises that overwhelm us with big portion sizes of the toxic food that we know and love. It is all very dreary.

The term *toxic foods* is a spin on the older term *junk foods— large portions* of high-fat, high-sugar, low-nutrient foods. Those foods and portions may overwhelm *us adults* because our regu- latory ability has been tarnished by life experience and our almost-continual efforts to eat less and less-appealing foods than we really want. But until we interfere, children are such good regulators that they do not have to be served a steady diet of nutritious low-calorie food in order for them to eat the right amount. High in fat or sugar? They eat less. Mostly low-calorie food? They look around for something else to fill up on. Big portion sizes? They eat until they get full and leave the rest.

A longitudinal study in the San Francisco Bay Area in California followed children from age 6 months to 16^1/$_2$ years. There were no differences in food selection between children who became overweight and those who remained slim. When compared with the others, the overweight children

- Ate no more calories
- Ate no more low-nutrient-density, high-fat, or high-sugar foods
- Were no more likely to have been formula-fed
- Were started no earlier on solid foods
- Were no more likely to have been given high-fat milk

While there appeared to be no differences in *what* the children were fed, there were differences in *how* they were fed. The histories of children who later became fat showed evidence of poor feeding practices. Feeding was less structured, parents were more likely to have worried about their fatness, and the children were more likely to have had feeding problems when they were younger.[6]

Plan meals around foods that *you* enjoy. Otherwise you will disinhibit: eat for virtue, then throw away the rules, and sneak for pleasure. Think of the foods you sneak off to eat, and then include them in meals: potato chips with the sandwiches, cookies or candy for dessert. We will focus on food selection in chapter 4, "Help Without Harming: Food Selection." If you need more help with meal planning, shopping, and cooking, read *Secrets of Feeding a Healthy Family.*

Lest we misunderstand each other, let us have a word about nutrition. There are those who feel I am flippant about nutrition and that in my writing and presentations I imply that "anything goes." I do take nutrition seriously, and I do expose people to the possibilities with food. What I *don't* do is deliver a lot of *shoulds* and *oughts.* I have found in my clinical work that supporting people in becoming positive and reliable about taking care of themselves with respect to food *absolutely* depends on honoring what they like and enjoy. I would not call that "anything goes," because I find that people generally do better nutritionally than they think they do. Most of the time, my task is helping them to realize that.

People eat what they like and what is rewarding to them.[7] People feel that going by the nutrition rules takes all the fun out of eating.[8] Putting people on a guilt trip about what they *should* eat acts as a barrier to eating consistently and well. Is there anyone in our culture who doesn't know that fruits and vegetables are good for them? Will still-again reciting the admonition to eat fruits and vegetables make a difference? Unlikely. But feeling obligated to eat them will make eating a chore, and *that* will undermine family meals.

In my experience, people do pretty well nutritionally when they honor their food preferences and are consistent about feeding themselves. They also learn and grow with respect to eating a variety of nutritious foods. That is as natural a process for adults as it is for children.

Provide Regular Meals and Snacks

If I had to settle for one piece of advice to give you about preventing child overweight, I would say, "have meals." Family meals are essential. From your child's birth, you are working toward including him at family meals. Once established, family meals are your cornerstone for parenting and feeding throughout your child's growing-up years.

Because you provide the structure of regular meals and sit-down snacks, your child will go to the table hungry, take an interest in the food there, and eat until he is satisfied. Then he will stop, knowing that there is another meal or snack coming when he can do it again. If you don't understand how empowering this can be, try it yourself.

Don't let your child graze for food or beverages—except water—between meal- and snack times. That includes even nutritious foods like crackers and cheese and fruit and nutritious beverages like juice and milk. Why not let him graze? Let me count the ways:

1. Grazing makes it harder for your child to eat the right amount (more about this later).
2. It makes him less interested in the nutritious food at meal- and snack time.
3. It makes him behave poorly at meals. Hungry children *eat* and therefore behave well.
4. It takes away his chance for the emotional and social learning at family meals.

5. Too-frequent consumption of even nutritious food can rot his teeth.

6. It is hard on the vacuum cleaner.

Make Eating Times Pleasant

Children (and the rest of us) need a positive emotional climate to do their best with eating. What one essential ingredient does your child need to have a pleasant meal? You! More than anything else, your child wants you to take an interest in him. Keep your child company, make easygoing conversation, help him get served, enjoy your own meal, then let him rise to the occasion. Don't nag, prompt, or bribe him to eat. Don't play games or cheerlead. Even when your child is a preschooler, school-age child, or adolescent and seems independent, he benefits from your companionship and attention at mealtime.

Your child will always do more and dare more with respect to eating if you are there. He will learn to behave well at mealtime and be braver about trying new foods. Being there is enough. Pressure doesn't work. Rewards and cheerleading don't work. Shaming doesn't work. Reasoning doesn't work. Giving lessons about nutrition doesn't work. What works? The presence of a trusted adult who doesn't interfere with what or how much your child eats.[9]

Turn off the television set and put down the toys, books, and games. Pay attention to your child. He needs to have his emotional needs met in order to do a good job of eating, and as far as he is concerned, *you* are the most important thing at the table. Don't make eating compete with other activities that are less important. If your child is distracted, he won't tune in on his feelings of hunger and fullness and may over- or undereat. The same holds true for *you* with *your* eating. Remember, the key word is *pleasant*. Family meals won't fix negative relationships, and they won't help your child if they are unpleasant. Don't use family mealtimes to scold, fight, or bring up negative topics. If mealtime is unpleasant and you can't fix it, seek help. It is that important.

Beyond the clear advantage to your relationship with your child, what do pleasant family mealtimes have to do with weight? To do well with eating, children need to have their emotional needs met. Otherwise, they may learn to eat more to try to take care of those needs, or eat less because they are listless and lonely.

Provide Mastery Expectations

Provided you do your job of feeding, your child will master eating at each stage along the way. Just as your child wants to eat, he wants to learn to eat more and more grown-up food in more and more grown-up ways. With the food and feeding situations you offer, you show him what *grown-up* is all about. You offer the nipple when he can cuddle and suck, semisolid food and then finger food when his mouth and fingers are ready, and table food when he can manage it.

As children get older, their table manners mature and they become more and more a part of the sociability of the family. The family table gives your child a mastery expectation. It says, "I know you can learn to behave nicely here and learn to eat this food." He will learn as fast as he can, in whatever way he can. You don't have to force him. Learning, growing, and mastering is what children *do*. Your child can learn to make conversation at mealtimes, and he can learn to listen while others talk. Dinnertime is a good time for family check-in. When he is small, you can have the "best and worst" ritual—telling the others at the table the best thing that happened to me today, and the worst. That helps your child learn to think about his day and bring a topic of conversation to the table that others might enjoy.

Pay attention to your child, but don't let him always be the center of attention. People actively participate by listening to others talk as well. Children can learn a lot by listening to grown-ups talk, as long as they aren't excluded or ignored.

Let Your Child Grow Up to Get the Body That Is Right for Him

Every child has within him the genetic blueprint for growth. Most of his size and shape grows out of that blueprint—it dictates whether he grows to be big or little, fat or slim, tall or short. Your child's internal signals of hunger and fullness, his natural inclination to move, and his body type are all intricately balanced, unique for him, and orchestrated to support his blueprint. Moreover, that orchestration is in dynamic equilibrium with the environment. Some days are hot, some cold. Some days he's active, some not. Some days a lot of luscious food is available, others it isn't. Provided you do your feeding jobs, he can compensate for it all.

It takes a great deal to overwhelm a child's growth tendency. Errors in feeding have to be repeated meal after meal, day after day, year after year in order to distort your child's growth. Otherwise, your child will simply compensate. In my clinical practice, I work with the casualties of such consistently poor feeding. The mother of one of my adult patients—I will call him Wesley—was a horrible cook, loaded up his plate when he was small with food he found revolting, and insisted he eat it all. He did. In the process, Wesley learned to put himself on automatic pilot. He tuned out his sensations of hunger, fullness, and pleasure and ate until he could eat no more. As an adult, he continued that pattern of mindlessly eating until he was stuffed, and he became obese.

We all make errors in feeding and parenting. The most successful parents detect their errors by being sensitive to their child's distress. Wesley's mother adhered to her agenda even though what she was doing made him miserable. Distorting a child's weight is possible only with that kind of determination and insensitivity. Accepting a weight agenda—or any agenda—for your child will make you parent in hurtful ways. If you worry about your child's weight, it is tempting to do *something* about it, if only to relieve your own anxiety. In doing something about it, you are more likely to bring about the very thing you want to avoid. Studies show that parents who worry about children's weight and try to get or keep them thinner raise fatter children.[6,10]

Resist weight agendas. Keep your nerve with respect to feeding, and let your child grow in the way nature intended. You may as well, because even the most ingenious schemes for manipulating energy intake and activity and forcing down body weight are but a drop in the bucket compared with your child's ability to regulate and grow. Ironically, the most notable outcome of such schemes is to cause *increases* in weight, not decreases.

TRUST YOUR CHILD'S EATING CAPABILITIES

After teaching him to overeat, Wesley's mother had the audacity to criticize him for being overweight. She was a tremendously controlling person, untroubled by contradictions in her own behavior. Control issues can make or break you. In any relationship, but particularly with respect to feeding your child, you must sort out the nebulous issue of control. Start with this: You make your choices and give your child his choices. If he wants his after-school snack, he must eat it right away when he gets home from school. If he is in a hurry to play and can't take time to eat, then he won't get to eat again until dinnertime. It is up to him. You say what you will do; there is a time you will offer food, a time you won't. Then he can choose to eat—or not.

The division of responsibility in feeding sorts out control issues. You can control only your feeding jobs. You can't control your child's eating jobs. This division of responsibility is *not* laissez-faire. You *must* hold the middle ground between being controlling on the one hand and throwing away all structure and limits on the other. Compared with a weight-loss regimen in which you get your child to eat certain amounts or types of food, holding the middle ground and trusting your child's eating capabilities may seem puny—tame—bland—unimpressive. Not so. Holding steady requires a leap of faith, steady nerves, and endurance. You have to hold steady for *decades*. I don't find that tame, bland, and unimpressive. I find it heroic.

To be capable with respect to eating, your child depends on you to do your feeding jobs. As she busied herself with her new baby, Tina's mother boasted to the home health worker about her 3-year-old daughter's independence. "She goes right to the refrigerator and gets what she needs," she enthused. "I don't even have to cook for her anymore." Tina's mother didn't know how important she was to Tina. The health worker knew—Tina had gained an extra 15 pounds in the last six months—moving her from the 97th percentile to way off the weight chart.

Without her mother's help, Tina was anxious and trying to relieve her anxiety with food. Maybe she was trying to grow up fast so she could be the big girl her mother thought she was. The story has a happy ending. With the health worker's encouragement, Tina's mother went back to providing for her, and Tina's weight leveled off.

Your child needs your support, but you must offer it without becoming controlling. Again, it is a matter of finding the middle ground. If you try to get your child to eat certain amounts or types of food, he will feel overwhelmed, put off, and rebellious. He may get caught up in a struggle for control that makes him lose track of his hunger, appetite, and satisfaction. He will defy you and undereat or comply and overeat. Either way, he will make errors in energy intake and weight regulation.

Your Child Wants to Eat

Children have built in to them the will to survive and the drive to eat. Even the sickest baby wants to eat and live. That drive can be blunted, but not obliterated—and it takes a lot to blunt the drive. Children's drive to eat is inborn, right along with their need to imitate their grown-ups. Your child wants to eat because he sees *you* eating.

If your child appears *not* to want to eat, don't ask, "How can I get him to eat?" Instead ask, "Why not?" What is going on that makes it appear that he won't eat? You may be too pushy. You are most likely to be too pushy in feeding if your child is small, was prematurely born, has grown poorly, or has been ill. You are to be forgiven for that, and you have lots of company. It's natural to try to help out however you can. But such help backfires. Children who are pressured eat less well, not better.

On the other hand, sometimes children eat poorly because they don't get enough support: The food isn't right for them, they don't get exposed to a variety of food, or parents don't give companionship at eating times. Sometimes parents do both at the same time. Researchers in the Western Massachusetts growth study observed that parents provided preschoolers structured meals and snacks. However, at those structured times they dictated what and how much children ate. Between times, children were allowed to graze—to help themselves with no limits to the refrigerator and cupboards.[11] The implications of this mixed-up approach to feeding, nurturing, and child development are grave. Children love their parents and depend on their presence to do more and dare more with eating—to push themselves along to learn and grow. However, when the Massachusetts parents were around, they spoiled eating by being controlling. To eat without interference, children had to go off on their own. What were the children learning? That to be your own person, you have to be by yourself.

What does this have to do with weight? We have already made the connection with errors in feeding and errors in food regulation. Here we will single out the topic of early childhood vulnerability. Because they are ill or small or seem to need help, children who seem fragile are often pushed to eat.[12] Those same children often get fat in later life. Why? Because their ability to regulate food intake—to tune in on and respond appropriately to hunger, appetite, and satisfaction—has been undermined.

Your Child Knows How Much to Eat
In our control-based culture, letting go and trusting your child to do his eating jobs is not easy. Trying to do it partway won't work either. Each child grows in the often surprising way nature intended for him. Your child was born with internal regulators adapted to his own physical requirements. He may be a relatively hungry child with a high energy need. Or he may have a relatively small appetite and not require much food to keep him going. Whether he needs a lot or a little, he knows instinctively how much he needs.

If you do your job—no more and no less—your child will automatically eat the right amount of food to grow and be as active as is right for him. Provided you don't try to control what and how much he eats—again, of what *you* have put before him—he can even overeat or undereat at times and still make up for these mistakes in food intake. He doesn't have to think about this process or use his willpower. His instinctive regulators of hunger and fullness even things out for him. As I said before, children can even regulate so-called toxic foods if parents do their feeding jobs.

Almost without exception, a child who is a "compulsive eater" or acts like he has no stopping place is not sure he is going to be fed. His grown-ups might be casual and unreliable about feeding him, may not have enough money to buy food, or may deliberately restrict his food intake to get or keep him slim. The child gets free access to food sometimes, but not knowing when those times will be, he eats as much as he can whenever he can. Those children tend to get fatter. The research backs up my observations. In the Framingham Children's Study, 9- and 10-year-old children were fatter when they were restricted sometimes and given free rein other times.[13] When mothers restricted, 9- and 10-year-old daughters were more likely to eat in the absence of hunger and be fatter.[14]

The process works the other way as well. In my clinical practice, I have frequently found that early struggles to get a child to eat more than he wants is the culprit in a school-age or teenage weight problem. Having a small, thin child with a small appetite may make parents into food pushers, catering, enticing, persuading, and even forcing him to eat. Children who have food pushed on them generally become turned off by food and are likely to undereat when they get the chance. Others give in to the pressure, ignore their feelings of hunger and fullness, and overeat and gain too much weight. Children who recover from childhood leukemia often gain too much weight in later life, probably as a result of struggles to get them to eat when they were having chemotherapy.[12]

Many parents restrict by forbidding their child to eat high-calorie "treat" foods. In a Pennsylvania study, school-age girls were first fed to make sure they weren't hungry. Then they were allowed to eat "forbidden" foods. The restricted girls ate more forbidden foods than did girls who were allowed to eat them regularly. Moreover, the deprived girls felt bad because they knew they were going against their parents' wishes.[15] It was as if the girls struggled with two people inside of them—the one who wanted to eat and the one who didn't. Such struggles undermine internal food regulation processes.

Chapter 4, "Help Without Harming: Food Selection," will focus on strategies for incorporating treat foods so they don't become forbidden. For now, here are a few suggestions:

- Serve chips with mealtime sandwiches every week or so. Make sure to have enough so each person gets his fill.
- Limit mealtime desserts to one serving each so dessert doesn't compete with other food.
- At snack time, every week or so, offer milk and a plate of cookies. Let your child eat as many cookies as he wants. At first he will eat a lot, but the newness will wear off and he won't eat so many. Have cookies and milk frequently enough to keep them from being a big deal.

The connection between food restriction and body weight is clear. Food-deprived children eat what they can, when they can, and they are likely to overeat and gain too much weight. In the world of eating disorders, this pattern is called *restraint and disinhibition*. While few of us are eating-disordered, negative and restrictive eating attitudes and behaviors are the norm in our culture. Since no one can restrict forever, people have to have ways of escaping. They take guilty pleasure in high-fat or high-sugar food, buy ice cream with no conscious intention of eating it, and embrace supersize portions as a market-condoned escape from deprivation. In brief, almost everyone has a greater or lesser pattern of restraint and disinhibition. We alternate between trying to eat less or less-appealing food than we really want on the one hand, and then overdo it by overeating on the other hand, generally on those foods we find appealing and have been trying to avoid.

Such efforts don't work for us, and they don't work for our children either. Parents who restrain and disinhibit teach their children to do the same. Once learned, inclinations to be inconsistent with respect to eating—swinging from one extreme to the other—can last a lifetime and can handicap a person's ability to eat the amount needed to maintain a stable adult body weight.

Your Child Will Eat a Variety of Food

From the time your child starts to eat semisolid and then solid food, if you offer a variety, over time your child will learn to eat a variety. His learning will be so erratic, however, that you may not recognize it. For weeks—or months—he will look at the food and watch you eat it. Eventually he will taste—and then take it out of his mouth. After many such tastes, he will swallow, and many swallows later, he will like it. Even then, he will only eat some foods sometimes. At meals, he will generally eat two or three food items—rarely some of everything that is put before him. For days, he will eat only bread or vegetables or meat. Then for no apparent reason he will switch and eat only something else. He will *love* a food, then abruptly go off it and not eat it for months. Very strange.

The positive benefit of such erratic eating behavior is that, *provided you do your feeding jobs,* over time your child will eat a variety and consume a nutritionally adequate diet. What is on the table and the emotional climate at the table have more to do with your child's nutritional health than what he actually eats on any given day. If mealtimes are pleasant and food is nutritious and appealing, a child will do well nutritionally.

What does this have to do with weight? Parents who are overly concerned about nutrition are likely to try to get their child to eat certain foods. They use a variety of pressuring tactics, from praise and rewards at the one extreme to downright coercion at the other. Parents might offer a child dessert as a reward for eating his vegetables, insist he take a bite of everything on the table, or make him stay at his place until he cleans his plate. Even positive pressure, such as praise or rewards, backfires because the child intuitively *knows* he is being pressured. Whether the pressure is positive or negative, he reacts by feeling overwhelmed, frightened, and often angry. Those strong feelings capture the child's attention more readily than do his feelings of hunger, appetite, and fullness. He gets upset, and the upset child loses track of his internal regulators and may overeat or undereat.

Your Child Will Learn to Behave Nicely at the Table

Your child will learn to behave nicely at the table. Honest.

However, being at the family table is a complicated business with lots to learn. It takes time and repeated effort. Teaching your child to behave in a civilized fashion at meals is part of your job in preparing him to go out into the world. He also needs to master mealtime behavior in order to get his emotional and nutritional needs met.

Four-year-old Ginny seemed to do well with eating as long as she stayed home. But her mother got a job, and Ginny went to the child care center, where she simply couldn't eat. She sat at the table and looked so woebegone that the teachers felt bad for her. At home, Ginny's parents continued to prepare what she liked, but as usual they didn't eat with her. They ate at their desks at work or ate in the car on the way home. While Ginny ate her peanut butter and jelly sandwich for dinner, her mother leaned against the counter and drank a cup of coffee. Ginny's father didn't get home until after Ginny went to bed. He made himself a sandwich, and her mother had a bowl of cereal during the evening if she got hungry.

Both parents grew up in homes where family meals had been a nightmare of food pressure, nagging, and fighting. Who would want to duplicate that? To do better for Ginny, they had to find a way of providing for her without coercing and traumatizing her.

What does this have to do with weight? One would predict that, uncorrected, Ginny's trouble with eating would make her undereat and be thin. As I have said before, Ginny feels anxious and afraid when she is exposed to unfamiliar food and unfamiliar eating situations. Her upset feels more powerful to her than her need for food—her hunger and appetite. As a consequence, Ginny doesn't know she is hungry. She just feels afraid and, at least for the time being, isn't able to eat unless she is at home and offered familiar food.

The other extreme is possible as well. Another child, perhaps a more compliant one, may learn to ignore his upset and eat in order to please his grown-ups. However, he will have the same problem Ginny has—his upset will interfere with his sensitivity to his hunger, appetite, and fullness. Lacking internal regulators, that child might overeat and get too fat.

Your Child Will Grow Predictably

Evaluating a child's weight is like nailing Jell-O to a wall. The problem is lack of consistency. Children are always growing and changing.

In the story of Mary at the beginning of this chapter and in figures 2.1 and 2.2, I introduced you to growth charts. Growth charts are simple graphs. At health clinic visits, your child's weight is plotted against his age. His height against his age is plotted, too, along with other assorted measurements. If all goes well, after some time the pattern that emerges for him will follow pretty consistently along one of the curves drawn on the charts, which are labeled numerically. Those are the percentile curves. It is the *pattern* that tells the tale. The pattern compares your child with himself over time and indicates he is growing consistently and well. The *numbers* on the curves compare him with other children his age. If he plots at the 50th percentile, for instance, he is about average in size—that is, about half of the children his age will be larger than he is, and the other half will be smaller.

Mary's *pattern* from birth to age 5 months, as shown in figure 2.1, was excellent: From one appointment to the next, she plotted consistently just above the 97th percentile. There is no value judgment to be made about her relative position. She was simply relatively large. She was heavier than 97 percent of other children. When she was 5 months old, her doctor made his error. He failed to understand the significance of her consistent growth and, instead, reacted to her large size. He thought her large size meant she was overweight.

It will be a great help for you to understand how to use a growth chart. Accurate judgments about your child's weight can be made only by comparing his weight over time with the percentile curves shown on the chart. It can be a huge relief to know that your large child who eats with enthusiasm or your small child of tiny appetite is growing consistently. You will trust the process, and you will hold steady with your job of feeding.

The story of Mary illustrates that there is another, *darker* reason for you to understand growth charts. You have to be able to *defend yourself and your child* from faulty growth assessments. Like Mary's doctor, health professionals often do not understand growth charts and may give you destructive advice based on your child's weight. Even when they are growing consistently, relatively large children—those growing at the 85th or 95th or 97th percentile or above—are often diagnosed as *overweight*. Small children—those growing consistently at the 5th or 3rd percentile or below—are diagnosed as having *failure to thrive* or showing a *constitutional growth delay*. Based on these faulty diagnoses, parents are encouraged to underfeed the overweight child or overfeed the underweight child. That intervention exacerbates the supposed problem it is intended to solve.

On the other hand, health professionals generally ignore blips in growth—small upward or downward divergences in your child's pattern of growth. Instead, they hope for the best and wait to intervene until growth divergence becomes established—until small blips turn into *big* overall changes months or years later. They are to be forgiven for that—barely—because diagnosing a child with overweight or failure to thrive is a serious business that calls out all sorts of grave and potentially disruptive interventions. Since most health professionals don't know about feeding dynamics, they don't realize how positive and accessible early intervention can be and how much parents and children can benefit.

When I see such blips, I ask these questions:

- How is feeding going?
- How would you like it to be different?
- How do you feel about your child's size and shape?
- About his weight?

Generally there is something going on in feeding or in the child's life that is affecting his growth. Caught early, the problem may be corrected easily.

HOW TO GET STARTED

The evidence is clear: Distortions in feeding create distortions in food intake and growth. Trying to get a child to eat more food than he wants can make him too fat. Trying to get a child to eat less food than he wants can make him too fat. Trying to get a child to eat certain foods or avoid certain others can make him too fat. Failing to provide a child with structure and support can make him too fat. It's all very daunting.

If you have discovered the error of your ways from reading this chapter, you have lots of company. Parents call or e-mail me from all over the world looking for advice about solving their child's feeding problems. In my many presentations to parents and child care professionals, I hear about lots of feeding problems. I hear about children who won't eat, those who eat too much, those who get stuck on the breast or bottle, finicky ones, ones who eat like there is no tomorrow, those who struggle so much with weight it handicaps their existence. It has been estimated that anywhere from 25 percent to 35 percent of children have feeding problems, and about 1 or 2 percent of children have problems so severe that their physical health is affected.[16]

For all feeding problems, the solution is the same: Establish and maintain the division of responsibility in feeding. That bit of simple but profound advice may be all you need. Here's another straightforward bit of basic advice—feed in a stage-appropriate fashion. (We will focus on stages in chapters 6, 7, and 8.) Stage-appropriate feeding works, even when it is applied to your own quirky child with his own quirky eating behaviors. Compared with what you have been struggling to do, establishing the division of responsibility may seem simple, and the idea that your child could become a competent eater almost too much to hope for.

Like other parents, you may feel the need of forgiveness for making mistakes. I can certainly give it—we all make mistakes, and you haven't damaged your child beyond repair. Young children change quickly and stay changed when their parents change—and stay changed. Older children may take longer to change, but they still depend on parents to make it possible. Adolescents are much on their own away from the family, and much of their food life is under their own control. They continue to depend on parents to provide meals and maintain structure and support with feeding, but they may or may not see the need to provide the same structure and support for themselves.

Changing on Your Own

Can you bring about change on your own, or do you need outside help? It depends. As I said earlier, change requires a leap of
faith and steady nerves. It also requires a lot of effort. You'll
need steady nerves when your child eats more after the restrictions are lifted and before his internal regulators help him
regain his equilibrium. The leap of faith comes in with trusting
that your child *can* learn to manage his eating. Providing structure and support is a *lot* of work.

Because I am a clinician, I have lots of stories of parents
who needed help to change. I hear less about parents who have
been able to change on their own. Erica, a small friend of my
colleague Pam Estes, is an exception. Erica was a big infant and
an enthusiastic eater. Since birth, her weight had plotted consistently well above the 97th percentile. Her parents worried but
believed it was wrong to restrict an infant, so they steeled themselves to let her eat as much she wanted. However, when Erica
was 7 months old, they could tolerate their anxiety no longer.
They became so worried about her large size and enthusiastic
eating that they began limiting her food intake. From then on, it
was fruit only for snacks, one helping only at mealtime, and
skim milk. From then on, Erica worried about her food, begging
for more, whining and crying. When she learned to talk, she
began singing a little song, "I'm hungry, I'm hungry." Despite
all the upset, food restriction wasn't working. Erica gained
weight rapidly, and by age 3 years her weight plotted *way* off
the growth chart.

Then Erica got a new baby sister, and Pam gave Erica's
mother a copy of *Child of Mine: Feeding with Love and Good Sense*.
Before long, Erica's mother called Pam. "I'm feeding them all
wrong!" she wailed. She resolved to change her ways, and she
did. A few weeks later, she called Pam again. "Keeping up with
family meals is a lot of work," she reported. "Get *Secrets of
Feeding a Healthy Family*," advised Pam. Pam is good for sales!

As of this writing, Erica is 6 years old. Her parents are
hanging in there with the division of responsibility in feeding.

Erica eats as much as she wants and forgets about food between times. She sings other songs now, none of them "I'm hungry." After first plummeting from way above the 97th percentile, her weight leveled off just above the 95th percentile. Judging from the consistency with which her weight follows along that percentile, Erica is growing in a way that is right for her. "It wasn't easy," says her mother. "At first she ate so much and I was so worried. It was especially hard because we changed the way we fed our son as well. He is small and slim, and we had been trying to get him to eat more. At the same time as Erica was eating more, he was eating less. For a time he seemed to stop eating altogether. He does better now too. Once he learned we wouldn't force him anymore, he took a greater interest in eating."

Get Help If You Need It

Establishing the division of responsibility may seem extraordinarily difficult to you. You may feel, for whatever reason, that your child is unique and needs a specialized approach with advice specifically catered to him and your situation. I do offer such help and advice, and I have trained other professionals to do the same. We can give good advice only after we have carefully evaluated the child and the situation. I describe that evaluation in appendix E, "Assessment of Feeding and Growth Problems." A detailed evaluation is called for if your child's growth veers abruptly upward or downward, if you worry a lot about his eating or growth, or if you and your child have ongoing struggles about his eating that you just can't resolve.

Long-standing feeding problems are complex and can grow out of oral-motor difficulties, medical problems, developmental delays, or family conflict. Often the problems grow out of the child's history—he was ill, temperamentally difficult, or exceptionally large or small. Parents have tried to compensate for their child's inclinations. In the process they have crossed the lines of the division of responsibility and tried to do their child's job of eating as well as their own job of feeding. Often, because struggling with the child's eating was so difficult, they have given up on family meals and have failed to provide their child with structure and support.

Despite all the complexity, parents of children with long-standing problems have generally been exposed to a piecemeal approach and offhand advice—much of it negative and counter-productive. Instead of giving still more ill-founded advice, I determine what is causing the problem and set up a treatment plan. In the best circumstances, I follow through on that plan with the parents. That is what happened with Leane.

Leane, Who Wanted to *Eat*

Leane's story is a cautionary tale with a happy ending. As you can see by figure 2.3, Leane was big—her birth weight plotted at the 97th percentile. To her parents, Leane's large size meant she was going to be fat for life. From the first, they tried to hold down the amounts she ate and stall her as long as possible between feedings. Naturally, Leane was fussy and unhappy. That made her parents feel bad, but Leane wanted the one thing they didn't want to give: more to eat. "She doesn't have a stopping place," they concluded wearily, as they struggled to distract her instead of feeding her.

If you look closely at figure 2.3, you can see that Leane's weight dropped drastically in the first month—from the 97th percentile to the 50th percentile. By age 3 months Leane's weight had climbed back up to the 75th percentile, and there it stayed. From the smoothness and consistency with which her data points followed along the 75th percentile curve, it appeared that things were going well during that time. However, some detailed history from Leane's parents told another story altogether. They had continued to be withholding with formula and bottle feeding, and the struggles around feeding went on. With solid food, it was the same—stop as soon as Leane was no longer ravenously hungry; don't let her stop eating on her own. They put off letting her join in with family meals because they anticipated she would eat everything she could get her hands on.

By age 14 months, Leane's weight began to accelerate upward from the 75th percentile. At age 17 months, it plotted at the 90th percentile; at 19 months, the 95th percentile; and by two years her weight was off the growth chart and still climbing. What happened? Leane got the upper hand. At around age14 months, she changed from being an immobile baby to being a mobile and aggressive toddler. She became so determined and resourceful about getting food—whining, tantrums, raids on the kitchen—that her parents simply could not withstand her pressure. Leane's weight gain showed she was eating too much. Her behavior said otherwise. She was *hungry*. At

FIGURE 2.3 LEANE WEIGHT-FOR-AGE BIRTH TO 30 MONTHS

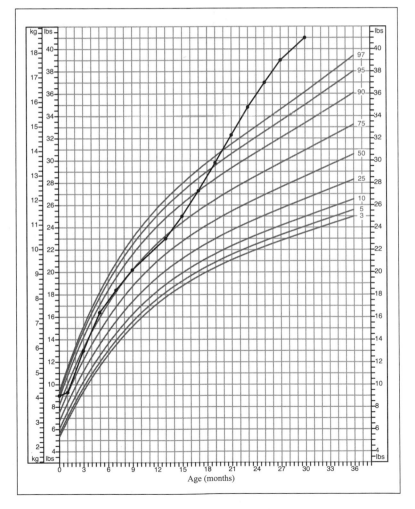

Age (months)

every meal Leane's plaintive call was "Is that all there is? Can I have more?"

When I first met Leane and her parents, they called her a compulsive eater, a bottomless pit. "Why does she want to eat all the time?" they lamented. "Why can't she be satisfied with so much less like other children?" "Because she is afraid of going hungry," I answered them. "She might manage to wear

---

FIGURE 2.4 IS YOUR BABY TOO BIG? DOES SHE EAT TOO MUCH

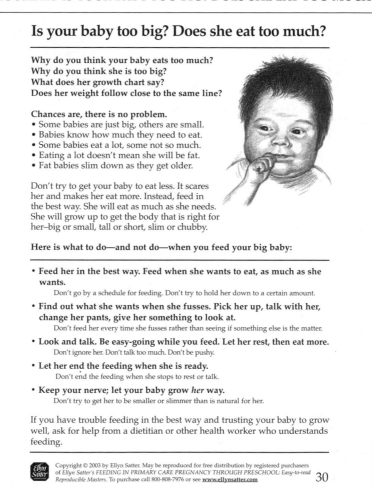

Is your baby too big? Does she eat too much?

Why do you think your baby eats too much?
Why do you think she is too big?
What does her growth chart say?
Does her weight follow close to the same line?

Chances are, there is no problem.
• Some babies are just big, others are small.
• Babies know how much they need to eat.
• Some babies eat a lot, some not so much.
• Eating a lot doesn't mean she will be fat.
• Fat babies slim down as they get older.

Don't try to get your baby to eat less. It scares her and makes her eat more. Instead, feed in the best way. She will eat as much as she needs. She will grow up to get the body that is right for her–big or small, tall or short, slim or chubby.

Here is what to do—and not do—when you feed your big baby:

• **Feed her in the best way. Feed when she wants to eat, as much as she wants.**
    Don't go by a schedule for feeding. Don't try to hold her down to a certain amount.

• **Find out what she wants when she fusses. Pick her up, talk with her, change her pants, give her something to look at.**
    Don't feed her every time she fusses rather than seeing if something else is the matter.

• **Look and talk. Be easy-going while you feed. Let her rest, then eat more.**
    Don't ignore her. Don't talk too much. Don't be pushy.

• **Let her end the feeding when she is ready.**
    Don't end the feeding when she stops to rest or talk.

• **Keep your nerve; let your baby grow *her* way.**
    Don't try to get her to be smaller or slimmer than is natural for her.

If you have trouble feeding in the best way and trusting your baby to grow well, ask for help from a dietitian or other health worker who understands feeding.

you down today and get more food, but she doesn't know if she can do it tomorrow or the next day. She has learned to eat when the eating is good. In order for her to get over that, you will have to reassure her that she can have enough too eat." Leane's parents were prepared for that answer because I had warned them ahead of time to expect it. The problem with Leane's weight wasn't that she didn't have a stopping place, and it wasn't that they were giving her the wrong food. The problem was that they had long ago misunderstood her normal growth patterns and restricted her food intake.

Consider how different things could have been for Leane and her parents if, right from the start, a health worker had asked questions about how the feeding was going, found out what was concerning her parents, and reassured them. The information in figure 2.4, "Is Your Baby Too Big? Does She Eat Too Much?" would have been very helpful to them. Help at any stage along the way would have made a *big* difference, and they would have benefited enormously from learning to do a good job with feeding throughout Leane's early months. *Years* of struggles around feeding would have been headed off.

But that didn't happen, the struggles continued, and as you can see by figure 2.5 on page 56, Leane's weight continued to go up and up. Leane's mother found me when she read *How to Get Your Kid to Eat . . . But Not Too Much* and was arrested by the idea that the interactions in the feeding relationship could make a child too fat. I first evaluated Leane and her family when she was $4^1/_2$ years old. After a careful assessment, I teased apart the story I just told you. Depriving Leane had caused the problem. Clearly, more deprivation was not the answer. Instead, I set up a treatment plan emphasizing the division of responsibility in feeding along with some finer points: (1) Put food in serving dishes on the table; (2) reassure Leane that she would get enough to eat; (3) include preferred foods at mealtime.

Because they lived hours away from me, Leane's parents decided to follow the treatment plan on their own. But Leane confirmed their worst fears and ate like there was no tomorrow—two and three helpings at meals, *lots* of graham crackers or toast at snacks. They could bear watching her eat that much for only so long; then they went back to controlling how much she ate. Predictably, Leane became miserable and food-preoccupied. Feeling bad about her misery, they again tried to establish the division of responsibility in feeding. As her mother said when she returned a year and a half later, "I know we made it worse with starting and stopping, starting and stopping. She

FIGURE 2.5 LEANE WEIGHT-FOR-AGE 2 TO 6 YEARS

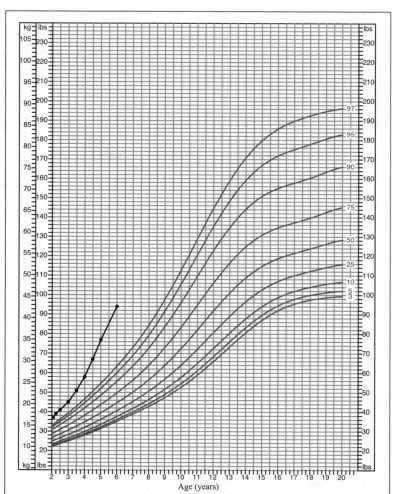

didn't know what to expect."

This time we arranged for follow-up appointments. Because Leane and her parents lived so far away, only the mother attended the sessions, but she did an excellent job of keeping the father involved with the plan. She began with strategic questions. "You say always to put bread on the table so she can fill up on that if she doesn't want to eat the other food. How much should we put on? (Her eyes widen as she watches me measure out a 6- or 8-inch pile.) That much bread! All right—we'll do it!" I told her that the issue wasn't *bread*, but *reassurance*. Leane needed to see the food there to know that she wouldn't have to go without.

Leane's parents needed my support to get through the scary times. "How can she eat so much?" her mother wailed at each office visit. "She's still afraid," I told her. "Leane doesn't know whether or not she can trust you to feed her the way you said you would. You said before you would let her eat as much as she wanted; then you went back on it. You have restricted her for a long time. She has learned that she has to eat while the eating is good. When she trusts that you won't take the food away from her, she will start to notice that she is full. Then she will eat like any other child—a lot one time, hardly anything the next."

Some detective work was needed to ferret out the ways Leane's parents were still being controlling and therefore were still causing Leane to fear that she might not get fed. "Do you mean I should remind her of her snack even when she has forgotten all about it?" "Yes," I said, beginning to sound like a broken record. "The issue is reassurance. Leane needs to know you will remember even if she doesn't, and she needs to choose. But warn her that if she decides to skip the snack and gets hungry before dinner, she will have to wait." The next session, Leane *had* chosen to skip her snack, then put up a fuss because she was hungry before dinner. Her parents knew exactly what to do, but they still needed my support for doing it. It was hard for them to ignore her hungry whining. Even in this backward-seeming sort of way, sticking to their guns about snack times was helping Leane learn to regulate her food intake. They were all learning that it wasn't so bad for Leane to be hungry for a while. There was another meal coming, and she could eat all she wanted then. Before, they had felt so ambivalent about restricting her food intake that they were inconsistent. They stood fast sometimes and gave in others. In the process, they taught her to fear being hungry and to use her hunger to manipulate them.

After three anxious weeks, Leane began to show signs of having eaten enough. She helped herself calmly instead of grabbing from the serving dishes. She began to relax and eat more slowly, rather than guarding her food with her arms and wolfing it down. By 6 weeks into treatment, she showed clear and consistent signs of having enough to eat. She stopped in the middle of a bowl of cereal. She asked for another sandwich, ate a bite or two, and then ran off to play. She asked for a *lot* of food and lost interest when she was reassured she could have it. She was right on the verge, in short, of eating like a normal 6-year-old. She still needed to waste food because that reassured her that there was plenty and she could have as much as she wanted. Over time, even that went away.

Leane didn't lose weight, but her rate of gain slowed down. Her weight began to parallel the top curve on the growth chart rather than accelerating rapidly upward the way it had before. If the struggles around eating had continued, her weight acceleration would have continued and she would likely have become much too fat.

CAN YOU DO IT ALONE, OR DO YOU NEED HELP?

I frankly don't know what allowed Erica's parents to institute the division of responsibility in feeding on their own while Leane's needed careful help. There were more similarities than differences between them. Both sets of parents loved their children and could see that what they were doing wasn't working. They both felt bad for their children. The children were about the same age when the parents started the change process— Erica was 3, and Leane was 4. Both sets of parents were dieters.

Like Erica's parents, you may be able to change on your own. Many of the parents with whom I have brief telephone conversations or, in fact, never even hear about do it alone. They read my books, they resolve to follow the division of responsibility in feeding, their child responds as I have predicted (after a while), and the problem is solved. On the other hand, your situation may be more like Leane's. Already at age 4 years, Leane's eating problems were well established and resistant to change, and her parents had grave concerns for her physical health. You may also need help to change if you feel a lot of pressure and concern about your child. For that help, look for professionals who have mastered the Satter Feeding Dynamics Approach. As I pointed out earlier in this chapter, people who recite the division of responsibility may or may not take a trusting approach to feeding. They may be giving permission but then taking it away, in which case the approach will fail.

How can you tell if you can or can't change on your own? Begin by establishing the division of responsibility in feeding. Don't *try* to do it—do it. As Yoda more-or-less said in *Star Wars: Episode V,* there is *doing* or *not doing*, there is no *trying.**

Consider Your Own Eating Attitudes and Behaviors
Doing your tasks with respect to feeding and trusting your child's eating capabilities will go best if you have healthy attitudes and behaviors about your own eating and weight. You certainly will find you have to become more responsible about feeding yourself before you can feed your child. You may need to get help trusting yourself before you can trust your child. On the other hand, you may be able to learn from your child. If you do your feeding jobs, keep your mouth shut and fingers crossed, and keep the look of incredulity off your face, your child will show you what healthy and normal eating is all about.

You will feel about your child the way you feel about yourself. Your child will feel about himself the way you feel about him. He will learn to eat the way you eat. If you criticize your own size and shape and continually try to change it, you aren't

---

* I have cleaned up Yoda's syntax somewhat. What he *actually* said was rather unintelligible.

showing your child what physical self-esteem is all about. If you worry about food, diet a lot, or avoid good-tasting food for fear you will overeat, you aren't showing your child what normal eating is all about. You are likely to restrict yourself at times and then eat to make up for it other times (and do the same with your child).

Whatever the cause, the task for you with yourself is the same as for you with your child: Feed yourself well, move in ways you find rewarding, and learn to love the body you *have*, not the body you *wish* you had.

YOU CAN MAKE A DIFFERENCE

To summarize, with respect to feeding your child well and raising him to get the body that is right for him, your tasks are twofold:

1. Be accepting of your child's size and shape.
2. Raise him well with respect to eating.

Rather than trying to change your child's natural body, it's much better to put your efforts into parenting well and feeling good about him. Help him develop in ways that *really* matter: good character, common sense, effective ways of responding to feelings, problem-solving skills, and the ability to get along with others. Even if your child grows up to be relatively fat, like children with other characteristics that make them distinct, relatively large children need better-than-average social skills in order to succeed.

Like the parents whose stories I have told in this chapter, you can make a difference. Follow through with your part of the division of responsibility in feeding and trust your child to do his, and teach him to enjoy and appreciate the body that nature gave him. You will be parenting responsibly and helping your child more than you can imagine. You will be helping without harming.

NOTES

1. Braet, Mervielde, and Vandereycken, "Psychological Aspects."

2. Davison, and Birth, "Weight Status."
3. Serdula et al., "Obese Children."
4. Wright et al., "Implications of Childhood Obesity."
5. Braddon et al., "Onset of Obesity."
6. Crawford and Shapiro, "How Obesity Develops."
7. Glanz et al., "Why Americans Eat."
8. ADA, *Nutrition and You.*
9. Birch, Johnson, and Fisher, "Children's Eating."
10. Birch and Fisher, "Mothers' Child-Feeding Practices"
11. Anliker et al., "Mothers' Reports."
12. Reilly et al., "Premature Adiposity."
13. Hood et al., "Parental Eating Attitudes."
14. Birch, Fisher, and Davison, "Learning to Overeat."
15. Fisher and Birch, "Parents' Restrictive Feeding Practices."
16. Chatoor, "Feeding Disorders."

WHY ARE FAMILY MEALS IMPORTANT?

- Meals support food regulation and appropriate growth.

- Meals make you a family.

- Meals support good parenting.

- Meals provide children with social and emotional support.

- Meals connect us to our history.

- Meals reassure children they will be fed.

- Meals teach children to behave well in polite company.

- Meals teach children to like a variety of food.

CHAPTER
3

MAKE FAMILY MEALS
A PRIORITY

A family is what you are when you take care of yourself. Whether your family numbers one or ten, meals are as essential for nurturing as they are for nutrition.

If I had lots of money and were in charge of a huge advertising scheme to solve the problem of child overweight, I would make the central theme *have family meals.* In the ads, I would show families eating together the way families today do—they would be opening cans and boxes and frozen packages—and quickly cooking and sitting down together to enjoy eating. They would be opening take-out packages and putting a meal on the kitchen table and eating together. They would be sitting down together at their favorite fast-food restaurant. They would be taking a pizza out of the oven, putting it on the breakfast bar, sitting down, and eating it together. I would have families making a point to turn off the television, and I might even have a child whining and the parent being firm about turning it off.

Of course, there would be some families cooking what we think of as a "home-cooked family meal," but they would be in the minority. I wouldn't want my ad campaign to give the impression that you had to go to enormous effort to feed your family. Parents today are *busy*, and they don't have time to cook the way previous generations cooked. Unrealistic standards make family meals way too hard and act as a deterrent.

The bottom line is that mealtime is essential for family time—it is about love, support, and connection. The structure and tradition of family meals gives you a framework on which to hang the foods and connections that you and your family need. Grazing won't give it; grabbing on the run won't give it. Meals provide us all with reliable access to food and provide children with dependable access to parents and to caring. Without meals, a home is just a place to stay.

This chapter is for attitude adjustment and for establishing the structure of meals and snacks. The next chapter is about choosing food and putting meals together. Everything you will learn in this chapter about food selection is summed up in Figure 3.1. The first point is most important: You must choose food you like. Food is rewarding when love and pleasure flow out of the kitchen.

Beyond this information, I am going to do with you as I do with my patients—actively withhold information about meal planning and food selection until you get the structure in place.

FIGURE 3.1 MAKING MEALS REWARDING

- Parents must choose food they find rewarding to plan, prepare, provide and eat
- Offer everyone in the family the same meal
- Put on four or five foods and let everyone pick and choose from what is on the table
- Put on two starches—always include bread
- Match familiar with unfamiliar food, favorite with not-so-favorite
- Teach and expect your children to behave nicely
- Understand enough about children's normal eating behavior to feel successful with feeding

Why? Because people think they can solve weight problems with the right menu. They impose that menu, everyone hates it, it sets family members off into sneaking and overeating, and family meals get lost. I once worked with a family that had boring, virtuous meals, and everyone had a food cache. The father's was the best—he kept Godiva chocolate in a locked desk drawer.

You *may* take a peek at the next chapter, but only if you can behave yourself and don't go off on a righteous-food-planning extravaganza. Remember that you are in for the long haul. To continue to have meals for 18 years *per child*, you must have food that *you* find rewarding to plan, purchase, prepare, serve, and eat. If it makes you sneak off to your food stash, you are being too rigid.

Now, let's turn to our work: getting family meals in place.

IN SUPPORT OF FAMILY MEALS

The societal deck is absolutely stacked against time with your family in general and mealtime in particular. Social norms supporting good parenting have eroded. Each set of parents in each family has to go against prevailing norms in order to preserve family time. My research tells me that parents think meals are important, they want them, and they strive to have them. A pep talk you don't need. But you *do* need to be reinforced in your determination to protect and preserve your family meals—and perhaps even reminded of your central responsibility to your family. When is soccer practice scheduled? At dinnertime! When are concerts and practices scheduled? Same! What is the expectation at many businesses? That you will work through dinner and get home after the children are in bed! Where are the social norms that say "family time—the family meal—is more important than all of this"? Gone! Nada!

If you are not having rewarding family meals, you can get them back. Some years ago, Oprah Winfrey conducted a family dinner experiment. Five families volunteered to eat dinner every night for a month, staying at the table for a half hour each time. At first, sharing meals was a chore, and the minutes dragged on. But by the end of the month, the families found their times together to be so rewarding that they planned to continue having family dinners. The greatest surprise to the parents was the reaction of their children. They treasured the dependable time with their parents. Not only do parents want to feel attached to their children; children want to feel attached to their parents.

Don't shop for rules or you will become as rigid and negative about "positive feeding" as with any other approach. Thirty minutes was a place for the families to start. Once they discovered the joy and reward of family meals, this guideline became unimportant.

FAMILY MEALS LET CHILDREN DO BETTER

Without broader social support, it is difficult for today's parents to remember how important they are to their children. You *are* important, and your importance extends *way* beyond being transportation and a checkbook. Children do better when they spend time with their parents and when they have a strong sense of family. Key to that connection is the family meal. Study after study shows that when teens have regular family meals—five or more per week—they achieve more and behave better.

Time spent with families at meals is more related to the psychological and academic success of adolescents than time spent in school, studying, church, playing sports, or doing art activities. Teens who had regular meals with a parent were better adjusted emotionally and socially, had better grades, and went further in school. They had lower rates of alcohol use, drug use, early sexual behavior, and suicide risk. The results applied for children of all ages, races, and ethnic groups as well as for those who had parents of all levels of education, ages, employment, income, and family structure. The results were the same for single-parent, two-parent, and extended-family homes.[1,2]

As you would expect, family meals contribute nutritionally as well. In fact, nutritionists use consumption of breakfast, milk, fruits, and vegetables as markers of nutritional quality and, in turn, measures of participation in family meals. When teens ate dinner with their parents, they ate better—more fruits, vegetables, and dairy foods. Dinner-eating predicted breakfast-eating.[3] A survey of sons and daughters of those followed in the huge, ongoing Harvard University Nurse's Health Study showed children and teens who participated in family dinner consumed less fat, soda, and fried foods and more fruits and vegetables, as well as more individual nutrients: folate, calcium, iron, and vitamins B6, B12, C, and E.[4] Interestingly, children whose families watched television at mealtime ate fewer fruits and vegetables, drank less juice, and ate more meats, pizza, salty snacks, and soda.[5]

Despite the clear emotional and nutritional advantages of eating together regularly, a high proportion of today's children do not participate in family meals. A huge Minneapolis / St. Paul, Minnesota study of 11- to 18-year-old students from ethnically and socioeconomically diverse communities found that a full third ate one or two meals, *at most*, with their families a week. Only one-fourth of adolescents ate seven or more meals per week with their families. As family meals and family connectedness went up, grade point average and self-esteem went up, and negative parameters went down: depression, suicidal ideation and attempts, and the use of cigarette, alcohol, and marijuana.[6]

PLANNED SNACKS ARE ESSENTIAL FOR FAMILY MEALS
Before I launch into a more-detailed discussion about the importance of family meals, I must remind us that for children, any consideration of structured, planned meals has to include a discussion of planned, sit-down snacks as well. In fact, when I talk about meals, I *think* meals-plus-snacks. I hope you will too. Planned snacks are the ace in the hole of the beleaguered parent. Notice the key words: *planned*; *sit-down*. Planned snacks are not food handouts. In fact, you give them *instead* of letting your child graze for food and beverages between regularly scheduled eating times.

To have family meals, you must avoid common pitfalls in feeding children: catering, trying to get your child to eat, your child not being hungry at meals or being so hungry it is painful for her to wait until it is time to eat. To avoid those pitfalls, provide planned snacks.

Consider this scenario. Your child gets up from the table

after eating little or nothing and is back five minutes later, begging. Say, "The meal is over, but snack time will be in a couple of hours. You can eat then." Many parents try to avoid this between-time food-begging by catering to their child at mealtime or pushing her to eat. Wrong approach. Her being hungry between times is *her* problem, not *yours.* Your problem is maintaining the structure and getting meals and snacks on the table.

It won't hurt her to go hungry for a while. It is the only way she will learn to take her meals seriously and to be businesslike when it is time to eat. Providing planned snacks keeps the consequences from being so high that you can't stand to administer them. Knowing another feeding is coming up in a couple of hours will let you step over her when she pitches her fit; it will enable you to hang in there for a couple of days while she finds out you aren't going to go back to the old ways. However, do not use snacks to put leverage on your child's eating at mealtimes, as in "If you want your snack, you had better eat your dinner," or "Since you didn't eat dinner, you can't have a snack." No, no, no! A snack just *is.* It is not a reward or a punishment for *anything.*

As children get older, they take more responsibility for choosing their snacks. However, the schedule doesn't change. "Eat your snack by four o'clock so you don't spoil your dinner" is a legitimate, staying-on-your-own-side-of-the-division-of-responsibility guideline for a school-age child or teenager. Of course, the time line depends on your child's school schedule and your family dinnertime. A mother approached me after a presentation complaining that now that her school-age daughter had a bike and money she was buying her own snacks—stopping at the convenience store to get ice cream and other goodies. I told her she couldn't control what her daughter purchased with her own money. However, she could set a limit: "Eat your snack by 4:00 so you don't spoil your dinner."

What would make her daughter do that, she wanted to know, when she couldn't supervise her? Your *authority,* I responded. Your daughter loves you and wants to please you. That is a reasonable limit and you have told her why. She will do what you say if you expect her to.

The same timing rule of thumb holds for teenagers: "Eat your snack early enough so you don't spoil your dinner." Learning to manage the timing and content of her snacks helps prepare your teenager for when she is out on her own. She can begin to think strategically about food selection. I will discuss that strategic thinking in the next chapter.

WHY FAMILY MEALS ARE IMPORTANT

You will need the courage of your convictions in order to buck social trends and preserve your family meals. In the best of all possible worlds, family-eroding social trends would change and you would get support for acting on behalf of your children. In the meantime, you will have to behave differently from other families. Why are family meals important? Let us count the ways:

1. Meals support food regulation and appropriate growth.
2. Meals make you a family.
3. Meals support good parenting.
4. Meals provide children with social and emotional support.
5. Meals connect us to our history.
6. Meals reassure children that they will be fed.
7. Meals teach children to behave at the dinner table.
8. Meals teach children to like a variety of food.

Meals Support Food Regulation and Appropriate Growth

Because this is a book about child overweight, I will begin by telling you what meals have to do with your child's ability to eat the right amount of food to grow well. After that, I will circle back around to consider the more basic and more important reasons for having family meals: good parenting and supporting the emotional welfare of every member of the family.

Regular and reliable meals provide the foundation for your child's energy and weight regulation. Grazing makes it hard for many, if not most, children to regulate food intake and body weight. Your child might be one of those grazers who eats more than she needs and gets too fat. She might eat less than she needs and grow poorly. She might be such a good regulator that she eats the amount she needs and grows consistently, no matter what. The catch is, you don't know which child you have. To support your child's food regulation and appropriate growth, you have to have meals.

In contrast, consider the way we eat today: We graze—we eat on the run, nibble and snack, grab and go, eat in the car, in front of the television, walking down the street, and while we wait in line. Compared with one or two decades ago, children aged 2 to 18 years get considerably more food from grazing and less from meals.[7] Both adolescents and young adults obtain 10 percent less of their energy intake at home and a corresponding 10 percent more at restaurants and fast-food places than they did 20 years ago. Overall energy intake has gone up; the increase has been in foods children eat outside the home.[8]

For your child to do well in *all* things, she *must* have structure and predictability. I quite realize that among those dedicated to grazing, being structured about eating is regarded as something of a perversion—as being rigid, perhaps, or overly preoccupied with food. Or being compulsive, and run by the clock. You are entitled to your convictions—when you are feeding just yourself. However, your child will simply not do well with grazing. For her to eat as much as she needs to grow appropriately, your child needs regular meals and sit-down snacks, and she needs you to sit and eat with her.

Meals Make You a Family
Parents are the backbone and architects of the family. Parents have to keep themselves healthy and strong in order to do a good job for their children.

Martin and Trudy were in a tizzy. Their 8-month-old-daughter, Rachel, was ready to eat from the family table, and they *had* no family table. After 2 months of happily eating baby cereal and pureed foods, Rachel made it clear in *no uncertain terms* that she expected something she could get her teeth into—all four of them! The problem was that the care Martin and Trudy devoted to feeding themselves did not *begin* to match the care they took with feeding Rachel. They waited to think about food until they got hungry, and then they grabbed it—pizza, hamburgers, French fries, and frozen snacks. You know the drill.

Why the tizzy? They did not think those foods were good for Rachel, and they didn't know how to cook anything else. Rachel, on the other hand, thought those foods were just fine and put up a great fuss when her parents failed to share with her. But how could they give those foods to Rachel?

Well, easily. My nutritionist friends cringe when I say this, but if pizza, hamburgers, French fries, and tacos are what parents eat, then that is what they need to feed their child. Nutritionally, those foods are not so bad and suffer mostly from lack of variety. Offering a child milk and staying away from soda saves those menus from being downright reprehensible. Rachel could eat everything, if they made a few modifications, like cutting up the hamburger, avoiding the hard French fries and substituting a burrito for the hard-shelled taco. The main problem with their eating style was its catch-as-catch-can nature. At 8 months, Rachel's eating patterns were becoming more regular. With a bit of foresight and planning, her parents could give her breastfeedings as snacks and arrange to have her arrive at the family table hungry and ready to learn to eat the food there. But first they had to *have* a family table. They had to become more regular in their own habits.

Basing their meal plans on their usual food choices gave Rachel's parents a place to start, and it bought them some time so they could learn to manage easy and tasty meals. If I could have turned back the clock for Martin and Trudy, I would have encouraged them to establish family meals from the first—from before they even conceived Rachel. Why? Because now they were playing catch-up and trying to parent at the same time. It is not easy for a pair of people to agree with each other on planning a menu, budgeting food money, sharing chores, and determining the mealtime schedule. At first, as with Oprah's families, all of this seems awkward and even unpleasant. For young parents, it can feel like playing dress-up, especially if they didn't grow up with family meals. Getting past the difficulty and awkwardness to a familiar and rewarding routine is best done with just the two of them.

Generating meals for themselves would have reminded Martin and Trudy that they were now grown-ups and a family.

Grown-ups do a good job of taking care of themselves. Family members look out for each other. Parenting goes best when couples take time for each other and have a good working relationship. Waiting until after they had Rachel to get all that in place was getting the cart before the horse. It left them feeling that if it weren't for her, they wouldn't be grown-ups and they wouldn't be a family.

Meals Support Good Parenting
Children do best—with eating and in every other way—when they are given love, structure, opportunities to learn, and limits. This is an *authoritative* approach to parenting. Children whose parents give both love and limits are most likely to become successful, happy with themselves, and generous with others. Children whose parents are overly strict are likely to be obedient but unhappy, and those whose parents are overly lenient and give few guidelines are likely to feel insecure and lack self-control.[9,10]

Ellyn Satter's Division of Responsibility in Feeding gives love and limits. It is an *authoritative* approach to parenting. The family meal is an integral part of the division of responsibility in feeding. Authoritative parenting with food allows children to eat the amount they need and to learn to like a variety of food. The parent who gives love and limits says, "It's dinner time, here's what we have, you may eat or not eat. No more until snack time." The overly strict parent says, "Eat it or else; clean up your plate." The overly lenient parent says, "What do you want to eat? When do you want it?"

Once family meals are established, assigning value to them and taking leadership will carry the day throughout all the years and stages of family life. Your child as an infant benefits from your taking care of yourself, keeping yourself healthy and strong, and recognizing your leadership role in the family. Moving through the stages from starting your child on solid food to teaching her to eat soft table foods falls into place when you have a family table your child is working toward joining. Between 10 and 18 months, your child completes the centrally important process of joining in with family meals. Becoming part of the sociability of family meals teaches toddlers to give up the infant's privileged position as the center of the universe. Preschoolers benefit from the benevolent leadership and reliable access to parents embedded in establishing and maintaining the division of responsibility in feeding. School-age children and adolescents continue to be in critical need of the nutritional and emotional support of family meals.

The pattern for family meals—for good or ill—is set during the toddler stage, when the toddler learns to participate in the meals-plus-snacks routine of the family—or not. Like other developmental tasks, if you miss the window of opportunity, the pattern is harder to establish later on. Getting your pre-schooler or school-age child back to the family table is possi-ble—but difficult. Getting your teenager back is possible—but only if she sees the need and is willing to be there. Your taking leadership with feeding continues to be important throughout the growing-up years. Your school-age child will work up to getting her own snack when she comes home from school and experiments at friends' homes with foods you don't purchase or prepare. Your teen will eat what she wants for lunch, snack where and on what she wants, and eat at friends' houses. But she will also cooperate when you say, "Get your snack early so you don't spoil your dinner." Even if she is the only one in her group expected home for dinner, do not be deterred. She will complain, but that is her way of seeking your support—as well as finding out if you really mean what you say. If your dinners are pleasant and offer a way for your family to connect, your teen will want to be there. Her friends will secretly envy her and may even show up for dinner!

Meals Provide Children Social and Emotional Support

Throughout your child's growing-up years, making pleasant and rewarding family meals your priority delivers more mes-sages and provides more emotional support than you can possi-bly know. Children treasure dependable time with their parents. Providing regular family meals reassures your child again and again that you will back her up. Your making meals reminds her that you make her a priority and that you want to give her your undivided attention. Expecting her at meals reminds her that she is a valued and respected part of the family.

As the Winfrey experiment showed, not only do parents want to feel attached to their children, but children want the same sense of attachment. Children feel attached to parents and to siblings when family meals are positive and rewarding, when everyone gets a chance to talk and listen, to share news of the day, and to have fun making conversation that is of interest to everyone. To preserve family meals as a source of *emotional* as well as *nutritional* support, it is essential to avoid lecturing and haranguing, including being controlling about what and how much *anyone* eats.

Finally, meals help *you* to remember how important *you* are, even when your child is older. Even then, as far as your child is concerned, the most important thing at the table is *you*.

Meals Connect Us to Our History

We are more fortunate than we realize to have a plentiful supply of clean, nourishing, and relatively low-cost food. Because our food—our most central of creature needs—can be acquired so readily, we tend to take it for granted. We are casual, jaded, and even negative about our food and about eating. Except for feast days like Thanksgiving, rituals and traditions around food and meals have eroded to the point that there are few left. We will gain from recovering them.

If we go back far enough into our family history, we will find that we all have traditions of eating and feeding that we can build on to help us in our current lives. All of our ancestors organized their lives around getting food. In every case, acquiring food and feeding the family have been priorities. In every case, some important person was in charge of the family cooking pot, and the character of meals was such that everyone ate together—children needed their grown-ups to cook for them and help them get fed.

Because of their strong tradition of revering and learning from elders, Native Americans offer a wonderful example of how we can all learn from and build on those traditions. When I am asked to present for groups of Native Americans, I arrange to first spend time with the elders. I say, "Tell us about the old ways with food and with feeding children." I also ask them what advice they have for young people today about feeding themselves and their children.

Because food and feeding is so full of memory for them, elders readily accept the invitation and they love to talk about their people's foodways. Their wonderful stories make it clear that the old ways with food and eating were joyful. People loved to eat good food, and they had an attitude of generosity and sharing. Food was closely linked to traditions—feasts, friends, and extended family. They knew they could travel, arrive hungry at someone else's home, and be invited in for a meal. Social and emotional connections were built on eating— on sharing meals. Their attitude in acquiring food was one of reverence—of giving thanks to the creatures, the land, and the spirits for providing. Because they had known hunger, they learned to be grateful, and they learned not to waste.

What did the elders recommend? That we remember that feeding ourselves and our children is centrally important. That we remember that feeding is about more than food—it is about love, support, and connection. Finally, and most important of all, that we get back to the old *feelings* about food that support- ed individuals, extended families, and communities—respect and reverence for the food.

It isn't easy to feel respect and reverence for a Big Mac, but it can be done. It's *food,* and we are privileged to have it. People have devoted their lives to putting that Big Mac in front of us, and we are privileged to have those people as well. We enjoy that Big Mac and find it sustaining, or we wouldn't be eating it. Joy and reward is part of eating and part of the emotional and spiritual refueling we get from our food—if we allow it—if we connect and pay attention and remain sensitive to how impor- tant it all is.

Of course, I am not recommending eating Big Macs three times a day or even every day. I am using that wondrous sand- wich as an extreme example of bringing reverence for food into our everyday lives. We don't have to go back to doing hunting, fishing, and gathering to regain that reverence. Certainly growing a garden or understanding where food comes from helps with connection and appreciation. But most fundamental of all is examining our *attitudes*. Those are the attitudes we pass along to our children. We can be mindful, joyful, and thankful as we choose, shop for, and prepare food, remembering the central importance of it all. We can be reverent with our food and pay attention when we eat it. It doesn't take any more time to tune in than it does to take food for granted (or even slander it) and wolf it down without noticing. But it makes all the difference— to us and to our children.

What does reverence for food have to do with your child's weight? Your child will pick up your eating attitudes and behavior. To know how much to eat, you have to treat your food with respect. You have to take time and pay attention when you eat—to the food and to your response to it. You have to notice how good the food tastes and feels in your mouth, how your physical self responds with a sense of peace and well-being. Don't let negative attitudes and feelings get in the way— castigating yourself that you shouldn't be eating it, rushing because you don't have time, eating on the run because you are busy doing something else. Your body will regulate if you let it—and if you help it.

Meals Reassure Children They Will Be Fed
Structure in all things reassures children that they will be taken care of. Imagine if we had to depend on another person to feed us—some person who has absolute control over the kitchen. Now imagine that person is predictable and regular in his habits. We won't have a single doubt that at a certain time there will be food on the table and that we can eat as much as we want. As a consequence, we can forget about food until the kitchen manager reminds us it is time to eat. We might even grumble and not want to be interrupted, ungrateful souls that we are! But grumble or not, we will know that we can go to the table hungry and eat until we are full. Then we can stop, knowing another meal or another snack is coming and we can do it all over again.

Now imagine the kitchen manager is casual or unpredictable, for whatever reason, about keeping track of the time and getting meals on the table. Sometimes he might forget about food altogether! How scary is that? Will we be able to forget about eating and attend to whatever we are doing? Not at all! We will think about food a lot—perhaps even constantly—and when we score with a meal or a snack, we will eat as much as we can. After all, who knows when the next meal or snack is coming and we can eat again?

What does this have to do with child overweight? Children arc an absolutely captive audience. They depend on regular meals and snacks to know they will get fed. If they don't know they will be fed and allowed to eat as much as they want at frequent and predictable times, they will eat as much as they can whenever they can. Their fear of going hungry will override their cues of hunger, appetite, and satisfaction and make them eat until they can hold no more. Consider 5-year-old Zack. At every meal, Zack ate until he threw up. He thought about food all thc time and constantly begged his parents for food handouts. Zack acted like he was starving, but his weight indicated otherwise. It was rapidly accelerating from his usual growth pattern. To all outward appearances, Zack had no stopping point and needed tight restrictions on his eating.

Fortunately, Zack's doctor, Francisco Carrion, a pediatric endocrinologist at Rockford Clinic in Illinois, was a good detective. He asked questions until he found out why Zack needed to eat so voraciously. Family meals were few and far between. Zack's extremely busy and frequently absent parents had meals whenever they got around to them, and mealtimes were all over the place. Worse, sometimes they might not have meals at all! "Have three meals and snacks midafternoon and at bedtime," instructed Dr. Carrion. The parents did as he advised, but found that having regular meals and snacks was no easy task. It meant totally transforming their priorities and their schedule. Two weeks later, when they got in to see dietitian Edie Applegate, the family had gotten themselves onto a meal schedule and Zack had stopped throwing up. His rapid weight acceleration stopped, and he went back to growing normally.

Children like Zack fear going without because parents are

inconsistent and unreliable with feeding. Others fear going without because weight-concerned parents deliberately restrict food intake. Still others fear going without because families simply do not have enough money to buy food. Whatever the cause, when they have to live with periods of food insecurity, children become food-preoccupied and prone to overeat when they get the chance. On the other hand, children eat as much as they need—no more and no less—when they are reassured in word and deed that they will get enough to eat. A nationwide survey showed that food-insecure girls ages 5 to 12 years who participated in the Food Stamp Program and the national school lunch and breakfast programs were 68 percent less likely to be overweight than food-insecure girls who didn't participate.[11]

Meals Teach Children to Behave at the Table
An important part of raising children is socializing them—helping them to be comfortable when they are out in polite company; teaching them to behave so they feel successful and others are comfortable being around them. Much of that socializing takes place at the family table.

Child care providers and Head Start teachers report that children come into their settings not knowing how to behave at mealtime. Among other school-readiness skills, Head Start teaches toddlers and preschoolers appropriate behavior at family-style meals. Barbara Turner, the Health and Nutrition Coordinator of Broome County Head Start in Binghamton, New York, says that in September, when new children come in, meals are chaotic and lessons are basic: Sit on your chair; eat off your plate—your *own* plate; use the serving spoon; say "no, thank you"; use words to ask and tell (don't whine and cry); keep your hands on your *own* body. Teachers have to be on guard with clean serving spoons to replace the ones children lick off. By the end of the year, teachers relax. Children set the table, are pleasant companions at mealtime, pass food to one another, attend to their eating, make conversation, and clear away after themselves.

When children feel comfortable and accomplished at the table, observes Barbara, they eat. Children's self-esteem is built on their accomplishments, and they take pride in and feel good about themselves when they are successful with mealtime behaviors.

Helping your child work toward those accomplishments is a long-term task with many steps. Even *getting* your child to the table requires learning. Your child has to be willing to have her play interrupted when eating is the furthest thing from her mind. She has to settle down enough to know she is hungry. She has to sit quietly long enough to eat. She has to get food into her mouth in a way that pleases you—or at least doesn't gross you out. She has to learn a dignified way of getting down from the table. She has to play quietly and let other family members finish eating. Whew! In order to preserve the tranquility of your own meals, you may be tempted to feed her separately or, like a lot of parents, resort to leaving out a dish of food for her to grab and eat on the run. But we are raising chil-

FIGURE 3.2 MEALTIME MOVES AND COUNTERMOVES

Your child's move	Your countermove
She says, "I'm not hungry."	You say, "you don't have to eat, just sit with us for a while."
She is too worked up and busy to eat.	Spend five minutes with her reading a book or washing hands.
She can't take time to eat.	Arrange for her to be hungry by avoiding grazing. Sit down with her.
She is too hungry to wait for meals.	Have sit-down snacks between meals.
She is too messy; she uses her fingers to eat.	Grin and bear it, cover the floor. Observe her concentration and creativity.
She is naughty at the table.	Let her down. She is full or she would eat—and behave!
She comes back right away, begging for a food handout.	Don't let her come back until the next meal or snack. Ignore her tantrums.
She doesn't eat "enough" at mealtime.	She may be grazing. Plan a snack for a specific time and stick to it.

dren, not dogs, so let's get to it. How do you manage all the challenges? Figure 3.2 outlines some time-tested strategies for helping your child behave at the dinner table.

Your child's moves entice you across the lines of the division of responsibility in feeding. Your countermoves keep you doing your jobs and resisting the temptation to do your child's. Your child is not just being perverse. Some of her moves come from childlike eating behavior, some come from her ongoing struggle for control. Children continually try for control—it's what they do. Remember, *your* job is feeding; hers is eating. Being firm about what you will and won't do and avoiding struggles for control is a continuous process. Struggles for control not resolved when your child is a toddler hang on into her older years.*

What does becoming competent with eating have to do with your child's weight? Everything! Competent eaters know how much they need to eat, and they know how to behave at the table. Throughout life, they can intuitively regulate food intake based on hunger, appetite, and satisfaction. They can take their eating competence out into the world and use it to learn to like the food there.

Meals Teach Children to Like a Variety of Food
Your child wants to please you, and she wants to grow up to behave in exactly the ways you behave. Your child wants to learn to eat and enjoy the foods you eat and enjoy. You know about the food that is in the world, and you get to choose what goes on the table. Your child's turn to choose will come later. Lots later.

In contrast, limiting the menu to food that your child readily accepts puts the least-capable person in charge of your family menu. It also seriously undermines her respect for you—and her desire to grow up. If you cater to your child, you will find yourself either cooking more than one meal or eating a steady diet of boxed macaroni and cheese, chicken nuggets, and hot dogs.

---

* For help feeding your child of any age, read the toddler chapter in either *Child of Mine: Feeding with Love and Good Sense* (chap. 8) or *How to Get Your Kid to Eat . . . But Not Too Much* (chap. 9).

We would like our children to eat more fruits and vegetables, to drink their milk, to eat some of everything that is put in front of them. They will and they do. But they do it in their own quirky ways that only an educated eye can detect. It all looks like food rejection:

- They look at the food and don't want it on their plate.
- They watch their parents eat it but don't eat it themselves.
- Eventually they might want the serving dish by their plate.
- They might want a small amount on their plate—but they do not eat it.
- After many meals, they may taste it—and take it back out again.
- After many tastes and take-outs, the food will be familiar enough for them to swallow it.
- After that, it will be on the list of preferred foods and they will eat it—sometimes.
- Even after they learn to like all the foods, they don't eat some of everything that is put before them.
- They eat one or two or three foods.
- Another meal or another day, they eat something different.

The key word is *erratic.* These common behaviors are very discouraging for parents, who interpret the whole routine as food rejection. It's not. It's a child's way of sneaking up on new food and learning to like it.

Research says that it takes children an average of 10 to 20 neutral exposures before they eat a food.[12] *Neutral* means no pushing, prodding, persuading, or cheerleading; no bribes or nutrition lessons; no little lectures about starving children *anywhere.* Pam Estes, a consultant for the Ellyn Satter Institute and resident of Indiana, tells of a mother who actually *counted* her numbers of offerings. After a while, she called Pam. "It's been 20 tries," she reported, "and she still hasn't tasted it. What do I do now?" "I don't know," responded Pam. "If you like it, keep having it." Months later, the mother called again. "Thirty-six," she announced. Pam's answer was exactly right. I hope that after running her experiment, the mother stopped counting. For some cautious children, it may take years of neutral food exposures, but eventually they will learn to eat most foods.

Parents who can't see the molasses-in-January progress get pushy. They try to hurry things along by being overly encouraging, by mandating "no-thank-you bites," or by rigidly insisting that their child eat. Such tactics don't work. Trying to hurry up the process slows it down. Children who are rushed and pressured are *less* likely to learn to like new food, not more.

What do typical patterns of learning to like new foods have to do with your child's weight? Again, it's that whole process of precipitating such strong feelings around eating that those feelings interfere with her sensitivity to her hunger, appetite, and fullness. Children have an intuitive sense of what they need to learn. When your child is not learning what she needs to learn, she feels anxious and upset. Getting into struggles with you about what or how much she eats creates a lot of internal conflict for her—she gets angry at you and feels ashamed of herself for being angry. Eventually, the conflict and negativity are associated with *eating*, and your child doesn't even need struggles to set those feelings off and undermine her feelings about eating.

APPLYING THIS INFORMATION
If your child is an infant, you can start off on the right foot. Beginning somewhere around the middle of the first year—or even earlier—you can include your child at family meals. She can be propped up in her infant seat to join you at the table, or you can pull her high chair over to the table after she has her solid foods. She will be thrilled to be there and will look forward to doing what you do with respect to eating. If, however, your child is older and you haven't been having meals and you have been crossing the lines of the division of responsibility and getting into some struggles about feeding, you have some repair work to do.

Since you are reading this book, it is likely you feel the need of some improvement in your child's eating habits. My message—one that not all parents are pleased to hear—is that your child's *eating* is determined by the way you *feed*. Children have a regrettable habit of behaving exactly as we teach them to behave! If you have been controlling the *how much* and *whether* of your child's eating (or trying to), your child will let you (or let you try) and will then find ways of getting around you. If you have had an open kitchen policy, then your child will likely be a grazer and grabber, eating only the easiest-to-like food and not taking much interest in meals or in learning to like more-challenging food. If you have been limiting your child's food intake, she will behave like she can't get filled up.

But, not to worry. We all make mistakes—the name of the game with raising children is to give it your best try, find out if it works, and then tinker. Children have a wonderful way of changing when their parents change—provided their parents really *mean* it. The younger the child, the more rapid the change.

How to Start Having Family Meals

The bottom line is the family meal. The most important task is to have and maintain family meals. How to get there? Agree on a course of action with your partner and with other grown-ups who feed your child. Then talk with your child and follow through.

Allow me to illustrate. Lydia found me by reading *Secrets of Feeding a Healthy Family*. She was particularly troubled by her daughter Wylie's rigidly finicky eating behavior. Eight-year-old Wylie ate only about 5 to 10 food items, counting cookies and candy, and became extremely upset when she was expected to eat food she didn't like. Lydia understood where Wylie was coming from, because she herself was extremely sensitive to new or surprising tastes and textures and enjoyed few foods. She backed way off with Wylie—so far, in fact, that she stopped having family meals.

As you would predict, Lydia had been forced to eat when she was small. However, she was forced in such a seemingly nice way that she hadn't been able to resist. Her mother was a grand and adventurous cook and could not understand how her cautious daughter could not positively *celebrate* her spicy, highly flavored food. In fact, Lydia's mother was deeply hurt when others didn't eat and enjoy her cooking. Lydia loved her mother and didn't want to hurt her feelings, so simply not eating the food was out of the question. No wonder she grew up dreading and avoiding family meals.

When Lydia started her own family, she made a few regrettable attempts at family meals. After that, she resorted to keeping easily prepared food in the house and let individual family members prepare what they wanted, whenever they wanted it—peanut butter sandwiches, cheese and crackers. One of the parents might make a pizza, boxed macaroni and cheese, or chicken nuggets and leave some out on the counter for the others to help themselves.

After she read *Secrets of Feeding a Healthy Family,* Lydia assigned herself the task of having family meals. As she told me, she stocked up on canned fruit and vegetables and prepared her campaign. "Wait a minute," I said. "Not so fast! Start out with what your family *currently* eats. First get the structure of meals in place; then worry about expanding the menu." Like many others, Lydia felt that having meals meant you had to have puritanically *nutritious* food—whether you liked it or not.

It was a bit of a stretch for her to offer pizza for one meal, boxed macaroni and cheese for another, chicken nuggets for still another, but she did. She also applied some of the menu-planning strategies listed in figure 3.1. She followed my suggestion to always put bread and butter on the table. In fact, bread and butter became her staple—she predicted Wylie would eat bread if all else failed.

Lydia talked the proposed changes over with Bryant, her husband. At first he thought the plan was daft. Bryant agreed to it, however, when she explained that it was a starting place. They needed to learn, first of all, that family meals could be rewarding. Later on, they would get bored eating the same foods all the time and be more receptive—or at least not as resistant—to less familiar food.

The next step was to talk with Wylie and her brother, 10-year-old Murray. Lydia and Bryant needed to tell the children that there was a change coming, why, and what that change was going to be. They could say, "You know, we haven't been having family meals because we haven't wanted to put pressure on you to eat. But we decided we are missing out on having a

good time together at mealtime. From now on, we will have all
the same food we are having now, but we will have it at mealtime. We will put the food on the table, we will make sure that
there is always something that you generally like, we will eat
our own food, and we will leave it up to you to decide what to
eat and how much to eat from what's on the table. What do you
think of that?"

Murray was thrilled. He liked a lot of different foods, and
he wanted time with his parents. Wylie, however, didn't like the
plan at all. "Oh, no!" she howled. "Every time you decide to
have meals you make me eat acky green beans, and I *hate* green
beans!" "No, we won't. We have been reading this book, and
we learned that making you eat what you don't like is a bad
idea. Instead, we will put the same food on the table that we all
eat now. Then you can decide what you want to eat of what we
put out. We will do the same for snacks—we will put out the
food, and you can eat or not eat. But you can't keep snacking all
the time. We'll talk about foods you like and foods we are comfortable giving you. We'll put the snacks on the table for you
just like it's a meal. And just like at mealtime, you can eat as
much or as little as you like from what we have put out for you.
What do you think of that?"

Wylie was cool with that. "Does that mean I get to have
candy and Little Debbies for snacks?" she asked.

"Once in a awhile. Mostly we will have candy or Little
Debbie's for dessert at meals. We'll put your serving by your
plate and you can eat it when you want to at mealtime." That
was a bundle of good strategies. "Snack" doesn't mean "treat."
It means "little meal." Since Wylie had been allowed to graze to
get treats, incorporating those treats at mealtime would make
meals more important and rewarding. But she wasn't to be
allowed to fill up on dessert—a single serving would leave her
hungry enough to eat some of the rest of the meal or at least
give it a passing glance.

Despite her parents' sweetening the mealtime pot with
candy and Little Debbies, Wylie was not convinced. She was
reluctant to go to table, and she consistently asked, "I don't
have to eat anything I don't want to, right?" Many meals she

just ate bread and dessert and drank milk. It was hard for her parents to ignore her food refusal, but they persisted. Instead, they concentrated on making mealtimes pleasant. They made conversation with Wylie and Murray. In fact, they had to learn how. "How was school?" They asked. "Tell me one thing you learned today." "Who did you play with at recess?" they wondered. "Who did you sit with at lunchtime?" Family members took turns telling their highs and lows—the best thing that happened today, the worst thing. Often Lydia and Bryant talked with each other and the children listened. But they didn't ignore the children—they included them.

After two weeks, Wylie's resistance began to lessen. After a month, Wylie was going to the table willingly and enjoying herself there. Lydia was encouraged. "Meals are actually pleasant!" she exclaimed, seeming to not believe her own words. "We all look forward to them. We have a good time talking and spending time with each other. My son especially likes it. I think it was harder on him than I realized to not have meals." Thoughtfully, she added, "Wylie is trying some new foods. She had a bite of carrot and one of pineapple. Now she is up to three different brands of chicken nuggets—not just ones from Burger King. She is eating a cheese sandwich for lunch, not just peanut butter and jelly all the time, and twice she ate the school lunch peanut butter and jelly. I am doing what you suggested and noticing but not acting excited about it. But really, I *am* excited."

I was impressed—with both Lydia and Wylie. Wylie's progress meant that Lydia was being consistent and reassuring. Wylie was taking a chance with the school's peanut butter and jelly. Even though it seemed like more of the same, everyone makes a PB&J differently, and Wylie would have to adjust.

But there was trouble in paradise. "I am opening lots of cans," she tossed out as she rushed on to another topic. For me, the word "cans" raised visions of Wylie's dreaded green beans, so we want back to investigate. Sure enough, Lydia was pushing the menu. "Surely by this time we should be having vegetables at our meals, shouldn't we? What about nutrition?" In any other family, it wouldn't have hurt to put vegetables on the table and let family members ignore them. But remember, Lydia grew up in a family where ignoring unwanted food was simply out of the question. In this family, even putting the food on the table would feel entirely too much like pressure.

"Slow down," I warned her, "or you will go backward. It is better to move slowly and have lasting change than to move quickly and have no change. Someday you can open cans. But not now—it is too soon. Plan to have the same limited menus with the same familiar foods for at least six months before you begin—slowly—to expand. By that time your family will feel so comfortable with their food that they will be willing to experiment."

How Long Does Change Take?
At age 8 years, Wylie's learning to like new foods is likely to take a long time. She is coming along—she has gotten the message that what she eats or doesn't eat is her business. But it will take *months,* and if Lydia and Bryant waffle and slip and go back to their old habits—even briefly—it will take even longer.

The younger the child, the easier the change. Toddlers, for instance, come around quickly. Weathering the storm for 3 or 4 days and being consistent with setting limits will do the job. If you can continue to be consistent for another month or two, you will have achieved permanent change. Older children take longer. I figure it takes a preschooler or a school-aged child, on the average, about 3 months before she really trusts that parents mean what they say and that they won't go back to giving food handouts, pushing food, or any of the other old ways. Then the child will learn to behave in the new way.

The keys are realistic expectations and consistency. If the struggle goes on and on, at least one adult is being controlling or giving the child the message that they aren't really serious about letting her be responsible for her own eating. Two of my small patients were said to sneak food and overeat when they could. The parents acknowledged that they had been restricting the boys' food intake at mealtimes and pressuring them to fill up on vegetables. We established the division of responsibility in feeding. The parents said they were following through, not restricting and not pressuring, but the boys continued to whine and behave badly at mealtime. After careful questioning, it emerged that the father was hounding his 3- and 5-year-old sons about table manners. He insisted they neatly use their silverware and napkin, which is unrealistic for such young children. Were the boys fighting back or were they simply overwhelmed? Probably both. Their father's rigid expectations were making mealtimes miserable for them. They were sneaking to eat between times when they didn't have to deal with the interference.

Teenagers need to be committed to a family dinner in order to make significant change. However, even without wholehearted cooperation, you can take leadership. There are some good reasons for your teenager to participate in family meals, and you can lay them out for her—being able to be matter-of-fact about taking care of her food needs and manage her weight without too much trouble, having a chance to check in with the family on a regular basis, having better nutrition, having the opportunity to become more competent with eating before she leaves home.

Then think about what *you* need in order to take leadership with the family dinner. You need to have control of the kitchen—no teenager rustling around getting her own food. You need to have all family members at the table—no teenager watching television or talking on the phone while you are eating. You need to close the kitchen after dinner—no teenager getting in the way rustling up a snack while you clean up and put things away. Finally, you need to have control of the food supplies—no teenager raiding what you have planned for tomorrow night's dinner.

Then tell your teenager her what her choices are: You would like her to sit down and join in the family sociability. You will plan meals so she can find something she likes, but you won't cater the menu to her. She doesn't have to eat if she doesn't want to, but neither can she go out right after the meal and rustle up something for herself to eat. Your child may or may not join you at the table. Either way you have done all you can.

If you decide to change the way you handle feeding, be advised that before your child begins to eat more competently, her eating will get more distorted and extreme. Weather the storms, keep your courage, and do not go back to your old ways. You may need to consult with a feeding specialist to plan your strategy and get help maintaining your courage and commitment. You may also need outside help to catch yourself when you become controlling or when you let down on the structure.

You may benefit from help dealing with your feelings while you make the changes. You may feel so sorry for your child or so angry at her that you can't be steady and consistent with feeding. You may have been so worried for so long about your ill child that you fear she won't survive. You may be so afraid your child will be fat that you can't let go of control. In such circumstances, well-informed help for a few weeks while you make your changes can be a very good investment. It helps enormously when someone you respect confirms your definition of the problem, helps you plan strategy, and supports you though the transition to a new way of feeding. Improving the way you feed your child will pay big dividends in your family life, your relationship with your child, and your child's ability to grow up to get the body that is right for her.

NOTES

1. Hofferth, "How American Children."
2. CEAP, *Teens and Their Parents.*
3. Videon and Manning, "Influences."
4. Gillman et al., "Family Dinner."
5. Coon et al., "Relationships."
6. Eisenberg et al., "Correlations."
7. Jahns, Siega-Riz, and Popkin, "Increasing Prevalence."
8. Nielsen, Siega-Riz, and Popkin, "Trends in Food Locations."
9. Baumrind, "Current Patterns."
10. Elder, "Structured Variations."
11. Jones et al., "Lower Risk of Overweight."
12. Birch, Johnson, and Fisher, "Children's Eating."

FOOD SELECTION TO SUPPORT FAMILY MEALS

Your child wants to learn and grow with respect to her eating, just as with everything else in her life. She wants to join in with the rest of the family and eat what they eat. But she needs the opportunity to learn. Make minor adjustments in your meal planning to allow her to be successful. Make sure there is *something* on the table she recognizes—she will be braver about trying something new. But don't limit the menu to foods she readily accepts. That takes away her opportunity to learn.

Adjust your expectations as well. Particularly when she is very young, her eating will be erratic—some days she will eat a lot; others not much. What she eats one day, she won't another. Generally she will eat only two or three foods out of the variety offered on the table.

Plan Meals That Include Four or Five Foods

Four or five foods sounds like a lot, until you count them up:

- A protein source
- Two grains or starchy foods
- A fruit or a vegetable or both
- Milk
- Butter, margarine, salad dressing, other fatty foods

Be Considerate Without Catering

- Don't make (or expect) anybody to eat—even yourself.
- Let children (and other people) pick and choose from what is on the table.
- Pair favorite with not-so-favorite foods (for example, corn with liver).
- Pair familiar with unfamiliar foods (for example, bread with liver).
- Include enough fat (for example, bacon, salad dressing, butter).

CHAPTER
4

HELP WITHOUT HARMING:
FOOD SELECTION

The standard explanations for child overweight all have to do with food selection: too few fruits and vegetables, too much high-calorie food that is too readily available, too heavily advertised, in too-large portion sizes. The standard solutions grow out of those explanations—restrict fat and sugar, eat more fruits and vegetables, limit portion sizes. However, children are such good regulators that those explanations—and interventions—simply do not suffice. Until or unless we support them too little or interfere too much, children do an excellent job of regulating their food intake. Children don't get too-liberal access to food unless we give it to them. If we maintain the division of responsibility in feeding, emphasizing the structure of regular meals and sit-down snacks, children can't be tricked into overeating—or undereating—by the type or amount of food we offer them.

In fact, basing a child nutrition discussion on keeping children slim is a matter of profoundly distorted priorities. The *absolutely* far-and-away *most* important issue concerning child nutrition and food selection is supporting normal growth and development. It is allowing your child to grow up healthy and strong, with the size and shape that nature intended for him. You have to know enough about nutrition and child development to plan meals that allow your child to be well nourished and successful with eating.

This chapter on food selection is intended to support your family meals and help you maintain the division of responsibility in feeding. As a feeding specialist, I have found predictable family meals and sit-down snacks to be essential, not only for helping children to eat the amount they need to grow appropriately but also for allowing them to learn to like a variety of nutritious food. Families who have regular meals manage to cobble together nutritious diets, and their children eat well, even if their food selection is what I consider eccentric. But look who's talking—I expect you would consider the foods *I* choose to be rather eccentric as well!

I have most often found in my clinical practice that when children *do* have deficient diets, it isn't because of the foods they are offered but because of struggles between them and their parents about eating. Children eat poorly when parents cross the lines of the division of responsibility in feeding—when they try to get their children to eat certain amounts or types of foods.

To stay out of such struggles, and to continue to have family meals, you have to feel successful in feeding your child. To feel successful, you must understand enough about your child's quirky eating behaviors to be able to know he is eating normally and well. Your child will learn to eat the food you eat, but it takes him a long time to learn. In the meantime, knowing he *is* learning takes an educated eye. If you are consistent with family meals, over time your child will eat a nutritionally adequate diet. However, on any one day his food intake will look distorted and inadequate. In the course of doing feeding and growth assessments, I have calculated many bizarre and inadequate-looking diets and have found that over a week's time they average out to be nutritionally adequate.

If you understand this key point, you will be comfortable with offering everyone in the family the same meal—no catering to individual tastes, no short-order cooking. I will teach you some meal-planning principles to allow you to be considerate of the different preferences at your table without running a catering business.

You have to know enough about nutrition to be comfortable eating the foods you like. Studies show that *taste* is our most important influence on food choices, followed by cost, nutrition, convenience, and then weight control.[1] For you to keep up the day in, day out, year-after-year grind of family meals, your food has to be rewarding *for you* to plan, prepare, serve, and eat. Even if you consider the foods you eat to be reprehensible, remember that the most reprehensible family meal is unconditionally better than no meal at all. Well, there is *one* condition—the people at the table have to be nice to each other.

CONSIDER YOUR OWN EATING ATTITUDES AND BEHAVIORS

If you were in my office, I would begin by asking you what you generally eat and feed your family. Then we would build on that—preserving what you hold dear, adding on, not taking away, guarding your pleasure in eating, and being absolutely respectful of the food traditions you grew up with. As we have our imaginary conversation, we will likely discover that your eating attitudes and behaviors fit into one of three main categories:

1. I know I should but . . .
2. I'm already doing it.
3. Don't bother me.

I Know I Should But . . .

You might be ashamed to tell me what you eat. You have lots of company. Every two years, the American Dietetic Association (ADA) surveys consumers about their nutritional behavior. When asked about the degree to which they achieved balanced nutrition and a healthy diet, about a third of people responded, "I know I should but . . ."[2]

If you feel that way, I would be very gentle with you and give you lots of support and head-nodding. Eventually you would confess what you really like and what you really do put on the table. Those who respond "I know I should but" are caught on the horns of a dilemma. When they eat what they think of as "good," they feel deprived. When they eat what they think of as "bad," they feel guilty. The upshot is inconsistency—a variant of the restraint-and-disinhibition pattern I have mentioned before. They restrain by avoiding all the "bad" foods and then disinhibit by eating those foods to excess before they go back to restraining again. Studies that follow children over time find that they, like their parents, are fatter when parents restrain and then disinhibit.[3,4]

In *Secrets of Feeding a Healthy Family* I introduced 8-year-old Joshua, who went hungry all week and overate on the weekends. Joshua's erratic eating behavior grew out of his parents' restraint and disinhibition. In their attempts to eat in a "healthy" fashion, they were "good" all week and ate all the "forbidden" foods on the weekend. They were so "good" during the week, in fact, that Joshua had trouble getting enough calories. He was hungry most of the time. Like Leane and Erica, the food-restricted children we met in chapter 2, "Feed and Parent in the Best Way," Joshua lost track of his internal regulators and got too fat. He ate the goodies when he could get them, even if he wasn't hungry. His parents' restrained feeding is hard to identify because in our culture it is so common that it seems to be normal feeding. It is not. Normal feeding is providing the child with a variety of nutritious and appealing food, then letting him decide what and how much to eat based on his internal regulators of hunger, appetite, and satisfaction. To help you recognize restrained feeding, figure 4.1 gives a partial listing of the forms it can take.

Restrained feeding is highly individual. The foods I choose to eat might seem wildly extravagant to you, or excruciatingly restrictive. To arrive at *your* definition, keep in mind that if you have to take vacations from it, it is restrained eating. No more vacations. Find a way of eating and feeding that is pleasant and rewarding enough so you can eat that way all the time—weekends and vacations included. With respect to weight management, the bottom line is *intent*. If you are choosing particular

FIGURE 4.1 RESTRAINED FEEDING

- Imposing arbitrary limits: ounces of formula, helpings, portion sizes, a food pattern.
- Imposing hurdles: "You have to eat this before you can eat that."
- Avoiding certain foods: sweets, chips, snacks.
- Limiting the menu to drab, uninspiring food.
- Pushing low-fat, "healthy" food.
- Pushing low-carbohydrate or low-glycemic-index food.
- Hiding the salad dressing and butter dish.
- Asking "Are you sure you really want that?"
- Giving your child "the look."
- Your method?

foods or feeding in a certain way in order to get your child to eat less or to manage his weight, it is restrained feeding.

Consumers say that *taste* is the most important consideration guiding food choices.[1] Surveys didn't ask consumers how they *felt* about making taste the priority. Chances are, at least a third of them felt ambivalent about eating the foods they liked and disinhibited to eat those foods. Like Joshua's parents, they likely took vacations from their standards. The so-called forbidden food is not the problem; it is the *ambivalence* about eating it. Our task is to get rid of the ambivalence.

A real advantage of being a dietitian is being able to find nutritional worth in almost any food. I enjoy good food and don't take kindly to anybody else telling me what to eat or not eat. With my benevolent help in our imaginary session, you would most likely find—to your relief, delight, and perhaps even skepticism—that what you ordinarily eat is really not so bad, even when you go on food vacations. In fact, your food selection is likely to be pretty good. To completely neutralize your shame about what you eat, we could have some fun planning family menus with the foods you like. We might fill in a few blanks, but overall you would be doing just fine. Even if we decide together that what you enjoy eating is truly as terrible as you think it is—and how likely is that—you get most of your points for having meals. I have told you more than once in this book that with respect to your child's weight, the *way* you feed is far more important than *what* you feed. To keep having meals, build them around foods you enjoy.

I'm Already Doing It
On the other hand, you might come into my office firmly convinced, as are about a third of the ADA survey respondents, that you are "already doing it."[2] If you are in this group, you are likely planning meals around broiled fish and chicken, low-fat salad dressing and margarine, skim milk, fruits (fresh or unsweetened) and vegetables (*naked* vegetables—no butter, no sauce). My task would be to break through your virtue. You would probably feel you are on the side of the angels and might not take kindly to being told otherwise. I would have to gently but firmly tell you that, while I can understand your getting the idea that that pattern of food selection is excellent and desirable, and while that pattern may even be good for *you*, for your child it is not the best.

In *Secrets of Feeding a Healthy Family*, I introduced a pair of "already doing it" parents and their poorly growing 4-year-old daughter. Annie would eat only at the neighbor's house, where the family wasn't nearly as careful about nutrition as Annie's parents were. I told them, "You have done what you thought was best for Annie. Unfortunately, it has taken all the fun out of eating for her. Children won't eat what they are supposed to— they eat what tastes good. I would guess the neighbors use more fat than you do, and that makes their food taste better to Annie than what you make at home. Extremely low-fat food is not tasty food. Part of the knack wonderful cooks have for making good food come alive is using some fat. Fat makes food taste good. Fat also makes food seem more moist. Dry food gets stuck in children's mouths."

Annie's parents were loath to give up their restrictive eating. They were proud of their self-discipline, and truth be told, for them food restriction and avoidance were trendy. But they loved Annie and wanted her back at dinnertime, so they lightened up. The new approach worked. Annie took more interest in family meals and stopped reminding her parents how much better the food was next door.

Such parents restrain, but they do not disinhibit. Their children are restrained but disinhibit only when they can find a way around the restrictions as Annie did. Annie was resourceful for a 4-year-old. Research shows that until age 9 years, children whose parents restrained only and did not disinhibit didn't show the same pattern of overweight as children of parents who restrained and disinhibited.[4] The author of the research is continuing to follow those children to see what happened to them when they got out on their own. From working with such restrained children clinically, I would predict that once they become preteens or teenagers they begin to find ways around such unrelenting restriction.

Children whose eating is restrained by their parents lack internal regulators. When they get out on their own, their lack of internal regulators can distort their eating in a variety of ways. A child may imitate his parents and restrict himself in the same persistent fashion—or try to. Lacking grown-up experience, he may go to extremes in his attempts at restriction and get too thin or grow poorly. On the other hand, he may disinhibit and get heavier, like the treat-deprived girls in the research study who loaded up on forbidden foods when they weren't even hungry.[5] He will surely feel bad about it—and about himself for falling so far short of his parents' standards.

Don't Bother Me

Still another group identified in the ADA survey was the "don't bother me" group. A lot of eaters out there have simply decided—either consciously or unconsciously—that going by the nutrition rules is simply too much of a hassle. They are not even going to try. Back in the early days of the survey, the ADA was still asking questions that gave skeptics like me ammunition for pointing out that the current dietary rules are unnecessarily prescriptive, rigid, and negative. One of my favorite bits of data was that nutritionally the "don't bother me" group was doing just as well as the two other groups. Whatever their approach to seeing to it that they got fed, they were eating foods that gave them what they needed nutritionally. Undoubtedly they were eating what they liked, an approach that served them well.

Those "don't bother me" eaters do all right as long as they are on their own. However, as with those who follow other distorted patterns, they run into problems when they feed their children. Children simply do not do well with casual, offhand feeding. In chapter 2, "Feed and Parent in the Best Way," we met Ginny, whose parents' failure to have family meals handicapped her eating at child care. Ginny's parents had their own reasons for wanting to steer clear of family meals. They had grown up in "already doing it" households and had been forced to eat the drab food their parents provided.

With "don't bother me" parents, I have to be firm. Unless they are willing to have family meals, I simply cannot help them. Anything less than family meals is a disservice to the child and, in fact, amounts to neglect. About what goes on the table, I am more flexible. I advised Ginny's parents to begin by organizing their menus around what they currently feed Ginny—peanut butter and jelly sandwiches, boxed macaroni and cheese, cheese and crackers, hot dogs. With milk as the beverage and the addition of a few apple slices or carrot sticks, they would have a nice menu. But the main ingredient in family dinner would still be missing—sitting down together to enjoy the meal. Ginny's parents had to eat *with* her, not just *feed* her. Until or unless they did, Ginny simply wouldn't know how to cope with meals at child care or anywhere else.

Ginny's parents objected to eating the same things all the time like Ginny did. All right, then, I told them. You don't have to limit the menu to the foods Ginny eats. Put four or five foods on the table, and be sure to include one or two foods that you know Ginny usually likes. Have plenty of bread on the table. Generally, children can eat bread even when all else fails. Use fat to make the food taste good. But don't push Ginny to eat *anything*—not her favorite food, not the unfamiliar food. Ginny needs to know that she doesn't have to eat what she doesn't want to. She needs to learn to turn down or ignore food she doesn't want.

Since all of every menu at home was prepared especially for her, Ginny didn't even know how to ignore food at the child care center! She assumed she had to eat even unfamiliar or unappealing foods. Being able to say no would free her up to say yes. She could relax at the child care mealtime and, after several months, begin to sneak up on new food and learn to like it.

What Works for Children

None of these three approaches—being inconsistent, being overzealous, or not caring—works for children. To help their children, all three kinds of parents have to learn to adjust their approach to food and eating so they can settle down to the years-long task of consistently providing a pleasant family table. How can you make meals important for yourself and your child without getting caught in negative nutrition rules? How can you find a wise and responsible way of putting together family meals that is comfortable enough so you don't have to take vacations from it? How can you relax with your food selection without being neglectful? You can find the middle ground—that whole nebulous area that exists in the midst of the extremes we just reviewed. It is Ellyn Satter's Division of Responsibility in Feeding. You do the feeding, and your child does the eating.

Before I begin to discuss meal planning, I must again remind you that by family meals, I *mean* meals-plus-snacks. Planning and providing snacks is an integral part of meal planning. Toward the end of this chapter, we will focus in more detail on the philosophy and practicality of planning snacks.

MEAL PLANNING

Have food in the house and have a rough idea of what you are going to eat at any given meal on any given day. Anything less will scare you, whether you know it or not, and will make you feel you might not get fed. It will *certainly* scare your child. Put together each meal using what I call the *Mother Principle:* A meal needs to have (1) some protein, (2) a starch (different cultures have different starches, like grits or potatoes or plantain or rice), (3) a vegetable (or fruit, or both), (4) bread (or tortillas or biscuits), (5) some good source of calcium, like milk, and (6) some fat. At breakfast, milk may do double duty as the protein source. The fruit/vegetable may be orange juice. (We'll focus more on the Mother Principle in the next section.)

If you put together well-balanced *meals* and nutritious

snacks and maintain a pattern of three meals and two or more snacks, your child's overall *diet* will turn out to be well balanced and nutritious. You don't have to try to wrap your mind around a guide that lays out the food for the whole day. Keep turning out varied meals and snacks; keep mealtimes pleasant by eating with your child, not just feeding him, and by not getting pushy. Then everyone's nutrition will fall into place.

As you would with any good guideline, at times you will disregard even my stellar advice. You will throw together a sketchy meal with parts missing. Occasionally you will have what you consider a nutritionally worthless meal. Like some families, you may enjoy having popcorn and cocoa in front of the television for Sunday supper (which is pretty good nutritionally). Or when you go to the fast-food restaurant, you and your kids may miss your vegetables (if they drink milk instead of soda, they will do pretty well otherwise). As you can see by both examples, coming up with a truly worthless meal is pretty hard. And even if you do, it will happen only occasionally. It's your everyday meal planning that has the real impact on your family's nutrition.

The foods you choose for your meals, and how you prepare them, will depend on the part of the country you live in, your ethnic group or nationality, what you like, how you feel about cooking, and lots of other factors. You might consider a meal without tortillas or grits to be incomplete, or you might be convinced that a meal without potatoes isn't a meal at all. You might depend on baked beans to be your protein, or you might think baked beans are a vegetable you have along with your hot dogs. You might be in the habit of putting the protein and vegetables all together in a stir-fry or a curry, or you may add in the starch and have a one-dish meal like lasagna or enchiladas. On the other hand, you may feel that mixing the meat in with something else turns it into—something else that just doesn't do at all.

Whatever your mealtime tradition, or the tradition you borrow from another culture, it is likely to be trustworthy. Moreover, you are stuck with it, because that is what feels right to you. Based on the available foods, every society has, through trial and error, put together a nutritious diet and tested that diet over the centuries. If the diet worked, people survived at least long enough to reproduce. If the diet didn't work, they didn't. It is as simple as that. The diet wasn't just based on a whole bunch of rules that dictated what people *should* eat. It was based on what tasted good and what was available and satisfying. Cooks went to real trouble to make the food taste good because that is what people do—they strive to make everyday things beautiful and rewarding.

Given that time and energy are in short supply for most parents, remember that good cooking doesn't have to take a lot of time. In fact, it *can't,* or you simply won't be able to do it. Make yourself into a *thinking* cook, where you use your head instead of your time and effort. Do some advance planning, look for shortcuts, and let the grocery store work for you in getting ingredients ready. For ideas, see appendix D, "Cooking in a Hurry," and *Secrets of Feeding a Healthy Family.*

Following the guidelines in figure 4.2, let's plan a menu:

- Meat, chicken, or fish
- Potatoes or rice
- Corn
- Apple slices
- Bread
- Milk
- Butter

There, that wasn't so bad, was it? That is seven foods, and we didn't even break a sweat!

FIGURE 4.2 PLAN MEALS THAT INCLUDE AT LEAST FOUR OR FIVE FOODS

Four or five foods sounds like a lot, until you count them up:
1. A protein source
2. A starch, like rice or potatoes
3. Fruit or vegetable or both
4. Bread or what you eat for bread, like tortillas or biscuits
5. Milk
6. Butter or margarine

Breakfast is a little different. If you have cereal and milk for breakfast, milk is the protein. At breakfast, toast is the second carbohydrate, juice is the fruit. There, that's four. Let's try lunch: peanut butter and jelly sandwich (bread and protein), milk, apple slices. That's four. Figure 4.3 gives specific suggestions for quick and familiar meals that have at least four food

---

FIGURE 4.3 WHAT YOU LIKE CAN BE GOOD FOR YOU

What you like can be good for you

Good food doesn't have to be boring or a lot of work. Foods that you make at home, buy in the frozen food case or eat when you go out can be good for you. They can even give you vegetables! Take a look at the chart below to find out what you get from favorite foods. Fill in the blanks with foods you like.

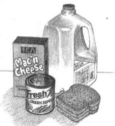

Here is what you get from your favorite foods:

	Protein	Vegetables	Grains	Milk
Pizza	√	√	√	√
Spaghetti with meat sauce	√	√	√	
Hot dog on a bun	√		√	
Tacos or burritos	√	√	√	√
Cheeseburger on a bun	√		√	√
Macaroni and cheese	√		√	√

Do you get the idea? Some foods have check marks in all the boxes. For other meals, fill in the blanks. Add vegetables or fruit. Have milk to drink.

Here are some complete meals:
• Spaghetti and meat sauce with cheese on top. Milk to drink.
• Cheeseburger on bun with tossed salad. Milk to drink.
• Hot dog on bun, raw carrots. Milk to drink.
• Macaroni and cheese, canned green beans, bread. Milk to drink.

items. If your child does not do well with put-together food, serve the hot dogs or hamburgers separate from the bun. Serve the spaghetti sauce as a side dish along with butter and Parmesan cheese. Serve the stir-fry separate from the rice. Add a bowl of peaches, even if they don't go with your menu.

In *Secrets of Feeding a Healthy Family* I give lots of recipes and menus with specific suggestions for adapting foods and meals to the young eaters at the table. Some of them look weird, like where I suggested scalloped corn for a vegetable when the main dish is mostaccioli with spinach and feta. Why? Since a one-dish meal can be sink-or-swim, other options are important. Scalloped corn is delicious and not challenging for children. Even if he skips the mostaccioli, a child can fill up on scalloped corn, bread, and milk.

Why emphasize the numbers of food items? To give a child variety to choose from and to increase his chances of being successful with the meal without your resorting to short-order cooking. A child won't eat some of each food that is put before him. He eats two or three food items. He might eat only bread and drink milk—for days and days. Then he might eat only vegetables and meat for more days and days. What tastes good to him one day does not another. We would be just as erratic if we paid attention as closely to the taste of food as a child does. We put ourselves on automatic pilot when we eat. We eat because we like it—or think we do—but also because we made it or paid for it or because it is good for us or to keep it from going to waste. Those reasons are lost on children. They eat because it tastes good, period.

A child's erratic, seemingly counterproductive nutritional behavior is more functional than it seems. Your child tires of even favorite food and chooses alternatives.[6] Over a week or two, his nutrition averages out nicely. He eats what he needs. He does, that is, if you do your job of meal planning—of offering four or five foods at a meal and then letting him pick and choose from what you have made available.

Embedded in this advice are some admonitions: Do not short-order cook. Do not put a jar of peanut butter or a box of cereal on the table for your child to fall back on. Such tactics tell him more clearly than words can say, "I don't expect you to grow up and learn to eat new foods."

Be Considerate but Don't Cater

Your child wants to be successful with his meals. Your job is to help him. However, do *not* stray into short-order cooking. Many a family meal project has foundered on the idea that everything on the menu has to please all the eaters all the time. To paraphrase Abraham Lincoln, you can please all of the eaters some of the time. You can please some of the eaters all of the time (generally the cook). But you can't please them all, all the time. Give it up. Striving for universal acceptance handicaps the eaters as well as the feeders.

Don't limit the menu to foods your child readily accepts. But don't be a sadistic menu planner either. One extreme condemns you to the day-after-day tedium of tuna helper, chicken nuggets, and hot dogs. Such catering does your child no favors because he doesn't learn to eat other foods. The other, sadistic extreme might be liver, boiled potatoes, and boiled cabbage. No butter. Of course, to be truly sadistic, you would have to force your child to eat the liver, even if he had to sit in front of it until bedtime. Figure 4.4 presents basic guidelines for finding a balance between the two extremes.

FIGURE 4.4 BE CONSIDERATE WITHOUT CATERING

- Don't make (or expect) anybody to eat—even yourself.
- Let children (and other people) pick and choose from what is on the table.
- Pair favorite with not-so-favorite foods (e.g., corn with liver).
- Pair familiar with unfamiliar foods (e.g., bread with liver).
- Include enough fat (e.g., bacon, salad dressing, butter).

Many families have a one-bite rule, or a "no-thank-you bite," meaning that children have to taste everything on the table. Those rules don't work, and they make children behave badly. Coercion takes away the child's initiative for pushing himself along to learn to like new food. Coerced children often respond—rudely—"I don't *like* it." With extremely challenging foods like liver or brussels sprouts, forcing even one bite is sadistic. Many children eventually learn to like those foods, but they must be allowed to do it at their own speed.

You could easily rescue that sadistic menu by putting bread and butter on the table. Let your child eat as much bread as he wants even if he doesn't eat anything else. To improve the menu still further, add bacon with the liver, substitute scalloped potatoes, and have corn for a vegetable. But to truly avoid mealtime sadism, you must allow your child to pick and choose from what you have put on the table. Let him eat as much as he wants even of the of bacon—provided he doesn't eat someone else's share.

Your child will learn to eat new food If you are like many of the parents I counsel about family meal planning, you will now raise two main objections: (1) "He won't learn to eat other food if I let him eat only what he likes"; and (2) "I don't want him to eat all that bacon—or butter."

Let's consider the first objection. Putting familiar and favored foods on the table helps your child do better, not worse, with learning to like new food. Children always do more and dare more if they have an out. Recognizing a food on the table reassures your child he can eat *something,* and that makes him braver about considering, tasting, and perhaps even eating what he doesn't recognize. Put yourself in your child's place. When was the last time you were offered a meal made up of totally unfamiliar, mysterious, unidentifiable food? How relieved were you to see something you recognized—maybe the rice? Did that help you to sneak a few tastes of the other food?

Your attitude is key to being considerate but not catering. You must reassure your child that he doesn't have to eat if he doesn't want to. You must also teach and expect him to be polite. No saying "yuck!" A simple "no, thank you" will do. For your child to be polite, you must take no for an answer. Children who are rude about turning down food have pushy grown-ups who won't take no for an answer.

Your child knows how much fat to eat Now let's discuss the implications of letting your child eat as much fat as he wants. If you do your job of feeding, your child will do his job of fat-eating as well. Don't try to manage your child's fat intake. That is crossing the lines of the division of responsibility. Instead, put butter, margarine, mayonnaise, salad dressing, gravy, and other fatty foods on the table and let your child eat as much or as little as he wants. Do the same with bacon; although, since bacon is generally prized by the whole family, you may not be able to let him eat as much as he wants, but only his share.

As long as you provide structure and support for your child's eating, his remarkable capability with food regulation will extend to fat regulation as well. From day to day and even meal to meal, his energy requirement varies a great deal. He grows more or less rapidly. He is more or less active. To provide for that wide variation in energy requirements, he eats more or less food. Most important, he eats more or less *high-calorie* foods—foods he has found from experience to be especially satisfying and to have particularly good staying power.[7] Most important among those high-calorie foods are fatty foods—foods like butter, margarine, mayonnaise, salad dressing, gravy—and bacon.

Think about it. After a fashion, we regulate too, even though our regulatory ability has been worn down and jaded by our own eating attitudes and behaviors. When you have missed a meal or two and are just *starved,* do you go for a salad? Probably not. You go for the sandwich and French fries (or you would like to)—admit it.

Of course, your child's ability is entirely intuitive. Unlike us, your child doesn't figure it all out and lay out a plan for his eating. He gets hungry, he eats, he becomes satisfied, he stops eating. There is no way we can anticipate when he will need more or fewer calories, more or less fat. However, we can support his varied energy needs by putting foods of a variety of caloric densities on the table and letting him decide how much or how little to eat.

Now that our nutritional fads are moving us from being obsessed with avoiding fat to being obsessed with avoiding carbohydrate, the fat arguments may be less important for you. However, let's lay the fat-avoidance message to rest anyway.

Children need fat. As I just illustrated, they need it for calories. As I will soon illustrate, they need it for staying power. They also need it for essential fatty acids. And they need it to make their food taste good. Toddlers eat butter like it is cheese, probably because the fat in their diets drops abruptly after they go off breastmilk or formula, and they need the extra fat. Breastmilk and formula have about 50 percent of calories as fat. The family diet, at best, typically has 30 to 35 percent. Toddlers intuitively make up the gap by eating butter. El Paso pediatric dietitian Ines Anchondo says her daughter Milagros makes up *her* fat deficit by eating avocados. After a while, even Milagros with her delicious avocados will adjust to the family menu and not eat so many. Then she, like other children, will eat an amount of fat that is somewhere between none at all and gobs.

Your child can't hop in the car and go to a fast-food place when he needs extra calories. You need to help him so he can eat as much fat as he needs. Keep in mind the division of responsibility in feeding. Put foods with a variety of fat concentrations on the table and let your child do the translating with his hunger and appetite. Figure 4.5 summarizes the principles for including fat in your family's meals. If he is particularly hungry and needs a lot of calories, your child will eat more fatty foods. If he isn't so hungry and needs fewer calories, he will eat less.

If you follow these general menu-planning guidelines, your child will eat on the average about 30 to 35 percent of calories

---

FIGURE 4.5 PLANNING FAT IN FAMILY MEALS

- Offer some foods that are low in fat: vegetables and fruit with no added fat, roasted or broiled low-fat meat, poultry, or fish.
- Offer some foods that are moderate in fat: vegetables and fruit prepared with 1 or 2 teaspoons of fat per serving or a fat-containing casserole or mashed potatoes.
- Offer some foods that are high in fat: salad dressing, butter or margarine, gravies and sauces, whole milk, or bacon.
- As with all other food, allow your child to pick and choose from the food you provide and eat as much or as little as he wants.

from fat. That is above the 30 percent upper limit recommended by the dietary guidelines. Being realistic about the fat percentage saves wasted effort. Children get around adults' efforts to manage them nutritionally. In a carefully constructed 2-year school nutrition intervention, children who were offered lunches containing only 25 percent of calories as fat actually ate 31 percent of their calories as fat. Children offered lunches that were 35 percent fat actually ate 33 percent of their calories as fat.[8] The schoolchildren picked and chose from the school lunch menu and ate the amount of fat they needed. For more about that research study, see appendix G, "Feeding and Parenting in the School Setting."

Don't Try to Dictate Portion Size

My audiences and readers want portion sizes. I hesitate to give them, because too often parents use them as a prescription and try to get their child to eat certain foods in certain amounts, which is absolutely what I *do not* want.

Instead, let's think of the amounts children realistically eat. For a toddler, think of finger-fulls, crumbs, and pinches. For young children, think of giving small helpings and letting them ask for as many more helpings as they want. A "small" helping is about a tablespoon per year of age. Or think of fractions of adult servings. Toddlers may eat about one-fourth of an adult serving—one-fourth of a slice of bread or piece of fruit, for instance. But remember, even those vague numbers are intended only to give a *rough guide,* not to tell you how much your child *should* eat.

Do *not* try to get your child to eat more or less than he wants *of anything* you have offered. What is the matter with trying to get him to eat more or less of something? It creates conflict and negativity around eating. Limiting a child's intake of a food he wants to eat or making him eat more of foods he *doesn't* want makes him upset and angry. Upset, angry children have trouble knowing when they are hungry and when they are full. They may undereat and grow poorly or overeat and get too fat.

Avoid even indirect methods of controlling portion sizes. Consider the dietitian who e-mailed me recently, wanting to know my opinion of her feeding tactic. She was limiting the amount of her toddler's favorite foods in the serving bowls so she could say "all gone" and he would go on to eat something else as well. The mother felt this was appropriate because she was "still allowing him to have more than one serving size." To her credit, the mother had a sneaking hunch I would tell her she was being controlling, and I did. I began by congratulating her for having family meals, and I meant it. Then I regretfully informed her that her tactic crossed the line into her son's right to decide whether and how much he ate. Moreover, I warned the mother that her son would catch on to her tactics before long and they would get into feeding struggles. And family meals would be spoiled. The problem was her *intent*. She was trying to get her son to eat a variety by seemingly running out of food.

In contrast to such creatively manipulative tactics, another dietitian at a conference wanted some advice about a fine point of controlling portions while avoiding restrained feeding. She wanted help examining the thorny issue of an insufficiency of green beans. One of her low-income families had hot competition for the green beans. Everyone loved them, and the parents didn't feel they could afford to open a second can so everyone could eat their fill. My recommendation was for the parents to portion them out—to themselves as well as to the children—and tell children that was all there was. As long as there were some other appealing food that children could fill up on, they didn't have to be allowed to eat all they wanted of the highly prized and more costly foods.

How is one situation different from the other? *Intent*. The green bean family experienced *real* scarcity, not *contrived* scarcity. The parents were not manipulating the children but dealing with reality. They were teaching their children to live with their economic circumstances at the same time as they reassured the children that they would be provided for.

Avoid Avoiding (Major Nutrients)
We are a nation of faddists. Five years ago, the fad was avoiding fat and eating a lot of complex carbohydrate. High-carbohy-

drate diets were all the rage, and pasta and bread were the politically correct foods. Now the fad is avoiding carbohydrate and eating a lot of protein and fat. Five years ago, a survey by the Food Marketing Institute found that for 59 percent of the respondents the primary nutritional concern was avoiding dietary fat. Only 12 percent of respondents thought the nutritional value of food was most important. Only 3 percent expressed the primary "desire to be healthy and eat what's good for us." By 2003, the concern about fat had fallen to 49 percent, concern about nutritional value remained the same, and the "desire to be healthy and eat what's good for us" had fallen so low that surveyors no longer included it in the report.[9]

I won't argue with people's values, but as I said earlier, for good health and supporting children's growth and development, the absolute priority is nutritional value: offering an overall healthy diet.

The passion for fat avoidance began eroding as the public began to catch on that restricting fat and eating lots of carbohydrate didn't automatically produce slimness. In fact, during the carbohydrate craze, people on the average got fatter, not thinner. The catalyst that turned public opinion most strongly against avoiding dietary fat was a July 2002 article in the *New York Times Magazine*. Gary Taubes, a science writer who had previously been almost completely ignored for his fine and responsible articles in *Science*, wrote a barn burner called "What If It's All Been a Big Fat Lie?"[10] That sensational and widely read article turned the tide from fat avoidance to carbohydrate avoidance. In another few years, I would lay even money that the Food Marketing Institute survey will show that concern about carbohydrate avoidance has replaced concern about fat avoidance. We will have replaced one destructive fad with another.

Neither fat avoidance nor carbohydrate avoidance is good for children, and both have social consequences. Beyond the fact that avoiding whole classes of foods makes it extremely difficult to eat an adequate diet, the weight-loss effect of carbohydrate avoidance is based on undermining metabolic processes and thereby distorting food regulation. The idea is to get the

dieter to go into ketosis—to accumulate an abnormal and undesirable by-product of fat metabolism called ketones—and thereby kill hunger and appetite. Such distortion is not good for
adults; for children it is much worse, and for pregnant women
it downright dangerous. Growing children—particularly the
unborn—are far more vulnerable metabolically than adults.
Disrupting their metabolic processes is dangerous.

What are the social consequences of avoiding a whole class
of foods—whether it is fat or carbohydrate? What does it do to
your meals with your mate, or friends, or extended family
when you are on a rigid diet? Isn't it hard to have guests or to
let someone else cook for you? How does avoiding carbohydrate—or fat—affect your ability to prepare family meals? Can
you prepare one diet for yourself and another for your family?
How capable will you be of preparing the rest of the family a
nice dish of scalloped potatoes when you are trying to stick to a
low-carbohydrate or a low-fat diet? How ambitious will you be
to seek out a lovely bread—and put a dish of butter on the
table—or make an appealing dish of (buttered) corn? Even if
you can manage to generate appealing meals, your avoiding
whole food groups will rub off on your child. He will notice,
and sooner or later he will eat the way you do.

Put Together Meals and Snacks with Staying Power
The truth is that you and your child need all three of the major
nutrients—protein, fat, and carbohydrate—in order to do well
with regulating food intake. Take a look at figure 4.6 on page
112. Protein, fat, and carbohydrate each has a role to play in
making a meal or snack rewarding while you eat it and in giving staying power afterward.

Let's work through a breakfast example. A sugar-only
breakfast would be fruit juice. Few other foods contain only
sugar—soda or Kool-Aid would qualify, as would Jell-O and
fat-free candies like gum drops or hard candy. They are not
exactly breakfast foods, but how many people do you know
who drink soda to jump-start themselves in the morning? As
you can see by the first up-and-down curve on the chart, sugar
calories get to you quickly, but they abandon you just as quickly.

FIGURE 4.6 SATISFACTION FROM CONSUMING SUGAR, STARCH, PROTEIN AND FAT

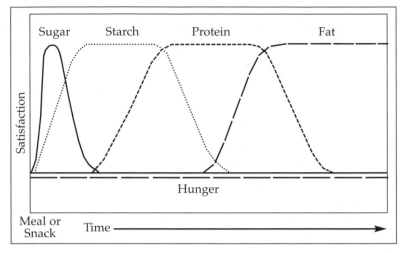

The quick fix and quick letdown is the basis for the idea that eating sugary foods makes children behave badly. Studies show that sugar consumption doesn't affect children's behavior or cognitive performance.[11] However, dietary imbalances do. Children who are allowed free access to high-sugar food and beverages experience a quick sugar fix and letdown, and hunger afterward. It is being *hungry,* not the sugar, that makes their behavior and intellectual performance worse.

As you can see by the starch curve, adding toast or cereal to the breakfast helps. Starch is essentially a time-release form of carbohydrate. It takes longer to digest and get into your blood-stream and gives a more sustained energy release than sugar. If the starchy food is all or partly whole-grain, it stretches out the curve—the timed-release quality. However, there is more to satisfaction than blood chemistry—there is the *aesthetic* reward as well. Toast and cereal also taste good and give something to chew. Increased blood sugar, chewing, and pleasure all contribute to the satisfaction you need to let you feel like stopping eating. Starchy foods are also bulky, and that bulk contributes by feeling substantial in your mouth and giving your stomach a pleasantly heavy and filled-up feeling.

Let's add skim milk for the cereal. As you can see from the protein curve, milk's protein gives still more staying power. Because protein molecules take a while to break down into the amino acids that get metered into the bloodstream, the protein curve takes a while to go up and stays up longer. Only a few foods provide protein without some dietary fat. Nonfat cottage cheese would qualify, as would egg white. Very low-fat fish is close. Generally, when you add protein to a meal, you add fat as well. Egg white is pure protein, but a whole egg has fat from the yolk.

Adding fat to the meal entirely changes the satisfaction picture. Choosing 2 percent or whole milk to put on cereal allows a cereal and milk breakfast to stave off hunger for an hour or two longer than the one that uses skim milk. As you can see from the fat curve in figure 4.6, fat added to the meal helps most of all to give the meal staying power. Fat makes the meal stay in your stomach longer. Because of the fat, the digestive process breaks down all the food more slowly and makes energy available over a longer time. Part of the satisfaction comes from biochemistry: Fat molecules take a while to break down into the fatty acids that are then metered into the bloodstream. The fatty acids stay in the bloodstream longer and extend satisfaction. Fat also makes food taste better and contributes enormously to the pleasure and reward from the meal. Pleasure and reward are essential to satisfaction. Chewing figures in here as well. Foods high in protein often require chewing.

From here on, you can figure it out for yourself. What happens to the curves in figure 4.6 when you avoid carbohydrate? What if you avoid fat?

Understanding figure 4.5 gives a basis for evaluating the low-glycemic-index diet, another up-and-coming dietary extreme primarily being promoted for weight loss. The South Beach Diet is essentially a low-glycemic, high-protein diet, and the Zone recommends a lower intake of high-glycemic-index foods. Foods are tested, one at a time, for their tendency to create a blood sugar pattern like the first curve in figure 4.5. The diet based on that testing emphasizes foods that test low, such as whole grains, and recommends avoiding foods that test high, like potatoes. Whole grains test lower and are therefore favored over breads and cereals made from refined grains, which test higher. As we learned from figure 4.5, the logic holds only if you eat the foods *one at a time.* Adding protein and fat increases the timed-release quality of the carbohydrate food. When you eat the starchy food *as part of a meal,* the starch in even refined-carbohydrate foods behaves like the second curve, not the first one—it has a timed-release quality. Adding other foods slows down the rate at which complex carbohydrate is digested and turns into glucose, a natural end product of digesting *any* carbohydrate.

Be Strategic About Eating in Restaurants

Seventy percent of families eat out at least once a week. If you can afford it, eating out is a way to have pleasant and relaxed family time and to get that all-important family meal. Keep in mind that the first priority is *having* a meal. The second is the *nutritional quality* of the meal—but you can have both. If you eat out only rarely, you can afford to throw nutritional considerations to the winds and let your child order only what he likes. If you eat out a lot, it's worth setting up some simple guidelines to encourage balanced meal plans without overloading his menu with fat and sugar. My suggestions in figure 4.7 are somewhat prescriptive, and here's why: When your child chooses what he wants to eat in a restaurant, he takes over your job of planning the meal. As a consequence, when he is young, you need to give him some rules to go by in choosing what to eat. When he gets into his school-age and adolescent years and has mastered food acceptance, he can go by his own rules. As with everything else, he has to earn the privilege.

KNOW ABOUT FOOD AND NUTRITION

Beyond the discussion of putting meals together, you need to know enough about nutrition to choose appropriately for your family and to protect yourself against fads and rumors. Not only that, but nutrition is *interesting,* if you talk about entertaining stuff rather than just drone on about what you *should*—or *shouldn't*—eat. *Don't* let this discussion send you off into a lot of self-critical thoughts and comments about your eating and weight.

Fruits and Vegetables Are Not Magic Bullets

Fruits and vegetables have a lot going for them, but eating them will not keep your child slim. You can't trick the body's regulatory ability. Trying to fill your child or yourself up on low-calorie foods like vegetables will not force energy intake down. It will simply turn everybody off to wonderful foods like broccoli and salad greens. I wish I had a nickel for every parent who has had meals spoiled by struggles about vegetables or for every long-term dieter who has told me he simply cannot *look* at another spear of broccoli or salad. Vegetables and fruits taste

---

FIGURE 4.7 FAMILY MEALS IN RESTAURANTS

- Try for three different food groups. You'll probably find that this happens automatically anyway. A hamburger and a bun with French fries would qualify, as would pizza (crust, cheese, and topping). A salad, bread, and milk would work, as would a taco (tortilla, meat, vegetables).
- Limit sweets to one per meal. If your child has a milkshake or soda for his beverage, that counts as his sweet. However, if he drinks milk or water, he can still have a sweet.
- Keep it down to one fried food per meal. For example, if your child has French fries and a hamburger, a fried apple pie for dessert would add up to too many fried foods. To have the apple pie, he would have to skip the French fries, and to fill up he might need a second hamburger. Grilled foods like burgers don't count as fried foods because they are relatively low in fat. French fries, chicken nuggets, and fish sandwiches are higher in fat because they are starchy and French-fried. The starch soaks up more fat.
- Keep dessert portions child-size, just as you would at home. That might mean splitting a dessert with someone else at the table, or ordering a sundae rather than a banana split.
- Don't feel obligated to order from the children's menus, which are typically very limited. Instead, consider the appetizers or a la carte menu. Split meals or plan to take some home from an adult portion.
- Lay out cost limits ahead of time, and then let your child cope. Order bread and let him fill up on that if he doesn't like what he ordered himself.
- Expect and enforce positive mealtime behavior. You owe it to the other diners.

wonderful, but not if you try to fill yourself or other people up on them.

Fruits and vegetables are important nutritionally—they give vitamins, minerals, phytochemicals, fiber. Include fruits and vegetables with meals, and over time your child will learn to like and eat them. Vegetables are more challenging to learn to like than fruit for most children. On the other hand, some children like vegetables and not fruit. The flavors in vegetables are strong, and the textures unusual. Your child will learn to like them if you prepare them regularly, dress them up with butter or sauces, eat and enjoy them yourself, and avoid getting pushy in any way. Put the fruits and vegetables on the table and let him decide what he will eat—and fill up on. Forcing him to eat anything—for any reason—will turn him off to it.

I am in favor of fruits and vegetables. However, I am *not* in favor of the conventional wisdom, which says that children are too fat because they eat the wrong food and if they eat the right food they will be slim. The fruit-and-vegetable enthusiasts explain the fattening effect of periodic food insecurity by asserting that people with limited food money choose filling, high-calorie foods that are low in nutrients. Actually, children who suffer from food insecurity eat no fewer fruits and vegetables than do those who live in families with plenty of money to buy food.[12] On the average, people with limited incomes purchase food more efficiently and get more nutrients per dollar than do people with more money.[13] The fattening effect of food insecurity comes from the fact that people who don't have enough to eat sometimes have a strong tendency to overeat when they have the opportunity. It is another variation of restraint and disinhibition.

Perhaps the logic is that children and other people who eat relatively low-calorie foods such as fruits and vegetables don't eat as much of higher-calorie foods, eat fewer calories overall, and are thinner. There is no evidence to substantiate that logic.[14] In fact, if *you* accept that logic, you have been dozing off while you have been reading this book. Think it through: Why doesn't this logic hold? It's important for you to get a firm grip on the thinking about normal processes of food regulation in order to keep from getting caught up in food restriction and dietary fads. Don't look until you figure it out, but the answer is in the footnote.*

Adults do seem to stop eating on fewer calories when they are offered lower-calorie food.[15] Adults eat more when offered large portion sizes.[16] However, the studies I just cited, done in a Pennsylvania State University laboratory, examined food regulation patterns only for short times—a day a week, or six meals in a row. Adults are easy to trick in the short term, but in the long term even adults compensate for eating less one time by eating more another.

What about children? Some preschoolers will eat more when they are offered a large portion size, but toddlers will not.[17] The difference is developmental. A preschooler will do your bidding when you say, "Clean your plate." He wants to please and can be shamed into doing what you want. A toddler won't. He is so committed to being his own person that he would rather fight than do your bidding with his eating. Unless or until grown-ups teach them to clean their plates, preschoolers regulate very well—even with large portion sizes.

In a classic study in the University of Illinois preschools, children demonstrated their food regulation ability. Preschoolers who were given either a high-calorie pudding or low-calorie pudding 20 minutes before a meal compensated with their lunch intake. Those who ate the high-calorie pudding ate fewer little sandwiches. Those who ate the low-calorie pudding ate more little sandwiches.[18] A few of the children did not compensate—they ate the same number of sandwiches no matter which pudding they ate. The difference was in the eating and feeding behaviors of the parents. Parents who were controlling of their own and their children's food intake had children who were less able to self-regulate.[19]

---

* Here is what I said in Chapter 2, page 34: "Until we interfere, children are such good regulators that they do not have to be served a steady diet of nutritious low-calorie food in order for them to eat the right amount. High in fat or sugar? They eat less. Mostly low-calorie food? They look around for something else to fill up on."

Milk May Be a Magic Bullet

It appears that with respect to your child's weight—and your own—drinking milk can't hurt, and it may even help. With respect to your child's bone health, drinking enough milk is absolutely essential.

I review the research about milk consumption in appendix J, "Dairy Products, Bone Health, and Weight Management." Here I will talk in more general terms. It is important for children to drink *enough* milk, but not *too much*. Children who drink too much milk fill up on it and don't eat the other nutritious foods they need. Toddlers, preschoolers, and school-age children need two to three cups of milk a day. Adolescents need three to four cups. Calcium-fortified beverages such as orange juice are not a substitute for milk. They replace milk's calcium, and perhaps even its vitamin D, but not its protein and its wide range of other protective nutrients.

Instead of milk, today's children drink sweet beverages like soda, fruit juices, fruit drinks, and sweet tea. Their bone health suffers, both in childhood and when they become adults. Children who get too little calcium are shorter; they have smaller, weaker bones and a greater number of broken bones. Teenage girls who drink more carbonated beverages and therefore less milk have more bone fractures. Women with low milk intake during childhood and adolescence have less bone mass in adulthood. Women are particularly vulnerable to poor bone health and fractures because their bones are smaller and because childbearing and breastfeeding sacrifice bone mass if dietary calcium is not available. Again, all the references are in appendix J.

Consuming milk and other dairy products may help with weight management. Studies show that both adults and children who drink milk are moderately slimmer than those who don't. Children who drank sodas and other sweetened beverages took in more calories and were fatter than children who drank milk instead. The caveat is that none of the research asked about structured meals and snacks versus grazing. When children and other people graze, they are likely to be heavier.

How do you get your child to drink milk? As with every

other food that is "good for" him, it is better not to try. The word to watch out for is *get*. You can't *get* your child to consume anything. He can only decide for himself to consume it. Do your part, and let him do his. Put milk on the table, have milk and water be the only mealtime beverages (juice for breakfast is all right), and drink milk yourself. If you won't drink milk, at least don't drink anything else your child would rather have than milk. While you wait for your child to drink milk, consider making your breakfast or snack-time juice one that is fortified with calcium. If your toddler is allergic to cow's milk, consider keeping him on soy formula in the cup. If he hasn't outgrown his milk allergy by the time he is 2 or 3 years old, consider one of the soy milk beverages. Read the label. To give milk's nutrients, a cup of soy milk needs to give about 8 grams protein, 2 grams fat, and about a quarter of the *percent daily value* for calcium and vitamin D.

Your child's milk intake will decrease abruptly right after he is weaned. Don't make a fuss about it—above all don't revert to the bottle or the breast—and in a few months he will get better at drinking from the cup and will drink more milk.

Does drinking milk help with weight maintenance? It can't hurt. It might help. Certainly with respect to the bone health of all family members, it can help a great deal.

Complex Carbohydrate Will Not Make Your Child Fat

Include bread with every meal so your child can eat that if he can't manage to eat anything else. Then include another complex carbohydrate with the meal, like rice, pasta, potatoes, or corn. Because complex-carbohydrate foods are tasty, not terribly challenging, and a vehicle for butter, margarine, sour cream, or gravy, children tend to like them and eat as many as they need. And so do we.

The bottom line? If you want to ignore everything I have said and go on a low-carbohydrate diet and your spouse will put up with it, it is up to you. If you are feeding a child, however, such a diet amounts to nutritional neglect. You cannot responsibly feed a child a diet devoid of any one of the major nutrients, whether it is protein, fat, or carbohydrate.

There is nothing about starch that makes it deserve its long-standing indictment of being fattening. I can only speculate that bread's presumed fattening effect comes from circumstantial evidence. As I said earlier, eating a lot of protein and fat makes you accumulate ketones and kills your appetite. You urinate a lot to get rid of the ketones as well as waste products from protein metabolism. That dehydrates you, so weight goes down. Adding back carbohydrate corrects the appetite loss and dehydration caused by metabolic havoc. Ergo, weight goes back up again. In fact, it goes back up at such a rapid and seemingly out-of-control rate that it is simply terrifying. Paying attention to only the carbohydrate-eating part of the sequence makes eating carbohydrate seem like the culprit. It's not. The problem is going without it in the first place. Why go there? Eat carbohydrate.

High-carbohydrate foods make vital nutritional contributions. Even refined breads and cereals, if they are enriched, are good sources of B vitamins, including folic acid, and iron. Whole grains offer fiber as well, along with additional vitamins and minerals. Use whole grains at most half the time—children who are offered too much whole grain have trouble getting filled up and getting other nutrients they need. Rather than being fattening, high-carbohydrate foods are essential for mealtime satisfaction. They are chewy, tasty, and bulky, so eating them lets you arrive naturally at a sense of feeling full. High-carbohydrate foods are moderate in caloric density, so they are easier to regulate—to fill up on without accidentally overdoing it. A gram of carbohydrate has 4 calories—the same as a gram of protein. Fat is higher—it has 9 calories per gram.

Since high-carbohydrate foods are relatively inexpensive, they make a better choice for filling up your family than high-protein foods, which tend to be more expensive.

Seek out good-tasting breads; eat rice, couscous, grits, and noodles if you like them. Use butter or a sauce to make starchy foods more interesting. Serve whole grains about half the time—again, if you like them. Eating whole grain all the time is not necessary and isn't even good for children. Too much of the fiber and other components in whole grain can interfere with children's iron and zinc nutrition.

Protein Will Not Slim Your Child Down

For a while, red meat was considered to be a nutritional culprit. Beef, pork, and lamb are back in favor now that high-protein diets are all the fad, and bakers are going broke instead of butchers. Why don't they just tell us, "I've had it! Get your own food!"?

A few years back the idea was that meat is bad for you. It is not. Now the idea is that it will make you thin. It won't.

However, red meat *is* good for you. National statistics that tell us what we eat and what nutrients we get from it indicate that from beef alone, on which we spend only about 7 percent of our calories, we get 18 percent of our protein; over 25 percent of our vitamin B-12 and zinc; 10 percent of our vitamin B-6, iron, and niacin; and significant amounts of thiamin. Red meat (and to a lesser extent, poultry and fish) contains a substance called meat factor, which improves iron nutrition. In other words, meat carries more than its nutritional weight.[20]

Enjoy poultry and fish In my defense of meat, I do not mean to slight poultry and fish. They, too, provide protein, vitamins, minerals, and some meat factor. Prepare poultry the way you like it—bake it, fry it, roast it, sauté it, put it in soups and casseroles. Do the same for fish. Most fish is low in fat, so consider the possibility of frying or baking it with a marinade. With baked or broiled fish, have a side dish that contains fat, such as potato salad or scalloped potatoes. Rice or baked potatoes don't work as well—unless you put sour cream on the baked potatoes.

Enjoy eggs It is safe enough to eat an egg a day or even 10 a week. Eggs are a mainstay of feeding a family. Eggs are easy to like, you can prepare them in lots of different ways, and they are an inexpensive source of high-quality protein. In addition to protein, eggs contribute important amounts of E, A, D, and B vitamins.

Eggs, like meat, are currently recovering from the negative press they got a few years ago. Egg yolks, as you undoubtedly know, are a rich source of cholesterol, which precipitated recommendations to avoid them. You don't have to avoid egg yolks because they contain cholesterol. Your body has to have cholesterol, and it manufactures it if you don't get it from the foods you eat. If you cut down your cholesterol intake, your

body manufactures more. If you eat more foods containing cholesterol, your body makes less. Cholesterol plays an essential
part in the makeup of the walls of all body cells and is a major
component of brain and nerve tissue. Your body uses cholesterol to manufacture essential hormones like estrogen, testos-
terone, and adrenal hormones.

A small percentage of people lack the biological feedback
loop that allows their bodies to make less cholesterol when they
eat more. For them, a low-cholesterol diet works because it
makes their blood cholesterol go down. If you have an exceptionally high blood cholesterol, see your dietitian. She will
instruct you in eating the right kinds of fats as well as in
restricting dietary cholesterol. It is worth a try to see whether
cutting down on cholesterol in your diet makes your blood cholesterol go down. If it doesn't go down, eat eggs. In my view,
we don't all have to go without eggs because some people are
cholesterol responders.

Enjoy dry beans and nuts Nuts and cooked dried beans—
legumes—are on the protein list as well. Legumes offer fiber,
minerals, and B vitamins and are filling, economical, and delicious. These vegetable sources of protein are mainstays world-
wide. An offshoot of the meat phobia was that people discovered beans, tofu made its way onto our tables, and we began to
use seeds and nuts as a protein source. But cooked dried beans
are high in carbohydrate, so the faddists may now shun them.

You don't have to be a faddist. Include all sources of protein and your diet will be the better for it. The greater your variety, the better your diet. Have beans as a main dish, as in red
beans and rice, or combine them with meat as in minestrone
soup. Have them as a side dish, as in wieners and beans—or
beanie wieners, as one of my families calls them.

Peanut butter is on the dry beans and nuts list. This mainstay for children has raised concerns recently because some
people experience life-threatening reactions when they eat
peanuts. Children are most likely to be seriously allergic to
peanuts if they have strong family histories of allergies of any
kind—not just food allergies. If someone in your family has
allergic reactions, keep your child away from peanuts and

peanut butter until he is 2 years old. If your family has no such history of allergies, he can start having peanut butter when he is a year old.

Lighten Up About Fats and Oils

The Food Marketing Institute survey I referred to earlier shows that we are starting to lighten up on our hysteria about dietary fat. However, since almost half of survey respondents still name fat avoidance as their number-one dietary concern, we still have to talk about it. In *Secrets of Feeding a Healthy Family*, I focus considerable attention on dietary policy in general and fat recommendations in particular. To arrive at the recommendations given in that book, I read more on the topic than I care to think about, consulted experts, and thought and thought. Here, I will tell you what I recommend. To find out *the reasons* for the recommendation, read *Secrets of Feeding a Healthy Family*.[21,22]

My recommendation? Lighten up and hedge your bets. Eating fat doesn't make you fat, provided you don't get into a restraint/disinhibition cycle. Unless you have a strong family history of heart disease, you can safely relax for both yourself and your child. Be moderate in your fat use, not restrictive. Use butter on vegetables or sauces on foods (if you enjoy butter and sauces). Put ranch dressing on the table and let your child use it as a dip for vegetables. My recipes in *Secrets of Feeding a Healthy Family* have 1 or 2 teaspoons of fat per serving, and they are still moderate in fat. Using a sauce or some butter or margarine in preparation of nutritious foods will make you and your child more interested in eating them. I endorse butter because its wonderful taste adds greatly to good food flavor. Because it carries so much flavor, you may end up using less than if you try to settle for margarine. If you prefer margarine, you have my blessings.

Put butter and salad dressing on the table, eat as much as you like, and let your child use them to make food taste good. He will eat more sometimes, less others. Even you, with your jaded sensitivity to your internal regulators, will tire of a steady diet of fatty foods. Your internal variety-seeking mechanism provides guidance for low- and high-fat food just as it does for other foods—if you pay attention.

Use a variety of fats. Emphasize monounsaturated fats, like olive, canola, and peanut oils in your cooking, frying, and salad dressings. Include polyunsaturated fats as well, like corn, sunflower, and soybean oils; just don't use them as much as the monounsaturated ones. If you use margarine, look for a margarine with the first ingredient a liquid form of one of the monounsaturated fats. Hardened, or hydrogenated, oils in margarine or vegetable shortening don't have the nutritional advantages of liquid oils.

Hydrogenated fats and foods made with them, and hydrogenated oils, like many store-bought cookies and crackers, contain *trans*-fatty acids. Use these foods moderately, but don't feel you have to avoid them altogether. Like a lot of other foods that are only marginally good for you, it takes a lot of trans-fatty acids to cause a problem.

DON'T TRY TO AVOID CONTROLLED SUBSTANCES

I get my best lines from parents. Not long ago, I presented to a parent group in Duluth, Minnesota. Robin—a prized associate from long ago—raised her hand to remind me of our history. She also had a question: "What about food like cookies, candy, potato chips and French fries?" she wanted to know. "In our house we call those 'controlled substances' and try not to let our children have them." The audience loved this turn of phrase, and I loved it too. How do you manage those wonderfully appealing, appallingly high-calorie foods that children see advertised over and over again on their favorite television programs? Aside from only letting them watch PBS (which is not such a bad idea), you need a strategy.

I will advise you as I advised Robin and the other Duluth parents: Don't set controlled substances up as forbidden fruit. If you do, your child will overeat on them when he gets a chance. Like the deprived girls in the laboratory studies who ate without hunger, and then felt bad about it, children who don't get to eat those foods at home are set up for overeating and too much weight gain. However, you also don't want to give your child unlimited access to those foods or they will spoil the nutritional quality of his diet and he won't learn to eat other nutritious food.

To find the middle ground, make controlled substances a routine part of family meals and snacks. For example, put potato chips on the table once or twice a week—or more—with the sandwiches. Have a large enough bowl so there are chips left over at the end of the meal. That way, you can be sure everyone has had enough. If this is new and chips have been a controlled substance, at first your child will eat a lot of chips and virtually nothing else. After a few meals, the newness will wear off and he will go back to eating his sandwiches and not so many chips.

Offer cookies and milk for occasional snacks. Put on a big plate of cookies—enough so there are some left over. At first your child may eat a lot, but soon the newness will wear off and he won't eat so many. Consider making cookies nutritious— peanut butter or oatmeal chocolate chip cookies, chocolate with nuts. Don't cheat by making cookies low-fat or low-sugar. They won't taste as good and your child won't trust you.

Desserts at meals are all right too, but limit the amount to a single child-sized serving. In fact, put each person's desert at their place when you set the table. Let your child eat it when he wants—before, during, or after the meal. Don't give seconds. Your child will discover he is still hungry after dessert and eat something else on the menu. Instead of eating something else, he might beg for more dessert and leave the table without eating anything else, but before long he will get the idea.

The alert reader will detect a crossing of the lines of the division of responsibility in this advice. Guilty as charged. The reason for the exception is that children will push themselves along to learn to like new food, but desserts have an unfair advantage over vegetables and other nutritious mealtime food. With a new sweet, you get one-trial learning. But learning to like new vegetables may take many exposures. It is all right to offer unlimited cookies at snack time because the cookies don't compete with other nutritious food.

Treat candy the same way you do other sweets. Your child needs to learn to manage sweets and to keep sweets in proportion to the other food he eats. Halloween candy presents a learning opportunity. Work toward having your child be able to manage his own stash. For him to learn, you will have to keep your interference to a minimum. When he comes home from trick-or-treating, let him lay out his booty, gloat over it, sort it, and eat as much of it as he wants. Let him do the same the next day. Then have him put it away and relegate it to meal- and snack-time: a couple of small pieces at meals for dessert and as much as he wants for snack time.

If he can follow the rules, your child gets to keep control of the stash. Otherwise, you do, on the assumption that as soon as he can manage it, he gets to keep it. Offer milk with the candy, and you have a chance at good nutrition. If you are doing a good job of feeding, a few days of eating a lot of candy won't impair your child's nutritional health. If you aren't, all the candy restriction in the world won't make any difference.

Ann Merritt, one of my reviewers, who is also an experienced parent and a pediatric dietitian, makes an observation about the importance of the way parents approach the subject of Halloween candy: "This advice should be in every parents' magazine every year. I have seen so many kids have Halloween ruined for them when parents are over-concerned about sugar." When you consider that for many children Halloween is their *very favorite* holiday, that is a serious concern.

MAKE WISE USE OF PLANNED SNACKS

Since snacks are little meals, apply the same planning strategies for them that you use for meals—except you can get by with two or three foods rather than four or five. A snack is not a treat. A snack is not a reward. Bring snacks out as reliably, matter-of-factly, and neutrally as you do meals. Have your child sit up to the table to eat his snacks. Let him eat as much as he wants. Don't let him run around the house to eat. It's dangerous, it's grazing instead of having a planned snack, and it makes a mess. Sit down and keep him company. Have something to drink or to eat. Make this a relaxing time for you and your child.

As your child gets older, into the school and teen years, let him take over the snack. Then start teaching the principles you use in planning snacks—including the one about timing.

Time Snacks Well

Good timing keeps snacks moderate in size and keeps them from interfering with meals. Time snacks to be not too early or too late. Offer your child a snack midway between meals. Give the snack long enough after the previous meal so he has time to get hungry but not *too* hungry, and long enough before the next meal so he has time to get hungry again. Children—and adults—may need more than one snack to make it from an early lunch to a late dinner.

Offer Protein, Fat, and Carbohydrate

Make snack food as nutritious and filling as meal food. A snack must be more than an apple or some carrot sticks. A satisfying snack that keeps your child from being hungry long before the next meal must contain protein, fat, and carbohydrate—the same as a nutritious meal. An apple or some carrots give only carbohydrate and few calories. As a consequence, they will soon leave your child hungry.

Appendixes in both *Child of Mine: Feeding with Love and Good Sense* and *Secrets of Feeding a Healthy Family* give snack suggestions. The short version is that any food that you consider appropriate for a meal is appropriate for a snack. At snack time, children are often more willing to try new foods than at mealtime. Maybe you can work in the servings of vegetables that are missing in the day's food totals. Consider serving them raw, perhaps with softened cheese spread to give protein and fat. Add a glass of milk, and you will have a filling and well-balanced snack!

Make Your Own Choices About Controlled Substances

Because they don't give many nutrients for cost and calories, foods defined by the advertising industry as snack foods generally fall into the category of controlled substances. Again, don't try to avoid controlled substances, but do use them wisely. If your child likes Twinkies and Ho Hos, fruit drinks, candies, and popsicles, offer them occasionally at planned sit-down snacks and improve the snack by offering milk with the snack cakes, cheese and crackers with the fruit drinks.

Foods that are more nutritious are better, but the bottom line is *structure*. Don't let me put you on a guilt trip. Guilt trips lead to restraint, which leads to overeating, which leads to excessive weight gain.

If you like foods like Twinkies and Ho Hos, fruit drinks, candies, and popsicles, ignore my nutritional hand-wringing and have them regularly. If you don't have them regularly, they will become the forbidden fruit on which everyone overeats when they have the chance. On the other hand, if you want to be moderate, buy a limited quantity—enough to give a child as much as he wants at a single snack but not so much that it forces you to be the gatekeeper in rationing out the leftovers. Children can satisfy all their nutritional requirements and still need more calories, so the extra sugar doesn't hurt.

With controlled substances, as with all other foods, if it *feels* like restraint to you, it *is* restraint. Restraint is a subjective and individual phenomenon. I don't crave Ho Hos and Twinkies, so not eating them doesn't feel like restraint to me. But deprive me of my potatoes and gravy, and *that* feels like restraint! Again, the bottom line is *structure*. Your child will gain too much weight if all the time and any time you let him have Twinkies and Ho Hos, fruit drinks, candies, popsicles, and other treat foods—or mashed potatoes and gravy for that matter. On the other hand, if you maintain the structure of meals and snacks *with any food,* your child will regulate.

MAKING USE OF THIS INFORMATION
Be careful with this information. I know from experience that no matter what I say to warn you or calm you down, you are right on the verge of packing for a guilt trip. "We should be eating healthy," you will say, forcing your eyes away from the French fries and making everyone have the salad instead. "Chili dogs can't be good for us," you will lament, and you will turn instead to broiled chicken breasts. "Baked fish—*that's* what we'll have," you will say. Then everyone will sneak back into

the kitchen to raid the ice cream.

There is nothing wrong with any of the foods I just listed. But if you get puritanical, you will undermine your meals. Eat what you like. Even the most reprehensible meal is far, far better than no meal at all. You must start by getting meals on the table with foods you like and find rewarding in combinations that are satisfying. If you do that, a year from now you will be actively courting foods you consider more nutritious. On the other hand, if you begin by forcing yourself to be virtuous about food selection, a year from now you will be right back where you started.

NOTES

1. Glanz et al., "Why Americans Eat What They Do."
2. ADA, *Nutrition and You.*
3. Birch and Fisher, "Mothers' Child-Feeding Practices."
4. Hood et al., "Parental Eating Attitudes."
5. Birch, Fisher, and Davison, "Learning to Overeat."
6. Rolls, "Sensory-Specific Satiety."
7. Kern et al., "The Postingestive Consequences of Fat."
8. Donnelly et al., "Nutrition and Physical Activity Program."
9. FMI Research Department, "Nature of Concern."
10. Taubes, "Big Fat Lie."
11. Wolraich, Wilson, and White, "Effect of Sugar on Behavior."
12. Knol, Haughton, and Fitzhugh, "Food Insufficiency."
13. Crocket and Sims, "Environmental Influences."
14. Rolls, Ello-Martin, and Tohill, "Intervention Studies."
15. Bell and Rolls, "Energy Density."
16. Rolls et al., "Increasing the Portion Size."
17. Rolls, Engell, and Birch, "Serving Portion Size."
18. Birch et al., "Children's Lunch Intake."
19. Johnson and Birch, "Parents' and Children's Adiposity."
20. Subar et al., "Dietary Sources of Nutrients."
21. Satter, "Children, Dietary Fat, and Heart Disease."
22. Satter, "Dietary Fat and Heart Disease."

STAGE-RELATED DEVELOPMENTAL PRINCIPLES AND FEEDING CONCEPTS

	Stage	Development Principle	Key Concept in Feeding
1	**BABY**		
	Newborn: **0–3 months**	Your baby needs help being calm and organized.	Your baby eats best when you pay attention to her and do what she wants.
	Infant: **2–6 months**	Your baby needs to connect with you.	
2	**OLDER BABY:** **5–9 months**	Your baby is getting interested in *things*.	Your baby eats solid foods best when she has a say in the matter.
3	**ALMOST–TODDLER:** **7–15 months**	The almost-toddler wants *very* much to do things for *herself*.	Your almost-toddler eats best when she feeds herself.
4	**TODDLER:** **11–36 months**	Your toddler finds out that she is a separate person.	Your toddler eats best when you teach her to participate in family meals.
5	**PRE-SCHOOLER:** **3–5 years**	Your preschooler wants to *learn, do,* and *please* you.	Your preschooler eats best when you provide both structure and support.

CHAPTER
5

OPTIMIZE FEEDING:
BIRTH THROUGH
PRESCHOOL

Your child's achieving and maintaining appropriate weight throughout her growing-up years is a matter of normal growth and development. She was born with the ability to eat the right amount of food and to grow consistently in a fashion that reflects her genetic endowment. Preserving and supporting those abilities as she grows up is identical to the process she used—or will use—in learning to smile and reach out, roll over, sit, crawl, walk, and run. The drive is within her. You support that drive by responding to her overtures, by being a spotter and role model, by avoiding interference, and by providing an environment that allows her to learn on the one hand and to be safe on the other.

Conversely, environmental distortions can interfere with her developing appropriate eating attitudes and behaviors, just as distortions can interfere with her development in other areas. Correcting those distortions restores normal growth and development. Children who are inadequately or unreliably fed become preoccupied with food and overeat when they can.

131

They only recover their ability to eat as much as they need based on their hunger, appetite, and satisfaction when they are reassured they will get enough to eat. Children who are forced to eat often become turned off to food and undereat. They recover their interest in eating only when parents restore the division of responsibility in feeding and let them decide what and how much to eat.

As you know, my approach to child overweight is built on *providing*, not *depriving*. Appendix B, "Satter Feeding Dynamics Approach: Child Weight Management," states the following:

- Child overweight can be *prevented* from birth by optimizing feeding.
- Child overweight can be *treated* by correcting disruptive influences and restoring positive feeding.

Optimizing feeding, in turn, depends on applying Ellyn Satter's Division of Responsibility in Feeding in a stage-appropriate fashion.

Before I launch into this chapter, I want to take a moment to address *your* emotional needs. My hope and dream is that you will read this chapter when your child is an infant. Given the subject area of the book, however, it is most likely that you will be reading it when she is older—when the stages that are the focus of this chapter are in the past. As a consequence, this discussion could feel like a critique of your mistakes with parenting.

As a parent, I know how you feel. I learned this information when my children were past these early stages. Looking back, I identify my mistakes, see how my behavior contributed to their dilemmas, and feel sorry. On the other hand, I realize I didn't do *too* badly because my instincts were good. I was tuned in to my children and trusted information coming from them. I have found the same is true for most parents.

As a clinician, I also know that in general parents have good instincts. Moreover, the best parents are tuned in enough to feel the pain I am talking about. They say, "Oh, my poor child, what have I done to you?" The not-as-good parents say, "What is the matter with that child? Why doesn't she just behave?" Good parents rarely get it right the first time. They do what they think is best, pay attention to their child's response, and then tinker.

As a clinician, I know that it is possible to correct mistakes in parenting. If you change your ways and keep them changed, your child will change right along with you. Of course, the younger your child is when you correct those mistakes, the easier the change. However, throughout your child's life, your changing will free your child to do the same. It will give her permission for greater possibilities.

This chapter summarizes the first six years of your child's growth and development as it applies to the issue of child overweight. For more detailed information and guidance about feeding and parenting during these critical first years, read *Child of Mine: Feeding with Love and Good Sense.*

WHAT EATING COMPETENCE LOOKS LIKE

Let's start with the end in mind. What does a child—or an adult—need to be able to do in order to maintain a reasonably stable body weight throughout life? To maintain positive nutritional status throughout life? Asked in another way, when your child is in her teens and approaching the time when she will leave home, what would you like her to be able to do with respect to her eating? What do *we* need to do in order to help her develop those capabilities?

First of all, your child needs positive eating attitudes. She will be relaxed about eating, enjoy it, and feel confident she can manage. Moreover, she will feel good about enjoying eating. She won't feel embarrassed that she likes to eat or apologetic about enjoying certain foods. She will behave decently when she eats and have good enough table manners so she can eat in public, even when she cares about making a favorable impression.

Your child will do best if she has good food acceptance skills—if her attitude about unfamiliar food is positive, or at least neutral—and she has ways of continually learning to like to new food. Unlike the 16-year-old whose parents found every steak house in Europe because he would eat nothing but steak, as she gets older she will enjoy more and more foods. She will feel good about eating and about being at the table. She will be able to remain calm when she is offered new food and be able to politely say "yes, please" or "no, thank you." She will take an interest in and be curious about new food. Since she will be able to defend herself—politely—against food she doesn't want to eat, she will know how to experiment with new food and learn to like it.

On the other hand, your child won't be a food snob. She will be able to eat food she is not particularly fond of when there is nothing else available, simply to get herself fed. In short, she will be able to feel comfortable with the food that is in the world outside your home.

Then your child needs good food regulation skills. She needs to be able to tune in on and trust her internal regulators of hunger and appetite as well as her experience of fullness and satisfaction to tell her how much to eat. She will be able to go to a meal hungry, eat with attention and enjoyment until she is satisfied, and then stop, knowing another meal or snack is coming and she can do it all over again. She will be comfortable with feeling hungry because she knows that she can eat enough to satisfy her hunger. She'll be comfortable with feeling full because she knows that's natural: she will empty out, and get hungry again.

As a result of her previous capabilities and your feeding in a regular and reliable fashion, your child will have good mealtime skills. She will conform to the structure of family meals and snacks. She will be able to tolerate her hunger and wait until mealtime to satisfy it. She will have mastered the social skills of sharing meals with other people—passing food to others, waiting for others to be served, making conversation, using her utensils properly, eating in a way that doesn't irritate other people or gross them out.

As she moves through her school-age and teen years, your competent eater will benefit from raising her intuitive eating capabilities to a conscious level. Growing up at your table, she has intuitively mastered food selection and regulation. As with any intuitive learning, it helps her if she knows what she knows. How does she know how much to eat? How does she learn to like new foods and get the nutrients she needs?

Finally, by the time she is in her late teens and ready to leave home, your child needs to know what *you* know. How can she provide for herself as you have provided for her? What does she need to do in order to be positive and reliable about feeding herself?

What This Has to Do with the Adult

Your eating attitudes and behaviors as an adult—positive or negative—began when you were an infant, were reinforced throughout the preschool years, and became consolidated when you began to learn as a school-age child to do for yourself what was done for you. If there were distortions, the younger you were when they began, and the older you were when those distortions were corrected, the more strongly fixed your counterproductive responses will be and the harder you will have to work to correct and manage them.

Moreover, we have found in our research* that the more competent adults are in their eating, the more competent they are socially and emotionally. Adults who have positive eating attitudes, have good food acceptance and food regulation skills, and can manage their food context are more self-aware, more trusting of themselves and other people, and are more comfortable with other people.

Our research corroborates what I have said all along: Feeding embodies the whole parent-child interaction. Children who are fed in a respectful, responsive, and developmentally appropriate fashion know what they are feeling, learn to respect themselves and others, and feel comfortable in the world. Assessing an adult's eating competence reveals not only that individual's history with respect to feeding but also his or her history with *relationships.*

Not surprisingly, our research also found that competent eaters do better with feeding themselves. They are more reliable about meals, they like a greater variety of food, they are less

---

* Barbara Lohse, a professor at Pennsylvania State University, and I are working together on this project. That research will be published by 2006—watch for it in the literature and on my Web site.

likely to be restrained eaters or bulimic, and they are more satisfied with their bodies.

You are your history We begin this chapter talking about the newborn, which may seem at a far remove from anything that concerns you today. However, you are living with your experience as an infant. Your ability to remain cool, calm, and collected in the midst of life in general and aggravation or excitement in particular was laid down in your first few months of life. With respect to eating, your ability to remain calm and tuned in to what goes on inside of you when you are stimulated by hunger and by the joyful anticipation of eating was formed in that earliest stage of development and reinforced—or moderated—by the stages that came after.

How do you experience hunger? Is it a positive sensation for you, and a delightful prelude to a rewarding meal? Or is it a negative, anxiety-provoking, even shameful prelude to a conflict-ridden and unrewarding eating experience? How do you experience satisfaction? Are you able to eat moderately without feeling deprived, on the one hand, and eat as much as you want without feeling like a glutton, on the other? The difference lies in whether, as a child, your hunger was respected and gratified or criticized and negated.

Consider how you experience eating. Do you enjoy it and find it rewarding? What was there about your early eating history that allowed you to have such positive eating attitudes and behaviors? On the other hand, is your eating so loaded up with shoulds and oughts that you feel deprived if you eat what you "should" and guilty if you eat what you like? Or maybe you are one of those people who don't enjoy eating at all, who consider it a chore that has to be done. What a loss! Eating is one of life's great pleasures! What could have happened to take away those rewards?

A word of encouragement: Change is possible at any age. With careful clinical work, adults can correct negative feelings about the self and seriously distorted eating attitudes and behaviors. It takes courage, determination, and hard work, but it can be done! However, as far as your child is concerned, it is far better to prevent such distortions.

Preserve Some Capabilities, Teach Others

Children develop their eating capabilities, step by step, throughout the growing-up years. Some of those capabilities are inborn; our job is to preserve them. Children come programmed with a drive to eat, they know how much they need to eat, and they can grow in the way nature intended for them.

Some eating capabilities are learned. Our job is to teach them. Children learn to remain relaxed when they eat, to manage the mechanics of eating, to try new food and learn to like it,

---

FIGURE 5.1 CHILDREN'S EATING CAPABILITIES

Children are born with these capabilities.
Your job is to *preserve* them:
1. The drive to eat
2. The ability to regulate based on hunger, appetite, and satisfaction
3. The ability to grow in the way nature intended

Children learn these capabilities step by step.
Your job is to *teach* them:
1. Remain calm at eating time
2. Be connected at eating time
3. Manage the mechanics of eating
4. Try new food and learn to like it
5. Conform to the family meal and snack pattern
6. Manage eating occasions with other familiar people—relatives, friends, school nutrition personnel
7. Choose from the standard school nutrition menu
8. Choose snack food at home from what you provide
9. Manage snacking times
10. With your guidance, choose food for snacks and then meals at restaurants, snack bars, convenience stores, and fast-food establishments
11. Increasingly understand their intuitive food regulation capabilities
12. Increasingly understand and refine their food acceptance skills
13. Independently apply food selection and meal- and snack-planning principles outside the home—at restaurants, convenience stores, and snack bars
14. Manage the schedule for feeding themselves, including participating in family meals
15. Plan family and independent meals
16. Prepare food

---

to conform to the family meal and snack patterns, and to eat in a variety of places with a variety of people. Figure 5.1 summarizes these capabilities.

CHILDREN KNOW HOW TO EAT AND GROW

From birth, your child knows how much she needs to eat in order to grow in the way nature intended. Preserving her ability to eat the amount she needs requires that you maintain the division of responsibility in feeding. For the infant, that means you follow her lead in feeding, paying attention to her signals to guide the feeding process with respect to timing, tempo, and amounts. Your being able to follow her lead, in turn, depends on *trust*. You have to trust that your child *wants* to eat, that she *will* eat the amount she needs, and that she will grow appropriately *for her.*

If, on the other hand, you become controlling, you will undermine your child's ability to eat the right amount to grow appropriately. Imposing your will and agenda on timing, tempo, or amounts will disrupt her response to her internal regulators of hunger and fullness and she may eat too much or too little.

Two Children Who Weren't Trusted

From birth, lack of trust distorts feeding and growth. Until trust is restored, the distortion persists and is compounded during each stage in development. Consider a couple of examples. In chapter 2, "Feed and Parent in the Best Way," on page 52, I told you Leane's story and showed you her weight-for-age growth charts. Leane's large size and robust appetite frightened her parents into thinking that she had no stopping place and therefore would be fat. They restricted her food intake *from birth* and caused the very problem they feared. She *lost* her inborn ability to eat the right amount to grow in the way nature intended her to grow. For almost the next 5 years, it was one feeding struggle after another: Leane's parents attempted to restrict her, she put pressure on them for food, and Leane continued to get heavier and heavier.

Leane's parents came to me for help. I found that her weight acceleration had been caused by all the factors I discussed in chapter 1, "Help Without Harming." Her parents had misinterpreted her normal size and shape and thought it was abnormal. They had instituted food restriction early on and in the process had undermined her ability to regulate food intake based on her sensations of hunger, appetite, and fullness. As a result, Leane had become so preoccupied with food that she asked for food whenever anything upset her—she had learned to eat in response to stress and was, in turn, stressed by not having enough to eat.

Leane's parents were relieved to have an explanation for their dilemma and worked hard to establish the division of responsibility in eating. They did their feeding jobs and gritted their teeth while they let Leane eat as much as she was hungry for. At first Leane ate a great deal and showed no signs of having a stopping place. But they hung in there, and after 4 to 6 weeks Leane started to eat like a normal preschooler—a lot one time, not much another; eager for snack one time, reluctant to take time another. Leane regained her sensitivity to her hunger, appetite, and fullness, and her rapid weight gain slowed down to parallel her growth curve.

Here is an example from the opposite direction. Five-year-old Ingrid had been relatively small when she was born. Despite her weighing 6 pounds, which is a good size, her parents quite naturally saw her as being tiny. The discharge physician and nurse reinforced that perception when they told them, "She is small. Because of that, you can't trust her to wake herself up to be fed. Wake her up and breastfeed her every three hours." That was poor advice. The way to prevent poor growth in the too-sleepy infant is to pay attention to her feeding cues and feed in the best way. It is *not* to impose structure.

But the advice was from people whom Ingrid's parents trusted, and that, coupled with their concern about her small size, led them to follow it. Feeding was a struggle. It was virtually impossible to wake Ingrid up to feed her, and she often didn't eat well. Her parents gave up on breastfeeding after a month, but formula-feeding didn't go any better. They spent long hours trying to entice Ingrid to take her bottle. She grew poorly, and at age 3 months the doctor recommended starting solids to try to increase her rate of growth. That was more bad advice. Better advice would have been to be more tuned in to the formula-feeding and wait to start solids until Ingrid showed signs that she was ready. Again, Ingrid's parents didn't know that. Feeding Ingrid solids was another struggle. They played games with her, and when she opened her mouth to laugh or make noises, they slipped in food. They ignored Ingrid's protests and hurt expressions and kept feeding until she cried.

By the time Ingrid was 6 months old, her parents came to positively dread feeding time. They felt bad about the way they were treating her, but they simply didn't dare to stop pressuring her to eat. They still had the impression that Ingrid was fragile and that she couldn't be counted on to do her part without being pushed. They were afraid if they stopped forcing that she wouldn't eat at all.

Ingrid continued to grow slowly when she became a toddler, and her doctor told them, "Get her to eat. I don't care how you do it." More bad advice. Better advice would have been to establish the division of responsibility in feeding and learn to understand normal toddler eating behavior. After a couple of weeks of eating less, Ingrid would have begun eating like a normal toddler. But they continued coercing her to eat, and she continued to protest and resist.

When Ingrid became a more-compliant preschooler, she finally gave in and ate. At first her parents were delighted with her weight gain. It wasn't long, however, until that weight gain became excessive, and the doctor told them to cut down on the amounts she was eating. More bad advice. Better advice would have been to establish the division of responsibility.

Like Leane, when she was an infant Ingrid *lost* her inborn ability to eat the right amount to grow in the way nature intended. During feeding, she got so upset and so caught up in the struggle with her parents that she was no longer aware that she was hungry. Her frustration and anxiety felt stronger to her than her need for food. Rather than doing her part, she resisted their attempts to force her to eat. When she finally gave in and ate in the way her parents wanted her to, she ate too much and gained too much weight. Then they restricted her, and she put pressure on them to feed her more.

Ingrid's weight acceleration grew out of the same four causes as Leane's: From birth, her normal size had been misinterpreted. Forcing Ingrid to eat more than she wanted made her insensitive to her internal regulators of hunger, appetite, and fullness. Eventually, she resolved the conflict with her parents by giving in to their pressure, whereupon she overate and gained too much weight. The basic problem was the same as it had been earlier—she wasn't tuning in to her internal regulators—but the outcome was different. Instead of undereating, she overate.

Ingrid's parents were not happy with feeding, and they didn't give up until they found a way to correct her eating problems. Once they got it all sorted out, the strategy for them was the same as for Leane and her parents: Establish the division of responsibility in feeding. Within the context of regular meals and sit-down snacks, they were to trust Ingrid to eat what and how much she wanted. Like Leane, she would start out by eating more than she needed before she would be able to find her equilibrium, but she *would* rediscover her hunger, appetite, and fullness and regain her eating competence.

Ingrid's problem, of course, started with the advice that her parents were given straight out of the obstetrical unit. While advice to be controlling with respect to feeding is common, it is totally counterproductive. In most cases, it is also unnecessary. Even small infants are capable of showing when they are hungry and when they are full, and their parents can depend on information coming from them to guide feeding. After that bumpy beginning, feeding became more and more distorted as Ingrid's parents and health workers tried to compensate for previous feeding errors. They started solid food too soon to get her to eat more and tried to control what and how much she ate when she was a toddler.

Nurses and doctors bristle when I tell stories like this, and I can understand that. Their motives are positive, even though they are the villains in the story. They were taught to give parents feeding schedules, based on the fact that some infants *are* too sleepy, *do* have trouble waking themselves up to eat, and *do* go back for their early health supervision appointments showing poor growth. Health care workers are often taught to advise

parents to start solids early to compensate for their child's fal-
tering growth, and to become coercive when their child refuses
to eat. Where I fault the health care professionals, however, is
that they settle for teaching feeding *lore* rather than seeking out
more authoritative and effective advice. Knowing how busy
and overwhelmed nurses and doctors are these days, I can even
understand *that*. However, I don't condone it.

The Early Stages Determine What Comes After

To avoid feeding errors, you have to know what to do instead.
A child works on a sequence of developmental tasks—homeostasis, attachment, separation-individuation, initiative, industry, identity. I will explain these terms in this chapter and the
following two chapters as well. Each stage provides the foundation for the achievements of the subsequent stages. A child's
ability to connect and fall in love in the attachment stage
depends on her ability to become calm and organized in the
homeostasis stage. Consider how connected you are able to be
when you are jittery and worked up on the one hand or overly
sleepy on the other!

While one or another task is primary in a given stage, a
child works on them all at every stage. Child development is
less like a stack of blocks and more like a jazz combo. One
instrument takes the solo, but the other instruments continue to
play in the background. When you are tuned in and responsive
to your newborn, you treat her as an individual with her own
needs and wishes. That gives her a jump start on the process of
separation-individuation that becomes primary when she is a
toddler. Infants who are respected and responded to are more
cooperative as toddlers.[1] They don't have as much to prove.

To cover child development and feeding from birth through
preschool in one chapter, I have had to make this brief, perhaps
too brief to give you the help you need. To learn more, read
Child of Mine: Feeding with Love and Good Sense. Keep in mind as
we go along that the age range for each of the child development stages is broad and the ages overlap. Some children are
younger when they get through a given stage; others are older.
Children with cognitive, neuromuscular, or oral-motor limita-

tions take longer. However, the sequence of change and the characteristics at each stage are the same for all children.

THE NEWBORN: 0 TO 3 MONTHS

Your baby's conscious existence—and your relationship with her—are centered around feeding. Thus, what happens in feeding becomes primary in her overall growth and development. Your newborn works to achieve *homeostasis,* a relatively stable state of equilibrium within herself and with the environment. The baby who has achieved homeostasis can be calm and alert at the same time. She is easy to be around. She is not easily upset, and when she *is* upset, she is relatively easy to read and calm down. To help her get to that point, your job is to figure out what she wants and to give it to her.

The trouble with Leane and Ingrid's feeding started at birth because their parents' agendas obliterated their receptivity to what the infants were telling them. Leane's parents ignored all but her most extreme hunger cues because they wanted her to eat less. Ingrid's parents ignored all but her most extreme fullness cues because they wanted her to eat more.

To achieve homeostasis, here is what your newborn must do:

- Begin to be interested in what goes on around her but not get so rattled she gets upset.
- Tune out excess commotion so it doesn't upset her.
- Regulate her sleep states.

Clearly, your baby needs your help in order to accomplish these tasks. What, then, must you do to help your baby achieve and maintain homeostasis?

- Trust your baby to know how much to eat.
- Understand and respect her sleep rhythms.
- Be willing and able to feed on demand.
- Learn to read and respond to her cues.
- Time care and feeding for her quiet alert state.
- Understand her temperament.

Your Baby Knows How Much to Eat

Tuning in on *when* and how *much* your baby wants to eat is essential to helping your baby be calm and alert. Trying to get her to eat less or less often, as Leane's parents did, will upset her, and she won't be able to remain calm and alert in general and during feeding in particular. The same holds true for trying to get her to eat more or more often, as Ingrid's parents did. You simply must trust that your child knows how much to eat and has an inborn wisdom about growth. She will grow in her own way in accordance with her genetic endowment.

Babies under age 6 weeks *can* be tricked into eating somewhat less or more than they need; after that, you can't trick them. When University of Iowa physician Sam Fomon fed babies either overconcentrated or overdiluted formula, babies over age 6 weeks compensated and grew consistently. The ones given overconcentrated formula ate less; those given overdiluted formula ate more. All the babies continued to grow at the same rate as they had when they were given formula that was appropriately diluted. The babies *under* age 6 weeks compensated, but not completely.[2]

Houston anthropologist Linda Adair followed a demand-fed boy's intake of formula and solid food from age 1 week to 9 months. Although the infant ate three times as much some days as others, and even though his food intake was lower than 90 percent of other babies, his growth was consistent and his size and shape were average. When he started eating solid foods, he took less formula and continued to regulate well.[3]

Babies eat best when parents pay attention to their feeding cues and do what their babies want. With some babies, it is hard to do that. For instance, parents of small babies intuitively get pushy with feeding. It is natural—small babies seem vulnerable, and parents want to help all they can. However, pushing backfires. In an Edinburgh, Scotland, study with small but still normal, well-born infants, formula-feeding parents tended to become overactive with feeding and their babies grew less well. Formula-feeding parents of average-sized infants did *not* get pushy, and their infants ate and grew well. Researchers also examined the growth of breastfed infants and found that both the small and average-sized infants grew well.[4]

Pushy feeding likely accounted for the difference in growth between the small formula- and breastfed infants. It is possible to get pushy with formula-feeding. Breastfeeding demands going by infant cues and makes being pushy more difficult. You can find a more complete discussion about food regulation and growth in *Child of Mine: Feeding with Love and Good Sense,* chapter 2, "Your Child Knows How to Eat and Grow."

There are other studies, but that is enough to make the point. From birth, children can regulate. However, their regulation depends on a parent who follows their lead with respect to feeding.

Understand Your Baby's Sleep Rhythms

Newborns sleep a lot. To do well, your baby has to learn to regulate her sleep. She has to wake up fully, stay quiet and alert long enough to eat, stay comfortably asleep when she is asleep, and make the shift from awake to asleep and back again with little commotion. Although she sleeps well, the baby who has achieved homeostasis doesn't sleep *too* much. She is able to wake herself up periodically and ask to be fed and stay awake long enough to eat as much as she needs.

Having an agenda for growth invariably goes with having an agenda for sleep. Both Leane and Ingrid were fed on a schedule—Leane to stave her off and get her to eat less, Ingrid to avoid too-long feeding intervals and get her to eat more. At times, Leane's parents tried to stave her off until she was upset and crying. At times Ingrid's parents tried to feed her when she wasn't hungry or even when she was sleeping.

You may want a schedule because you want predictability in your life. I understand that, but I don't encourage it. In the long run, a schedule will make your baby require *more* care, not less. She will eat best, sleep best, and go longest between feedings if you feed her when she is calm and wide awake.

To understand what *calm and wide awake* looks like, you must understand sleep states. When your baby sleeps, she cycles between quiet, or deep sleep, and active, or light sleep—often two or three times in a single sleep session. Then she begins to wake into a drowsy state—her eyes may be open, and she may fuss a bit. Picking her up, talking with her, and changing her diaper will wake her fully, and she will become fully awake and show she is ready to eat by sucking on her hands, fussing or making faces, and turning toward you when you touch her cheek. If she cries, you have waited too long. By then she is likely to be too upset to eat well.

Separate Comforting and Sleeping from Feeding

Separating eating from comforting and sleeping is intended not to make your baby go without eating, but to allow her to eat when she eats, sleep when she sleeps, and calm herself down when she is upset. After feeding, keep your baby company until she looks drowsy; then put her to bed and let her put herself to sleep. She may fuss a bit to get herself settled down, but not much. Don't feed her to help her fall asleep. That hooks eating with sleeping.

If you use food to help yourself sleep or to calm yourself down, you may have begun to form that tendency in your earliest infancy. While eating can be calming and eating for emotional reasons is natural, *having* to eat to calm down or go to sleep is a learned distortion. Feeding a baby to help her sleep teaches her that she *has* to eat to go to sleep. Feeding a baby to comfort her teaches her she *has* to eat to calm down.

Learn to Read and Respond to Your Baby's Cues

Paying attention and doing what your baby wants teaches her that the world is a friendly place where she is cared about and respected. Leane and Ingrid's parents unintentionally taught their children that they had to get upset or angry to make their parents listen to them.

Getting so you can be accurate and consistent about deciphering your newborn's body language can take *months*. For disorganized and unpredictable babies, it can take the whole first year. Here are some clues to get you started. Later, you will know your baby best and be able to identify her unique feeding cues. Hunger cues include sucking on her hands or turning toward you when you touch her cheek. Her eyes will be wide, eyes and face bright; she will look interested and positive and move her head, arms, and legs toward you. If she makes loud feeding sounds and fusses, she is *really* hungry, and you have waited too long to feed her. It will be hard to settle her down to eat well. Fullness cues include stopping nursing, relaxing, and extending arms, legs, and fingers. If she pushes away, arches her back, or cries, she is *really* full and you are trying to feed her too much.

THE INFANT: 2 TO 6 MONTHS

Very soon, your baby starts working on attachment—she adds on the rewarding task of being *connected.* Attachment is learning to love. She begins deliberately smiling and reaching out to you. She continues to work on being calm, and feeding will look much like it did during the homeostasis phase as you follow her lead and cuddle her to breast- or formula-feed.

You meet your baby's needs—and your own—by being smitten. Letting her captivate you puts the two of you on the same wavelength, where you can connect and joyfully talk, coo, play little reaching and tongue-thrusting games, and generally behave like an infatuated idiot. It is all very lovely.

Connecting with your baby has everything to do with supporting her normal growth and development and therefore preventing overweight. In order to eat well, your child at this and every other stage has to have her emotional needs met. All of the feeding behaviors that supported homeostasis now support her feeling loved. Your baby feels important and loved when you let yourself be guided by her feeding cues. Don't worry about spoiling at this stage—you can't spoil a little baby. You *can* spoil a toddler, but we will come to that presently.

Sleeping Affects Eating

When she is somewhere between 2 and 6 months old, parents begin longing for their baby to sleep through the night. Much misuse of feeding is made in the name of sleeping. Parents feed their child to help her sleep or put her to bed with a bottle. Since formula digests more slowly than breastmilk, formula-fed babies sleep through the night first, on the average at around age 16 weeks. Breastfed babies sleep through eventually, although often not until they are weaned.[5] As long as they know this is a normal pattern, breastfeeding parents do not seem to mind. Starting solid foods doesn't help babies to sleep better at night or last longer between feedings.[6]

You can avoid sleep problems starting at birth by teaching your child to put herself to sleep. Why does it help? Because babies don't sleep through the night any more than we do. They just get to the point where they are not hungry at night, so they don't need to wake us up to feed them. Instead, they put themselves back to sleep. Babies who learn to go to sleep when they are fed, rocked, or walked don't put themselves back to sleep. They wake us up to feed, rock, or walk them. They are doing what we taught them to do.

Co-sleeping parents have a whole different take on the night-sleeping issue. Some parents and professionals feel strongly that keeping the baby in the bed with parents is essential to nurturing and to safety. Professionals who support co-sleeping feel that it prevents infant sleep problems and is safer. They say that as long as babies sleep on a firm surface with sober nonsmoking parents, they are at decreased risk of sudden infant death syndrome (SIDS). The grounds for that thinking is that babies who co-sleep don't sleep as deeply, they wake up more easily and more often, and they can be more closely supervised by parents.

Infants who co-sleep do have significantly different sleeping and breathing patterns. They spend less time in quiet, or deep sleep, more time in active, or light sleep, and tend to nurse more frequently for shorter time periods. As a consequence, co-sleeping infants are likely to wake up more frequently at night than are those who sleep alone.[5]

As far as I am concerned, there are no shoulds or oughts. You must consider your own needs as well as your baby's needs and choose the manner of sleeping that is right for you.

THE OLDER BABY: 5 TO 9 MONTHS
After this all-too-short and intensely connected time, at around age 6 months, your baby's attachment will begin to merge with

the beginnings of separation-individuation. How can you tell? Instead of being exclusively preoccupied with you, she will start to take an interest in the outside world. Soon she will be ready to start experimenting with solid foods. Look again at the developmental tasks listed in figure 5.1. To her beginning mastery of remaining calm and connected at eating time, your child will add the tasks of (3) managing the mechanics of eating and (4) trying new food and learning to like it.

Separation-Individuation

The child working on separation-individuation learns to experience herself as separate, a process that continues to be primary until she is about 3 years old. Because we can't know what it is like for the infant *not* to feel separate, it is hard to understand this concept. Imagine being surrounded by a thick fog, so thick that you can't perceive familiar outlines and can't even see the corner of your house 3 feet away. This gives a sense of somehow being one with the environment. You can tell if something is there only by bumping into it. There are no clear boundaries. With separation-individuation, gradually the fog lifts and boundaries become defined. You become separate from the fog and from the unseen landmarks.

The fog lifts for an infant as she becomes mentally more aware, physically more capable of having an impact on her environment, and more invested in having that impact. In attending to her cues with respect to feeding, she has had control all along. Now she begins to find out she can deliberately exert that control. She starts small. She begins by taking an interest in what lies beyond her mother and other primary care providers. As she moves beyond the older baby into the almost-toddler stage, she begins to care deeply about doing things for *herself*. When she gets to be a "real" toddler and becomes mobile, she establishes her autonomy by moving and exploring, challenging and defying, and continually testing her limits.

Spoon-Feeding

You support separation-individuation by starting solid foods based on what your baby can *do*, not on how old she is. Waiting until she is ready will give her the sense of being in control of the process. Again, you offer the food, she decides to eat—or not eat. She will be more willing, not less, to experiment if you take no for an answer. Children always do and dare more when they have an out. In addition, feeding in this trusting fashion will continue to support both homeostasis and attachment. Following her cues will help her stay calm and organized as well as feel loved and accepted.

Spoon-feeding and introducing your child to new food takes self-restraint. The spoon offers more leverage, and the food offers an agenda—getting your child to eat it. It is easy to become controlling. In order to be trusting when you begin spoon-feeding, you need to

- Wait and watch for your child's signs of readiness
- Have good technique
- Understand her process of learning to like new food

Your child will be ready to start solid foods when she can sit up straight in a high chair on her own or with gentle support, open her mouth when she sees the spoon coming, close her lips over the spoon, and swallow. She will also show her readiness socially, by beginning to take an interest in what lies beyond you. She will abruptly come off the breast or shove away the bottle, sit bolt upright, and watch what is going on around her.

Feeding can be lots of fun when your child is ready. It can be unpleasant and dead boring if she is not. Your baby will eat solid foods best if you wait until she is ready, let her say yes and no, and let her eat at her own tempo to keep her in charge of the feeding.

- Seat her up straight in the high chair, maybe propped up with pillows.
- Sit directly in front of her and hold the spoon about a foot away from her mouth.
- Wait for her to open her mouth. Start by putting a little on her lip. Put familiar food in her mouth.

- Feed the way she wants to eat: little or much, fast or slow.
- Stop when she shows she is done, even after just a taste.
- Give her another chance another day.

Your child may be cautious about spoon-feeding and new tastes and textures. She needs time to learn—even 10 or 15 tries to learn to like new food. Eventually, she will like most of what you offer. On the other hand, she may take to solid foods abruptly and enthusiastically and scold you for not feeding her fast enough. It's all normal. Trust. You don't have to be like the mother who interpreted her son's passionate response to cereal as a sign of an abnormal interest in food and therefore a precursor to obesity.

Balancing nipple-feeding with solid foods depends on the stage of learning. At first, your child is likely to be more willing to experiment with solid foods if you take the edge off her hunger by giving part of a breast- or formula-feeding. As she learns to eat solid food, she can have her nipple-feeding along with, or after, the solids-feeding. Later still, you can skip the nipple-feeding and give her expressed breastmilk or formula in a cup.

Avoid controlling tactics like prying your child's mouth open with the spoon, tricking her to open her mouth, or slipping food in when she isn't looking. Being overbearing precipitates feeding struggles that teach both infants and parents to dislike feeding time. Feeding struggles, in turn, undermine food regulation and appropriate growth. Children who are upset and angry when they eat can't be sensitive to their internal regulators of hunger, appetite, and satisfaction.

Leane and Ingrid's parents' well-meaning agendas caused trouble at this stage as well. Leane's parents stopped feeding before she was fully satisfied. Ingrid's parents made her eat when she didn't want to. Ignoring all but their children's most emphatic feeding cues got in the way of both connecting and individuating. Both children were deprived of the self-respecting sense that they could get things to happen. That sense is fundamental to a child's experiencing herself as loved, on the one hand, and separate on the other.

Ann Merritt, parent, pediatric dietitian, and reviewer, speaks for all parents with her observation: "As parents, we don't realize how profound the feeding relationship is—how important it is for emotional development. If we could remember that, maybe it would be easier for us to put our agendas on the back burner."

Feeding for Emotional Reasons

While the tendency to use food for emotional reasons is most strongly put in place when a child is a toddler, it begins at birth and intensifies for the older baby. Eating can be calming, and eating occasionally for emotional reasons is natural. However, *having* to eat to calm down or to go to sleep is a learned distortion. The problem lies in *misusing* feeding as a way of connecting or as an alternative to connecting. Certainly, it is important to be connected while you feed. However, feeding when a child wants to smile or play or when she fusses for company teaches her to use food for emotional reasons. Feeding for the wrong reasons also befuddles the child's experience of herself as separate because it presents her with an impossible choice: To experience herself as separate, she has to give up connecting. To connect, she has to ignore herself and her own wishes. It is better to sort out her cues, play when she wants to play, and comfort when she needs to be comforted.

Restricting Leane's food intake left her unsatisfied in *all* ways. Although they did it inadvertently, Leane's parents taught her to use food for emotional reasons by underfeeding her so she was constantly hungry. Playing, talking, and comforting never fully satisfied her because what she wanted and needed was enough to eat. Eventually, her need for food became fused with her need for love and companionship. When she became mobile, she gratified her food cravings, ate too much, and gained too much weight.

Ingrid's father used her love of playing and connecting to get her to eat. He talked and laughed with her, then slipped in a spoonful of food when she opened her mouth to talk or laugh back. Being pressured to eat first turned her off to food and made her prone to undereat when she got the chance. Later on, she learned to disconnect from her discomfort and give in to the pressure and overeat.

THE ALMOST-TODDLER: 7 TO 15 MONTHS

Your key task for your almost-toddler is to recognize and support her need to do it *herself*. She wants to feed herself and begins to master one more task from figure 5.1: (5) *Conform to the family meal and snack pattern.* By now, she is working on quite a list: (1) remaining calm at eating time, (2) being connected at eating time, (3) managing the mechanics of eating, and (4) trying new food and learning to like it.

Your almost-toddler's need for separation-individuation will take the form of caring deeply about feeding herself. She started working on learning to like new food as an older baby. Now, growing out of her passion for feeding herself, she will eat almost everything, including marbles, pennies, and LEGO bricks. She is ready to join in with the family meals by feeding herself soft table food. Toward the end of the first year, parents begin to make judicious use of snacks to allow the child to go to the family table hungry but not famished and therefore ready to enjoy the food there.

The almost-toddler's desire to *do* makes her enthusiastic about chasing food around on her high-chair tray, capturing it with her awkward little fingers, and getting it into her mouth by whatever means she can manage. Until she could make her fingers work, a friend's grandchild put her face down to the tray and swept food into her mouth! A child in this stage looks *determined* when she eats.

The almost-toddler is ready to begin the transition from the demand feeding of infancy to the structured feeding of childhood. She is, for the most part, ready to eat pieces of soft table food, and therefore ready to join in with family meals. As earlier, to do well with eating, the almost-toddler needs her emotional needs to be met. Now that is the need to do it *herself.* Understandably, unsuspecting parents think she is still a baby— or they *want* her to still be a baby—and try to feed her. Affronted, the infant who has right up to this moment been happily allowing herself to be fed suddenly refuses to eat and will go back to eating only when she is allowed to do it *herself.* Parenting is a constantly shifting game with ever-changing rules!

Whether they knew it or not, Leane and Ingrid's parents had trouble with this stage as well. Since neither set of parents could give details, I will extrapolate from observing other children. I was reminded of Leane when I watched a teaching video of an 8-month-old. Instead of demanding to feed himself, as I would expect at his stage of development, he passively allowed himself to be fed semisolid food. It seemed that being chronically hungry made him unwilling to take chances with the source of supply. I was reminded of Ingrid when I watched a video of a 10-month-old who wanted to feed himself. His clearly devoted mother tried to feed him, but he refused and grabbed for the spoon and grabbed for the food. He wanted to eat, but he would go *without* eating rather than let his mother feed him.

Feeding Problems and the Almost-Toddler

The almost-toddler and toddler stages appear to offer more than their share of pitfalls where feeding is concerned. To navigate these stages without mishap, you must understand your child and correctly interpret her behavior. Recently, I spoke with an alarmed mother who told me that her 8-month-old wouldn't eat. Until recently he had been eating solid food with great enthusiasm. Abruptly, he had begun refusing his food, grabbing the spoon, and demanding to eat what his parents were eating. She tried to feed him soft finger-food, but he gagged.

In desperation, the mother had increased her pressure to spoon-feed her son semisolid food, and he in turn had increased the vigor and emphasis of his refusal. "Does he like to feed himself?" I asked. "For instance, does he like Cheerios or toast strips or crackers?" "Yes," she responded. "But he gags when he eats them and he doesn't have any back teeth for chewing, so I haven't been letting him have them."

The mother was looking for the wrong developmental signs. The *right* signs were her son's insistence on feeding himself and his ability to eat with his fingers. In fact, he was saying, more clearly than words could express, that he was ready to join in at the family table and eat soft pieces of table food.

Getting teeth was unnecessary—he wouldn't get molars for another 10 months, and in the meantime he could gum his food. Gagging was normal—an essential part of the process of learning to eat. Rather than first positioning a piece of food between her toothless jaws to mash it, the inexperienced eater sends it straight down her throat. Her gag reflex sends it right back up. It is all part of the learning process, and with more experience, she won't gag as much. Gagging is protection against choking. How can you tell whether a child is gagging or choking? If she can breathe, she is gagging.

Uncorrected, this all-too-common struggle for control can persist and distort feeding for *years.* Correcting it is an easy fix. Everything was in synch—the little boy had the desire to feed himself and the skills to back it up. He just needed to be given the chance.

For the almost-toddler, family meals become critically important in supporting eating competence. If you haven't started already, have meals *now.* There is simply no way around it, and no way that your child can do a good job of eating if you are not doing a good job of feeding yourself and the rest of the family. To strengthen your resolve, go back and read chapter 3, "Make Family Meals a Priority." To get help being realistic about planning meals, reread chapter 4, "Help Without Harming: Food Selection."

Weaning from the Breast or Bottle

Weaning at the appropriate time and in the appropriate fashion is essential for allowing your child to develop eating competence. An almost-toddler who is too heavily dependent on the bottle or the breast doesn't learn to eat. A toddler who is stuck on the bottle or breast goes backward with her eating capability, getting so dependent on nipple-feeding and so limited in her mealtime skills that her growth is likely to be distorted.

Weaning doesn't have to be hard or traumatic. In fact, you start the process of weaning when you introduce solid food. You finish when your child stops taking the breast or bottle. Actually, your child weans *herself* as she takes more and more interest in eating solid foods and in feeding herself and therefore loses interest in nursing. You can quietly omit first one mealtime nursing and then another and she will never miss it. Substitute the cup at mealtimes. Put formula or expressed breastmilk in the cup—if you don't mind having the breastmilk wasted. Otherwise, for mealtimes, whole milk in the cup is all right. Notice I said *in the cup*—never *in the bottle*. She won't drink enough from the cup to cause problems. In fact, at first you will worry about how little she takes. Don't make a fuss about it, and after several months she will increase her milk intake.

Build on your child's increased regularity with eating to move her toward nipple-feeding at more-or-less predictable times. Don't make her be famished, but do let her get hungry enough between times to have a substantial meal or snack. Letting your child breast- or formula-feed on demand could mean that she doesn't have a chance to get hungry—she just tops herself up.

You might find yourself having a breast- or formula-feeding approximate snack time by offering it midway between meals. Or you might find that you and your child move quickly to more grown-up sit-down snacks. Either is fine. Just keep the nipple-feedings away from mealtime. For heaven's sakes, *don't* let her carry around a bottle or a tippy cup. That will disrupt her eating and is all too likely to disrupt her growth as well.

The Almost-Toddler and Weight Regulation

What does the almost-toddler's potential for feeding problems have to do with weight? With Leane it was obvious. Restricting Leane made her preoccupied with food and prone to overeat when she got the chance. With Ingrid, it was less obvious, but the connection was there nonetheless. Forcing Ingrid made her revolted by food and prone to undereat when she got the chance. All the forcing overwhelmed her sensitivity to her internal regulators of hunger, appetite, and satisfaction, and she made errors in regulation, first undereating and then overeating.

In previous chapters, I have written about the San Francisco study that followed children from age 6 months to 16 1/2 years to identify differences in upbringing between teenagers who became overweight and those who remained slim. The overweight adolescents had more feeding problems when they were little.[7] Some of their parents likely restrained their feeding. The researchers found that teenagers were fatter when their parents were concerned about obesity in early life. Other feeding problems included food refusal, excess finickiness, or bizarre food habits.

Researchers also found that teenage fatness increased when toddlers' feeding times were not structured—which brings us to our next developmental stage: the toddler.

THE TODDLER: 11 TO 36 MONTHS

Your key parenting task for your toddler is to teach her that she is part of the family. With feeding, you teach her to conform to the family meal pattern. When she was a baby, she was the center of the universe. You dropped everything and fed on demand. Now you teach her she is no longer the star. She can learn to wait a short time to eat, she can join in with the sociability of family meals, and she can learn to behave well enough at the table for you to enjoy having her there. Parents often feel bad about applying these expectations and depriving their child of her starring role. The toddler can be reluctant to give it up as well. However, it is a *necessary* loss, and one that allows the child to do well and have rewards in the next stages of her life.

Your toddler gets seriously down to the business of finding out she is separate from you. At the same time, she gains a more precise sensitivity to herself. Of course, all this has an impact on her eating. A toddler has endless mobility, energy, and curiosity, and absolutely no judgment. It is as important to her to be treated like a separate person as it was when she was an infant. In fact, if you treated her with respect and understanding when she was an infant, she will be a lot more accommodating now. However, living with a toddler is still a challenge.

Your child has always responded well to your paying attention to what she wants. Now she is able to be a lot more assertive about seeing to it that her wishes are respected. She says no a lot, because by saying no she can establish for herself that she is in control of what happens. Her whole small world and all the actions she can perform with her newly mobile body are open to her. She is at once thrilled at the process, dedicated to exploring and manipulating, determined to do it her own way, frustrated at not being able to do everything she sets out to do, and profoundly afraid of being alone and losing contact with you. Little wonder she is hard to live with!

Your job is to give limits without controlling, to give autonomy without abandoning. With feeding, your job is to maintain the division of responsibility, doing your jobs of selecting the foods that are offered, maintaining the structure of meals and snacks, and then turning over to your toddler the prerogative of deciding what and how much she will eat of what you have put before her.

Control issues are all-important. The problem is that control is nebulous and hard to define, especially since we live in such a controlling culture and since nutritional and medical advice tends to be controlling. Not to worry. Your toddler will teach you. She can smell control a mile away and will react when you get controlling. I tell my audiences that if they have problems with being controlling, they need to rent a toddler!

Don't be controlling, but don't go to the other extreme either, throwing away all limits. Not having limits is so frightening for a toddler that she will unconsciously increase her negative behavior to force you to take charge.

Feeding the Toddler

Compared with the almost-toddler, who is exuberant about eating almost everything as long as she is allowed to feed herself, the toddler becomes skeptical of anything *she* doesn't recognize, even if *you* know she has had it many times before. Combine your toddler's increased skepticism about new food with her natural slowdown in her rate of growth. Throw in the enthusiastic and often relentless exploration that makes her loath to take time to eat. Mix it all together, and you have a child who has seemingly lost interest in eating.

Your toddler's skepticism is actually a more mature and self-preserving behavior than the almost-toddler's indiscriminate eating. It could be that the toddler has matured mentally enough to distinguish new from familiar food but has not matured enough to gain familiarity in any other way but tasting. Some things *could* be bad for her, and sneaking up on new food is a survival tactic. Of course, you won't offer anything bad for her, but reassuring her will cut absolutely *no* ice. She has to find out for herself.

To help your toddler join in with family meals, plan the timing of sit-down snacks so she can arrive at the table hungry but not famished. She has to be composed enough to take an interest. She will continue to work on the same five tasks as the almost-toddler: (1) remain calm at eating time; (2) remain connected at eating time; (3) manage the mechanics of eating; (4) try new food and learn to like it; and (5) conform to the family meal and snack pattern. However, it will seem that she has suffered a relapse with number four: trying new food and learning to like it.

The toddler's skeptical attitude toward new food and caution about trying it once again booby-traps concerned parents into getting pushy with their feeding. Parents can't understand why their heretofore happily eating child suddenly becomes so picky.

Avoid Common Pitfalls
To parent a toddler, you must find the middle ground between being permissive and being domineering. Check yourself. You are being too controlling if you

- Expect your child to be predictable about eating *anything*
- Expect your child to eat a certain amount
- Expect your child to eat what she did some other time
- Expect your child to eat what she tells you she will eat
- Get by on only three meals a day

You aren't providing enough structure and support if you

- Wait for your child to ask before you offer food
- Give her a snack whenever she wants one
- Let her stay at the table when she behaves badly
- Short-order cook for her

- Let her have juice, milk, or other beverages besides water whenever she wants them

Maybe you find yourself on both sides of the fence—being too controlling with some things and not providing enough structure and support with others. Being inconsistent is confusing to your child and will make it hard for her to do well with her eating.

If you are taking the lead with having family meals, feeding your toddler will go relatively smoothly. If you are not, feeding is littered with pitfalls. The timing and menus for meals and snacks have to be *your* idea, because your busy toddler will know she is hungry only when she collapses.

Today's standard way of feeding toddlers is anything but optimum. Some parents leave little dishes of food at toddler level so their toddler can grab and run all day long. That deprives her of the socialization of the family table. Others search for the magic food that will make their child eat. In Tennessee studies, Jean Skinner and her students found that 70 percent of parents prepared alternative foods for their toddler if she didn't eat the first thing that she was offered.[8] That approach engages the toddler in playing "jerk the parent around" rather than attending to eating. Many parents generate meals on demand, waiting for their toddler to ask for food before they begin to rustle it up. By then it's far too late. Overly hungry toddlers collapse and refuse to eat.

In defense of young parents, those are the most common patterns of feeding that parents pick up from each other, from misguided advisers, and even from advertising. Some parents cater because they don't want to hurt their child. They were overcontrolled as children, and they swear not to repeat that misery. In the short term, these common patterns avoid hassle. In the long term, these patterns profoundly undermine family meals. Toddlers who don't get the guidance and limits they need become more and more demanding and cranky. If all goes well, eventually parents are forced to do what would have been better done in the first place—teach the child to participate in the meals-plus-snacks routine of the family.

What do these patterns of grazing, short-order cooking, and meals-on-demand have to do with your child's weight, especially as a school-age child and teenager? Once established, your child's doing her own thing with respect to eating will hang on. Unless you make some changes, you will raise a dictatorial, finicky child who is anxious and ambivalent about her eating. Her conflict and negativity will undermine her ability to tune in on her hunger, appetite, and satisfaction. She may eat more than she needs to make herself feel better—or to defy you. She may eat less than she needs because she lacks social and emotional support for eating—or to defy you. She will experience so much inner and outer conflict that she won't be sensitive to her hunger, appetite, and fullness.

At this stage, distortions in feeding became even more apparent for Leane and Ingrid. Once she became mobile, Leane began running raids on the food supply—getting into cabinets and the refrigerator. She used her toddler aggressiveness to relentlessly hound her parents for food. When they gave in to her, she ate as much as she could hold because she never knew when she could wear them down again. Ingrid, on the other hand, used *her* toddler aggressiveness to resist her parents' feeding attempts all the more energetically.

Misusing Eating for Emotional Reasons

The real loss for a child who learns to misuse food for emotional reasons is the lack of emotional development. The overweight that could grow out of such a pattern is only a symptom. If *you* have a pronounced tendency to misuse food for emotional reasons, it was likely most strongly put in place during the toddler period.

Let's make a distinction. Eating for emotional reasons is not bad or wrong. It is one of the ways we celebrate or comfort ourselves. However, we *misuse* eating for emotional reasons if eating is the only or the predominant way we deal with feelings, or if we eat unthinkingly whenever we are upset. Learning to misuse eating can start at birth, when feeding is used to comfort, distract, or entertain. However, that learning is cemented into place during the toddler period.

The toddler goes through a process called somatopsycholog- ical differentiation. Let's break that down: somato = body; psy- chological = emotional; differentiation = learning to distinguish one from the other. Somatopsychological differentiation occurs when the toddler learns to distinguish among her feelings and differentiate her feelings from her sensations. Is she angry or hungry? Sad or cold? Full or tired? You have helped her to dis- tinguish all along by paying attention to her cues, sorting out their meaning, and—most of the time—applying the proper solution. If she was angry, you let her yell. If she was bored, you kept her company. If she was tired, you put her to bed.

Continuing to make those distinctions with your toddler helps her to identify those feelings and sensations for herself and apply the proper solution. Eventually, you help her learn to talk about what is bothering her. On the other hand, if you feed instead of tolerating anger, feed as a sop for boredom, or feed when your child is whiney or tired, those feelings and sensa- tions *don't* get sorted out. In later life, it will be hard for her to know what she is feeling and apply the proper solution. Instead, she will eat.

Why would you feed instead of dealing with a toddler's feelings? Have you ever lived with a toddler? They are the most energetic and disputatious little beings who have ever been put on this green earth. Little wonder that parents resort to food handouts just to get a moment's peace!

While I understand giving food handouts and letting a tod- dler cruise for food, I do not condone it. The short-term solution is tempting, but you—and your child—will pay for it in the long run. Her eating behavior will get worse—lots worse. Her pleas for food will become relentless. Her refusal to eat at meal- time will become vociferous. Better that you follow the division of responsibility in feeding and maintain the structure of meals and snacks. That will remove the temptation to dole out food in the midst of mayhem. If it's not time, you don't feed, the associ- ation doesn't get made, and both you and your toddler learn to tolerate her feelings.

What does this have to do with weight? Stress is certainly a part of life. I have reassured you before that we all use food for emotional reasons, and there is nothing wrong with that. However, failure to effectively accomplish somatopsychological differentiation means a child will learn to reflexively and routinely relieve emotional upset with food. She will eat without ever bringing her feelings up to a conscious level. When such a child experiences too much stress or stress that goes on and on, she is at risk of eating too much and gaining too much weight.

THE PRESCHOOLER: 3 TO 5 YEARS

After living with a toddler, living with a preschooler feels like sailing into tranquil waters. When she was a toddler, your child found out that she was a separate person from you. Now that she has done that, as a preschooler she can go back to being cooperative—most of the time. She can remember what you tell her and manage her own behavior. Her language is better now, and rather than *learning to talk* she is *talking to learn*. Rather than using the toddler's unrelenting process of trial and error, she can talk with you to find out about the world and think about what she will and won't be allowed to do.

Therein lie the pitfalls. Not having to supervise your preschooler *every single minute* may make you feel that you aren't as important as you used to be. Not so. Your guidance and support is as important as ever before—with feeding as with everything else in your preschooler's life. Your preschooler's capability and compliance can lull you into being casual and nonchalant about feeding. Because she is reliable enough to eat on her own, you can forget that she needs you to eat with her, not just feed her. Because she wants to please you, you can shame her into doing what you want. You *can* coerce her to eat—and to overeat.

The division of responsibility in feeding is as important for your preschooler as it was when she was younger. In some ways, it is *more* important, because your preschooler thinks you are the best, depends on your presence to do well, and wants to be just like you. She works on initiative—on learning and doing, on trying things out, on beginning to understand, on imitating and trying to please you. If she can achieve and please, she feels great. If she can't, she feels ashamed and guilty. She will do your bidding when you say "clean your plate," or "eat your vegetables before you can have dessert," or "you have to take 2 (or 3 or 10) more bites," or "surely you like that—you grew it in your garden!"

What's the matter with the garden bit? Preschoolers *can* gain familiarity with food and *are* more likely to eat if they help cook it or grow it. But cooking or gardening backfires if parents have an agenda—if they cook or grow a garden with their preschooler to *get* her to eat. That's pressure, the child will be on to it in a flash, and she will eat less well, not better.

Make Choices About Parenting

Your key parenting task with your preschooler is to provide both structure and trust. You have been parenting all along, use the relative composure and predictability of living with a preschooler to make some deliberate choices about parenting. In a classic, often-quoted and often-confirmed piece of work, Diane Baumrind, a child development specialist at the University of California, Berkeley, observed 134 children, 3 and 4 years old, in nursery school to see how comfortable they were with themselves and how well they did with other people. She then observed them with their parents. Children whose parents gave both love and limits were most likely to become successful, happy with themselves, and generous with others. Children whose parents were overly strict were likely to be obedient but unhappy, and those whose parents were overly lenient and gave few guidelines were likely to feel insecure and lack self-control. Baumrind called these three parenting approaches *authoritative, authoritarian,* and *permissive.*[9]

The words *authoritative* and *authoritarian* are much alike but carry far different meanings. Authoritative means *decisive* and *reliable.* Authoritative parents have rules, then give the child leeway within the rules. Authoritarian means *dictatorial* or *overbearing.* Authoritarian parents have lots of rules and make children do what they want or else. Permissive parents let almost anything go until they can no longer stand their child's negative behavior. They blow up, then feel bad and try to make up for it.

The division of responsibility in feeding is an authoritative approach to parenting—you take a strong leadership role but also give your child scope for acting on her own wishes. For your toddler, maintaining the division of responsibility was essential for staying out of eating struggles. For your preschooler, maintaining the division of responsibility is necessary to allow her to experiment and learn and grow. It is also necessary to keep from hurting her feelings and distorting her eating attitudes and behaviors.

As with Leane and Ingrid, restrained feeding becomes a marked problem for the preschooler. She has enough autonomy to go against her parents' wishes and get food, enough emotional maturity to feel guilty and ashamed about it. Uncorrected, her conflict and anxiety about eating can get stuck and undermine her ability to do a good job with eating.

Preschoolers, Food Regulation, and Food Acceptance
Preschoolers continue to be excellent at regulating food intake, but outside interference can make them lose that regulatory ability. In a Pennsylvania State University study, preschoolers ate more when presented with larger portions. In contrast, toddlers ate the same amount, no matter the portion size. The researchers interpreted their results to mean that preschoolers become less capable of regulating food intake and thus can be made to overeat by offering them large portion sizes.[10] This interpretation overlooks the feeding relationship as well as child development principles. Large portion sizes alone won't make a child overeat. Large portions plus *feeding pressure* makes preschoolers, but not toddlers, overeat. Preschoolers are compliant. Toddlers would rather fight than submit.

The preschooler recovers lost territory with food acceptance as she becomes less skeptical about new food and is therefore relatively willing to try it and learn to like it. She can learn about new food by talking about it, helping cook it, and helping grow it in the garden. For tips about including your preschooler in food preparation, see *Secrets of Feeding a Healthy Family.* Each menu has an "Involving Your Children" feature.

By this time your child has capability number 5, conform to the family meal and snack pattern, well in place. Now she adds the sixth capability from the list in figure 5.1: manage eating occasions with other familiar people—relatives, friends, school nutrition personnel. Please note the wording in number 6: It does not say "eat with other people"; it says "manage eating occasions." This goes back to the food acceptance competencies we focused on early in this chapter. To participate comfortably in meals and snacks, children need to know that they don't have to eat what they don't want to eat, and they need to be able to refuse food politely. For a child to be able to say yes to new food, she has to be able to say no. Children who can effectively manage eating occasions eventually learn to like a variety of food. Trust that your child wants to learn and grow.

Preschoolers feel proud when they can please their elders, guilty and ashamed when they can't. When her parents began restricting her eating, Ingrid, like Leane, became preoccupied with food and overate when she got the chance. Leane and Ingrid could not manage eating occasions in a way that pleased their elders because they were being asked to do the impossible—to make themselves go hungry. By the time they were preschoolers, extended family, friends, and school personnel had been deputized to withhold food. But both children were so driven by hunger and the fear of going without that they had become resourceful about sneaking food and wearing down their elders. Of course, they felt bad about it, but they simply couldn't help themselves.

THE LARGE INFANT, TODDLER, OR PRESCHOOLER
Leane and Ingrid, and their parents, have taught us to feed well, resist interference, and catch problems early.

To feed well, maintain the division of responsibility in feeding. Your large infant, toddler, or preschooler is entitled to depend on you to do a good job with feeding and to be trusted to do hers with eating—and growing. Your large child is entitled to like her body and *not* be made to feel that there is something wrong with her. Your large child is entitled to go to the table hungry, eat until she is satisfied, and then stop, knowing another meal or snack is coming and she can do it again.

To protect yourself and your child from interference, understand normal growth. Jump ahead now to read chapter 10,

"Understand Your Child's Growth." Understand the difference between *high normal* weight and weight *acceleration*. Know that your child is growing well if her weight consistently follows a particular percentile curve. Know the difference between a normal and an abnormal growth adjustment. Understand that the large child is more likely to slim down than remain heavy. The research shows that 75 percent of overweight infants and toddlers and roughly 60 to 75 percent of overweight preschoolers are no longer overweight by the time they are adults.[11] Even if your child does *not* slim down, if her growth is consistent, it is likely to be normal *for her*.

To further resist interference, be skeptical of media headlines and consternation about obesity in the very young child. In their attempts to identify biological causes for overweight, researchers are scrutinizing younger and younger children. You will hear their speculation about causes of child overweight—everything from factors during pregnancy to the fat infant's having too many fat cells to mysterious hormonal changes. When you consider that most young children slim down on their own, the consternation about early overweight and speculation about causes simply don't make sense.

Hindsight is always 20-20. It is easy to look back and identify times when Ingrid and Leane's parents could have fed differently and avoided their pain and struggle. It's not so easy when it is happening to you. Here are some guidelines to help you catch your problems early. You are likely to need help with feeding when any of the following are true:

- Your child's growth (at any age) veers upward or downward abruptly.
- You and your child struggle a lot about her eating.
- You have tried lots of ways to resolve the problem, but you can't.
- You worry a lot about her eating or growth.

Don't let problems drag on. An early fix is an easy one. Ask for an appointment with a dietitian or other professional who clearly understands Ellyn Satter's Division of Responsibility in

Feeding and evidence-based recommended feeding practice as I have taught in this chapter. Help is out there. Keep looking until you find it.

If all goes well with feeding during the preschool years, a child arrives at her school-age years with her eating competence intact. She has a positive attitude toward eating. She has good food acceptance and food regulation skills. She has the tools and capabilities to master what comes next. On the other hand, when the first stages in feeding are distorted, the child's eating capability is undermined. Each stage to follow becomes increasingly distorted by misguided attempts to compensate.

As we leave the preschool years and turn to the school-age and then the teenage child, we reap what we have sown. Will we be able to build on the child's eating competencies, or will we have to make up for past errors? The good news is that even for the school-age child and the teenager, the capabilities are still there, waiting to be tapped. The child still needs parents to take reliable leadership with feeding. The division of responsibility in feeding still applies.

NOTES

1. Stayton, Hogan, and Ainsworth, "Infant Obedience."
2. Fomon et al., "Influence of Formula Concentration."
3. Adair, "Infant's Ability to Self-Regulate."
4. Crow, Fawcett, and Wright, "Maternal Behavior."
5. Johnson, "Helping Infants to Sleep."
6. Mackin, Medendorp, and Maier, "Infant Sleep and Bedtime Cereal."
7. Crawford and Shapiro, "How Obesity Develops."
8. Skinner et al., "Mealtime Communication Patterns."
9. Baumrind, "Current Patterns of Parental Authority."
10. Rolls, Engell, and Birch, "Serving Portion Sizes."
11. Serdula et al., "Obese Children."

UNDERSTAND AND PARENT YOUR SCHOOL-AGE CHILD

Your school-age child is learning to function independently. He has much to learn and a long way to go, and you must provide support without controlling and provide autonomy without abandoning.

Your Child's Growth and Development
- He systematically learns and masters. He needs to achieve in order to feel worthwhile.
- He internalizes your values and functions independently; he thinks he knows it all.
- He works on physical capability by practicing and playing with friends.
- He can reason logically, organize himself, categorize, and think about thinking.
- Friends become very important, and he works out ways of getting along with them.

How to Parent Your School-Age Child
- Teach and guide. His industry and eagerness to learn will prompt you.
- Talk and listen; consult and support to work out expectations and limits.
- Give independence as he demonstrates responsibility.
- Work behind the scenes with other adults and outside opportunities.

How to Parent Your School-Age Child with Respect to Feeding
- Retain leadership with family meals and food selection.
- Give guidelines for food away from home and time limits for snacks.
- Accept suggestions for menus after he masters food acceptance.
- Help him to know what he knows about his intuitive eating capabilities.

CHAPTER
6

OPTIMIZE FEEDING:
YOUR SCHOOL-AGE
CHILD

Your school-age child's ability to eat the amount he needs to grow in a way that is right for him builds on the achievements of the earlier stages—or suffers the consequences of earlier failure to achieve. For your child to continue to do well with eating, you must continue to do well with feeding. You must continue to manage the *what, when,* and *where* of *feeding* and trust him to do the *how much* and *whether* of *eating.*

In the previous chapter, I emphasized that from birth through preschool you can prevent child overweight by feeding in a tuned-in, stage-appropriate fashion. The same holds true for the school-age child. Doing your feeding jobs and supporting your child's eating capabilities allow him to continue to grow appropriately.

If all has gone well earlier, your school-age child's innate eating capabilities have been preserved. He takes an interest in eating, eats as much or little as he is hungry for, and grows the way nature intended. Now he begins to integrate those capabilities: He makes them his own, puts them more strongly in place, and applies them in the outside world. Your continuing to do your feeding jobs will help these *learned* eating capabilities to stay in place:

1. Remain calm at eating time
2. Be connected at eating time
3. Manage the mechanics of eating
4. Try new food and learn to like it
5. Conform to the family meal and snack pattern
6. Manage eating occasions with other familiar people

The school-age years revolve around beginning to prepare for the adult world. Either consciously or unconsciously, the school-age child realizes he is growing up and must someday leave his family. That task is a daunting one, but your child, in time, will want to do it anyway. As with younger children, the drive to grow up, learn, and do does not have to be put in place. It comes with being a child. His drive to learn and grow is an older version of the drive for separation-individuation—to establish autonomy—which began when he was 6 months old.

During the school-age years, your child gradually starts learning to do for himself, not only with eating but also with everything else in his life. You help him by gradually doling out tasks and responsibility as he is able to manage. You challenge him without overwhelming him, provide support without controlling, give independence without abandoning. Still working from the list in figure 5.1, "Children's Eating Capabilities" (page 137), here is how your school-age child, with your guidance and support, gradually prepares himself to take adult responsibility with food selection:

7. Choose from the standard school nutrition menu
8. Choose snack food at home from what you provide
9. Manage snacking *times*
10. With your guidance, choose food for snacks and then meals at restaurants, snack bars, convenience stores, and fast-food establishments

11. Increasingly understand his intuitive food regulation capabilities
12. Increasingly understand and refine his food acceptance skills

With your blessings and under your guidance, your school-age child gradually begins taking over *your* job of choosing food for him. He starts small, with school lunch and afternoon snack. As an adolescent, he works up to understanding enough about food selection, planning, shopping, and cooking to provide for himself after he leaves home.

Parents most often present their child for treatment of overweight during the school-age years. Now that the school-age child is more out on his own and has greater access to food, food-restriction tactics that worked before may not work any longer. With the younger child, you might be able limit access to certain foods to control the amount he eats, but not anymore. In my clinical practice, I find that starting with the school-age child, struggles around feeding graduate from being merely irritating to being pitched battles. Furthermore, parents find that their child's chubbiness—either long-standing or newly emerging—becomes impossible for them to ignore.

A CHILD WHO GAINED TOO MUCH WEIGHT

On the telephone, Haley's mother told me that 10-year-old Haley had "gained a huge amount of weight—shot up off the scale." The mother's intensity and her observation that struggles about Haley's eating had gone on for *years* prompted me to recommend a careful assessment. Haley's parents, like those of other children with long-standing feeding problems, had been exposed to a piecemeal approach to the problem. In the process, they had been given lots of advice, and more advice wouldn't help. They needed someone to look at their situation in detail, to consider all the issues, to provide an explanation for Haley's unstable weight, and to make a plan for resolution that covered all the bases.

Haley's parents could see the merit of such an approach and collaborated with me on the evaluation. I reviewed Haley's medical records from birth, replotted her weight, calculated a 7-

day food intake, watched videos of three family meals, had her parents fill out a questionnaire on parenting, and interviewed Haley and her parents in my office.

Haley's weight-for-age record from 2 to 10 years (shown in figure 6.1), showed that after remaining stable at the 75th percentile from age 2 ¹/₂ to 7 years, her weight over the following 3 years had accelerated from the 75th to the 95th percentiles.

FIGURE 6.1 HALEY WEIGHT-FOR-AGE 2 TO 10 YEARS

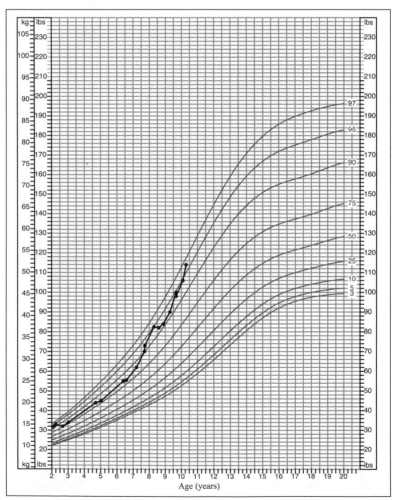

While Haley's weight had increased, it had *not* shot up off the scale. That statement said more about her mother's weight pre-occupation than about Haley's weight per se. However, to give credit where credit is due, her mother's action may have pre-vented a more drastic weight gain.

My records showed that when Haley was 8 ½ years old, her weight increase and reportedly out-of-control eating led her doctor to advise that she "eat less fat, more fiber, more fruits and vegetables" and that food that adhered to these guidelines be sent to the sitter's for Haley to eat when she was there. Haley's weight dipped down a bit and then continued to rise. When Haley was 10, the dietitian recorded "strange food crav-ings—mother finds half-eaten sticks of butter and jars of honey. Haley dislikes the healthy food her mother prepares for her." The dietitian emphasized healthy eating, following the Food Guide Pyramid. That time, Haley's weight didn't even dip down before it climbed even faster.

The videotapes of family meals showed feeding to be extremely restrictive and meals to be unpleasant and full of con-flict. Haley's parents kept after her about what and how much to eat, and Haley was sullen, angry, and oppositional. By now her parents were preparing a drab and unappealing low-fat, high-fiber, high-carbohydrate, high-fruit-and-vegetable diet that Haley detested. Haley's parents limited her portion sizes, kept butter and salad dressing away from her, pushed her to eat salad, and forced her to eat food she loathed. Haley's parents asked the sitter and school nutrition staff to restrict as well, instructing them to limit Haley to certain foods in certain amounts. Haley got around them all, taking multiple portions from the food lines, trading food with other children, eating for-bidden food at friends' houses, spending her allowance at the local convenience store, and sneaking food at home.

Even allowing for sneaking, Haley's average daily calorie intake was only about 2,300 calories—65 percent of recommend-ed amounts. Children with high BMIs generally eat less, not more, than children of average weight.[1] Haley's "bizarre food cravings" for honey and butter actually represented a sophisti-cated tactic that children instinctively use to maintain their energy balance. Haley was *hungry,* and her parents were trying to get her to undereat. Under those circumstances, children automatically choose food of high caloric density (high in fat or sugar) to supply needed energy.[2] Of course, in response to her fear of going hungry, Haley was overeating, but the basic problem was food *restriction.* Until that was corrected, her bizarre eating would continue.

Haley's food cravings were also a measure of the degree to which her needs were not being met and her desperation to try to meet those needs on her own. Haley was all bluster and anger, but on some level her parents were hurting her feelings. To a child, not getting enough to eat feels very much like not getting enough love.

Haley's problems were social as well as nutritional. Haley's parents never came right out and said it, but their attitude was clear: There was something wrong with *her.* As would any other child, Haley felt that being flawed where her weight was concerned meant she was flawed in *all* ways. Children don't distinguish among their characteristics. To a child, being regarded as being flawed in *one* way means she is flawed in *all* ways. Haley felt bad about herself, and it showed in the form of a great big chip on her shoulder. Her belligerence, as well as being labeled an out-of-control eater, made her the perfect target for teasing. Rather than helping her to find ways to work things out with other children or handle the teasing, her parents agreed with her tormenters that she was too fat. If she were thinner, she wouldn't be getting teased, and it was her own fault for failing to adhere to their dietary prescriptions. Little wonder she had a chip on her shoulder.

Haley's current doctor and dietitian simply did not realize the impact of their food recommendations. Ironically, they were trying to be moderate—they were trying *not* to deprive. The problem was their *intent.* Their recommendations to eat more fruits and vegetables and cut down on high-calorie foods were intended to make Haley eat less and lose or maintain her weight. If Haley followed those guidelines and lost weight, she would have to go hungry. She wasn't about to do that.

So Haley's mother imposed the guidelines, and Haley reacted by being furious and rebellious. Another, more compliant child would have tried to restrict herself. I have found clinically that those children are no more successful, and they feel ashamed and bad that they can't live up the expectations put on them by their parents and other grown-ups. Deep down, all the children feel hurt that their parents don't like and accept them just the way they are.

Essentially, the question Haley's parents and health professionals asked was, "How can we stop Haley from gaining so much weight?" I asked a different question, and I arrived at a much different conclusion. I asked, "What is interfering with Haley's natural ability to eat the amount she needs to grow consistently?" To answer, I investigated her earlier history with respect to eating and weight. That investigation revealed that her food intake had been restricted since she was an infant, that from the beginning food restriction had destabilized her weight rather than slimming her down, and that more of the same was *not* the solution.

Haley Was Large from Birth

As indicated by figure 6.2, Haley had been large from birth. Although her weight-for-age had plotted consistently at the 95th percentile, at the 10-month visit, Haley's physician observed "weighs too much." In response to the physician's comment, Haley's parents began restricting her food intake. Restricting made sense to Haley's parents because they were dieters—her mother rigid, her father off-again-on-again. By age 12 months, Haley's weight dropped to the 75th percentile. But the physician noted, "tendency to obesity," stimulating Haley's parents to restrict even more.

I hope that Haley's 15-month, 50th percentile plotting was a measurement error rather than frank starvation. However, she *was* being forced to undereat. Once she became mobile, she got the upper hand. According to the clinical record, at 16 months her mother complained that Haley had a "voracious appetite." Haley's aggressive food scavenging overcame her parents' attempts to withhold, and Haley's weight accelerated to above the 97th percentile. Food restriction had made her preoccupied with food and prone to overeat when she got the chance. At that young age, she and her parents had developed a cyclical pattern around Haley's eating. Her parents restricted and forced Haley to undereat. She got around them with her relentless begging and food-supply raiding, and overate.

Food restriction and struggles around eating, however, weren't the worst things happening with Haley and her par-

FIGURE 6.2 HALEY WEIGHT-FOR-AGE 2 WEEKS TO 32 MONTHS

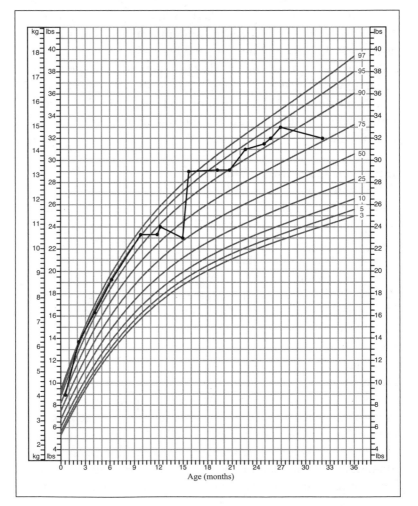

ents. Haley's parents were so intent on slimming her down that they didn't realize the cost to them all of underfeeding Haley. Keeping Haley chronically hungry undermined their relationship with her, and undermined Haley's social, emotional, and nutritional development as well. Rather than nurturing and providing, her parents deprived. Rather than being able to develop autonomy within reasonable structure and limits, Haley continually struggled with her parents for food. Because Haley was always hungry and unhappy, harmonious relationships and rewarding parenting were simply out of the question. In the process, Haley learned that she was an obnoxious child, and she learned to use food for emotional reasons.

When Haley was 18 months old, her nutritional fortunes improved. The family moved, her new physician was relaxed about her weight, her mother was in school, and her father took charge of feeding. Over the next 4 $^1/_2$ years, Haley's weight stabilized at the 75th percentile. But the good times didn't last. When Haley was 6 $^1/_2$ years old, the family again moved. Her mother took over the task of feeding and reimposed restraint. Haley immediately began gaining weight. Since she had learned as an infant to fear food deprivation, she rapidly reverted to food preoccupation and overeating. Stress from the move exacerbated her tendency to overeat, and she rapidly gained weight.

Preventing an Iatrogenic Condition

Haley's was an iatrogenic condition: The pursuit of thinness had made her gain too much weight. I have defined the word *iatrogenic* elsewhere. The narrow meaning is "physician-induced," but of course, lots of people and programs nowadays are culprits in promoting food restriction. Haley's mother was certainly responsible for contributing to the problem. Her physician's comments combined with her own weight preoccupation set her off on a relentless campaign to force down Haley's weight. Haley's father didn't fully approve of depriving Haley, but he went along with his wife rather than standing up for Haley.

Clearly, child overweight is far easier to prevent than to treat. In this case and in many others my colleagues and I see in our practices, prevention involves avoiding interference with the child's normal growth process. Arbitrarily defining Haley as overweight simply because she was growing at the 95th percentile led both Haley's early pediatrician and her parents to distort Haley's feeding and in the long run made her fatter, not thinner. The fact that 10-month-old Haley was growing so consistently and showed so much internal integrity about her growth was lost on the pediatrician, who apparently felt obligated to follow medical guidelines and diagnose Haley as overweight.

Ironically, her mother's resultant preoccupation with Haley's weight and attempts to slim her down likely deprived Haley of the *natural* slimming typical of infants, toddlers, and preschoolers. The large infant and toddler have a 75 percent likelihood of slimming down, and the large preschooler nearly that. It is only at age 9 to 11 that the likelihood of retaining child overweight increases to over 50 percent.[3]

In the context of today's concern about child overweight, Haley's parents needed help recognizing Haley's growth integrity and ability to regulate food intake. Her first pediatrician could have been tremendously helpful to them by pointing out that although Haley was large, she intuitively knew what she was doing. She was eating the amount she needed and growing consistently. The second pediatrician didn't make an issue about weight—he deserves credit for that. But he missed the opportunity to point out Haley's consistent growth and reassure her parents of her ability to regulate food intake. Since they didn't receive that reassurance, they were left with the perception that she was a voracious eater with a tendency to gain weight. That perception set her up for the later struggles that caused her weight acceleration.

Haley's parents loved her and wanted the best for her. They were persistent in getting the help that they needed and brave about taking a detailed look at themselves in order to help their daughter. It was too bad they had gotten started down such a destructive path all those years before. It would have been better for them to ignore the pediatrician's advice and continue to go by Haley's feeding cues, but that's not easy. Going against the doctor's advice leaves parents uneasy. Even 10 years ago, taking such a wise and responsible course of action would have left them with the guilty fear that they were condemning Haley to a lifetime of overweight.

Understanding Haley's Problem

The answer to the question "What happened to undermine Haley's considerable ability to regulate her food intake?" went back to those same four causes presented in chapter 1, "Help Without Harming":

1. Misinterpretation of her normal high weight as overweight
2. Trying to get her to eat less and weigh less
3. Poor feeding practices
4. Stress

Growing out of her physician's and parents' misinterpretation of her normal growth pattern, Haley's parents restricted her food intake by trying to get her to eat less food and lower-calorie food. That more or less worked when she was an infant. But when she became a mobile and aggressive toddler she began to insist on having more food than her parents wanted to give her, and she began to get into the cupboard and refrigerator to get her own food. The constant struggles around eating distorted her learning about eating—they made it hard for her to know how hungry and how full she was. In addition, having food be such a constant concern also meant she learned to use food for emotional reasons. She strongly associated food with feelings—when she was upset, she tended to eat whether she was hungry or not. During a time of high stress, she ate more as a way of taking care of herself.

The good news was that, given positive feeding, Haley could recover the capability with food regulation and growth that she had demonstrated twice before, from birth until age 10 months and from age 3 to 6 1/2 years. Her parents had to establish Ellyn Satter's Division of Responsibility in Feeding and trust Haley to do her part with respect to her eating. For them, trusting Haley was the hard part.

To get their relationships sorted out so they could manage the division of responsibility in feeding, they first had to go into family therapy. Haley's mother was a highly controlling person. Her need to control made it virtually impossible to give Haley autonomy with her food intake. Haley's father deferred too much. He needed to learn to take a more active leadership role with his family. Haley did her part to keep the conflict going. She played one parent against the other, and her extremes in eating provoked her mother's tendency to be controlling. She had to stop that and learn other ways of getting her needs met.

The Feeding and Eating Plan

Once the family was functioning well enough to enact it, the feeding plan was ready and waiting. Both Haley and her parents had jobs to do. These were the parents' jobs:

- Establish and maintain the division of responsibility in feeding.
- Particularly emphasize structure: regular meals, and snacks at set times.
- Provide good-tasting, enjoyable meals and snacks.
- Identify and discontinue restraint tactics.
- Give Haley strong permission to eat what and how much she wanted to eat at regularly scheduled eating times.
- Provide rewarding food for snacks, including "forbidden" food.

Haley's jobs were to recognize her own tendencies to eat as much as she could get, whenever she could get it, and know that those tendencies would continue for a while, even after her parents had stopped restricting her. Haley had some emotional tasks as well. She was intensely involved in guerrilla warfare with her parents—mostly around eating. She was furious and rebellious. Pointing out to her parents the error of their ways quite naturally left her feeling vindicated and self-righteous. She wanted to make them pay for what they had done to her.

With some help, however, Haley was old enough to discover what she was feeling and why she was feeling that way. She could learn to talk about those feelings, not just take them out on her parents. Putting it all together, these were Haley's tasks:

- Go to the table hungry and eat until you are satisfied.
- Pay attention while you eat.
- Ask parents to include the "forbidden" food you like.
- Sneak up on new food and learn to like it.
- Let parents know when they slip up, but be patient.

In the normal course of events, Haley would eat a lot for a while. She would particularly eat a lot of foods that had been forbidden in the past. After a few weeks, she would begin to trust that her parents really *would* let her eat as much as she wanted. Then she would begin to discover her feelings of hunger and fullness and be guided by those cues in regulating her food intake.

For parents, getting through the transition when a child eats more to compensate for past restriction takes steady nerves and a leap of faith. It is hard to watch a child eat what seems like way too much without feeling like putting on the brakes. In cases like Haley's, I find that parents benefit from several weeks of follow-up to help them make their changes.

Finding Your Own Way to Change
Perhaps you identify with Haley and her family or with some of the other children introduced in *Your Child's Weight*. You may or may not have someone to help you sort things out and resolve your problems. Haley's family can help you find a direction.

Haley's mother had a whole repertoire of restraint tactics that had become so automatic that they were unconscious. She could have written figure 4.1, "Restrained Feeding" (page 95), and undoubtedly could have added a few other tactics as well. Haley could help her mother detect those tactics, because she knew when she was being deprived of the amount or type of food that she wanted. Such deprivation made her feel like defiantly eating more, not less. In fact, when Haley's eating went out of control, it was a sure sign that her parents were restraining her. Haley's parents also had to be firm in looking at their own *intent*. If their intent with *any* feeding tactic was to get Haley to eat less or to lose or maintain her weight, it was restrained feeding.

Lots of details come up as parents and children make the transition to the division of responsibility from interfering with the child's prerogative with *how much* and *whether*. What do I do about this or that situation? I tell parents, "You can't be sure your child gets enough to eat unless there are leftovers." Bread becomes an issue. "Always put plenty of bread on the table so your child can fill up on that if all else fails," I instruct. "How much bread?" they want to know. "That much!" They come back the next week. "All he ate was bread," they report. "One meal, he ate five slices." "That's fine," I say. "He's the one who gets to decide." Of course, the possibility always exists that the child is eating lots to get a rise out of the parents. Children who have been in long-standing battles with parents don't give up those battles overnight. Part of the solution for parents is to ignore the provocative eating. Another part is for parents to say to the child, "You may eat all the bread you want. However, you do need to be clear with yourself why you are eating it. Is it because you want it, or because you want to bug us?"

We deal with the situations in detail, but I have found a good rule-of-thumb question to be "What would you do about this situation if you were not at all concerned about your child's weight?" That rule of thumb came to me with a mother who was struggling through a similar situation and wanted to know what to do when her son lined up with the other children at a picnic—like all children everywhere—and started loading up his plate with desserts. "Should I just let him do that?" she wanted to know. Momentarily stumped, I finally blurted out (as I said before, some of my best answers have been blurted), "What would you do if he were just any other kid and you weren't concerned about his weight?" She thought hard. Finally she said, "I would have made them all stop. Those kids were eating all the brownies, and I wanted some for myself." Great answer! Another rule of thumb with children is you get to protect your own rights!

Haley's parents asked themselves the same question about school lunch. What if she were just any other kid? They realized they had to lay off all the food-restriction deputies—the babysitter, lunch ladies, and friends' parents. Then they told Haley,

"You may have as many lunches as you are hungry for. However, we hope you will eat because you are *hungry*, not because you are showing off or trying to get back at us."

SCHOOL-AGE CHILDREN KNOW HOW TO EAT AND GROW
My message throughout this book is "It is better to prevent than to treat." I hope Haley's example helps you realize what *you* have prevented by maintaining the division of responsibility in feeding. Now, we turn from problems to prevention.

Haley was capable of regulating her food intake, but that capability had been undermined by restrictive feeding. Provided you have done nothing to undermine his capabilities, your school-age child still knows how much he needs to eat in order to grow in the way nature intended. His ability to regulate, however, still requires that you maintain the division of responsibility in feeding. For the school-age child, that means you maintain the structure of meals and snacks. You still respect his prerogative to decide how much and whether he eats of what you provide. It is still your prerogative to insist "Eat your snack by (insert time here) so you don't spoil your dinner." Respecting his right to decide depends on *trust*. You have to trust that he wants to eat, that he *will* eat the amount he needs, and that he will grow appropriately *for him*.

THE SCHOOL-AGE CHILD: ROUGHLY 6 TO 11 YEARS
The struggles with Haley and her parents both complicated her development and postponed it. Children can't achieve their necessary developmental tasks when they are preoccupied with getting enough to eat, focusing their energy on struggles with parents around eating and weight, and learning that life problems can be solved only by getting thinner. Restraining Haley's eating was hard for Haley's parents as well. Parenting the school-age child is challenging enough without imposing struggles around food. Rather than giving trust and supporting appropriate autonomy, parents who strive to get their child to lose or even maintain weight have to control and spy.

Yours is a balancing act during the school-age years. You maintain structure and limits, provide backup and support, and gradually dole out responsibility as your child is able to handle it. You increasingly work behind the scenes as your child devotes his energy to achieving in school, in relationships with friends, and in other activities.

During early school-age, say from age 6 to 8 years, your child is like a more sophisticated preschooler. He is positive, wants to learn and do, thinks you are the greatest, and wants to please. Those traits persist for the 8- to 11-year-old. However, for the older school-age child, those positive traits get leavened—or perhaps you would say liberally spiked, with traits that make him somewhat *less* available and appealing.

You and your school-age child either begin to reap the benefits—or pay the price—for all that has gone before with feeding. He works on self-management and takes on the behaviors of his grown-ups. If you have maintained the division of responsibility in feeding and have modeled internal regulation of your own food intake, he can simply carry those capabilities into his outside life. His self-control with eating is *intuitive*—it is deeply embedded within him. He knows how much he needs to eat, he grows in a way that is right for him, and he is able to sneak up on new food and learn to like it.

Family meals are as important now as they ever were before. Go back and reread the discussion in chapter 3, "Make Family Meals a Priority," about how profoundly children benefit from family meals. To recap: Children who have regular family meals—five or more per week—achieve more, behave better, and do better nutritionally. Time spent with family members at meals is more related to psychological and academic success than time spent in any other activity.

Most studies on the positive benefits of family meals have been done with adolescents, but keep in mind that if you want your adolescent at the table, you have to keep your school-age child at the table. He is likely to be cooperative because school-age children still want times to be with family. If he doesn't get regular family meals now, by the time he is an adolescent, he will give up on them.

Again, summarizing from chapter 3, the trend is away from family meals. Between ages 9 and 14 years, the fraction of children who eat daily family dinner drops from one-half to one-third. Breakfast-eating drops from 99 percent to 85 percent, fruit consumption decreases by 41 percent, vegetable intake by 25 percent, and soft drink consumption triples.

INDUSTRY

The developmental task for the school-age child is *industry*. Your school-age child wants to learn and master. In contrast to the preschooler, who tries things out for the pure joy of it, the school-age child brings a certain diligence to his endeavors. He wants to achieve and to carry tasks through to conclusion. If he achieves, he builds a self-perception of one who can learn and do. If he does not or cannot achieve, he develops a sense of inferiority—a feeling that he is not quite good enough.

Attempting weight loss is particularly destructive for the school-age child because it is a task that cannot be achieved. Haley's experience is not unique. Even in energetic, highly funded multidisciplinary programs, weight-reduction efforts do not work. Children lose modest amounts of weight and soon gain it back.[4]

Your school-age child constructs his ability to cope. He models himself on you and other important adults and internalizes your attitudes and expectations. You no longer have to be physically present to provide and enforce values and limits. Your authority is enough. Your child *gives* you authority because he wants to please you—and because you earn it. Haley acted belligerent, like she didn't care. Deep down, however, she felt bad about herself for being so unsatisfactory to her parents. Your child takes your values and limits into himself and either makes them his own or rejects them. Some of this process is conscious, as he works on self-control. However, most of it is unconscious, as he strives to comply with—or defy—what you have taught him.

Ten-year-old Haley could gain insight on her anger and desire to take revenge on her parents because, as a school-age child, she could learn to understand herself and to explain her behavior in terms of complex motivations. With increased self-knowledge comes increased self-criticism. The school-age child

blames himself for his shortcomings and has only a limited ability to see that his weaknesses in some areas are balanced by
strengths in others. His self-esteem, which is likely to have been
high earlier, gradually drops until it hits a low point at about
age 12. Then it gradually increases again.[5,6]

Your school-age child works on physical capability. His relatively slow, smooth, and consistent growth during these years
gives him control over his body and the physical activities he
sets out to master. His slow reaction time, limited coordination,
and social immaturity make him best suited for simple cooperative games like kickball, dodgeball, hide-and-seek, king-of-the-
mountain. Children who dance or do gymnastics typically do it
for the pure joy of movement. Games that adults organize, like
soccer, football, or basketball, require more physical and social
skills than the most school-age children can muster. Trying to
force or coach competitive sports before the child is ready can
sour him on the activity and likely tarnish his feelings about his
body and his abilities overall.

At first, the school-age child dabbles; then he chooses. He
starts by trying out a number of activities and developing a range
of skills. Toward the end of school-age, he distinguishes the activities he likes and is good at. Then he devotes himself to gaining
skills in those activities. However, being ready to choose is part
of the continuity of development and can't be hurried.

Your school-age child develops cognitively. He can reason
logically about concrete issues, organize himself to learn better,
categorize similar objects, arrange objects in order of size, and
develop mnemonic devices to help himself remember. He will
not be able to reason abstractly, however, until he is an adolescent. He thinks he knows it all, or definitely more than you, his
teachers, and all other grown-ups do. This attitude is so common
that it has a name: *cognitive conceit*. It forms the basis for books
that are enormously popular with school-age children, like the
Harry Potter series, that portray most grown-ups as bumbling
and out of touch and children as brilliant and resourceful.

Haley's weight-based difficulties with her friends were particularly painful because the school-age child joins a society of
friends. Friendships *seemingly* become more important than

relationships with parents and family. Your child begins to understand differences in personality among people and uses that understanding to get along with others better. He gains skills in resolving conflict and can see situations from another's point of view and can therefore be sympathetic.

The school-age child often gets chubby just as he leaves this stage. Like the bird who fattens up to prepare itself to migrate, he appears to be storing energy to provide for the rapid growth of puberty.

PARENTING THE SCHOOL-AGE CHILD

As during every other stage of development, parenting the school-age child well requires both love and limits. You have to observe and correctly interpret your child's behavior. Some of your child's traits prompt you in the right direction. Your child's industry, eagerness to learn, imitating and learning from you, logical thought processes, and ability to reason will prompt you most pleasantly to teach and guide. During the school-age years, adults in every culture begin teaching children to take on the tasks of the grown-up world. In *Childhood and Society*, Erik Erikson termed this process *systematic instruction*.[7] Your teaching tasks are all the better because your child loves it when you teach him how to cope and remembers what you teach him. I happily remember one of my own successes: My school-age daughter was worrying about going on a field trip. "I don't know anyone," she fretted. "How will I find a friend?" "Look for someone else who is alone and introduce yourself," I suggested. She was relieved and equipped, the approach worked, and she remembers and uses it almost 30 years later.

In contrast to characteristics that prompt good parenting, some of your school-age child's behaviors and attitudes will positively lead you astray. What are you to do with a child who acts independent, is convinced he knows more and better than you do, and seemingly values friends more than family? See through it all and keep on parenting—that's what. As with the toddler's disputatious experimentation, it is difficult to identify the survival value in a school-aged child's alienating the people he depends on, but that is exactly what he does. In his considered opinion, your school-age child can manage on his own! Of course, that is totally bogus, but many parents accept their child's pretentiousness as guidance for parenting. They stop having family meals and declare an open kitchen.

Think about this stage from your child's point of view. He is dealing with the daunting realization that he will soon have to go out on his own. How do his cognitive conceit and preoccupation with friends help him? The answer, of course, is embedded in the question. Like the Lion in the *Wizard of Oz*, these qualities give him courage. Your greatest unkindness would be to take him at his word. On some level, he knows he still needs you enormously, and he is absolutely unprepared to manage on his own. Only with continued learning and achievement will he be ready.

The school-age child is bright but naive. He thinks he knows all and can do all. Your job is to know better. You are as important as ever. Your work is behind the scenes, providing the same structure, limits, backup, and support that you always have. If all goes well, you become your child's consultant—his sounding board. You ask the questions, raise the issues, refrain from laying down the law, and help him find his way.

FEEDING THE SCHOOL-AGE CHILD

Haley's problems with eating and weight started with her parents' efforts to slim her down when she was an almost-toddler. For a time, her parents crossed the lines of the division of responsibility in feeding. However, when Haley became a preschooler, her weight stability indicated they did better with finding the middle ground between being permissive and being domineering. That stability persisted until she was 6 1/2 years old. It was only when her parents intruded on her prerogative of *what* and *how much* she ate that she again began gaining weight.

The division of responsibility in feeding is important throughout the growing-up years and continues to be critically important for the school-age child. You continue to provide the *what, when,* and *where* of *feeding;* your school-age child continues to manage the *how much* and *whether* of *eating.* However, the middle ground begins to shift, as he gradually takes over some of the *what, when,* and *where* of feeding *himself.* Figure 6.3 helps define that middle ground with the school-age child.

The bottom line is your *attitude* and *intent.* You are being controlling if your attitude is that your child can't control himself. You are being restrictive if your intent is to get your child to eat less and/or lose or maintain weight. You may think you are being sneaky and oh-so-clever about your restrictive tactics,

---

FIGURE 6.3 MAINTAINING THE DIVISION OF RESPONSIBILITY WITH THE SCHOOL-AGE CHILD

Check yourself. You are being too controlling if you

- Make your child eat certain foods, like vegetables
- Dictate his portion sizes or use other tactics to control the amount he eats, like giving him "the look"
- Expect him to apply nutrition principles to decide what and how much to eat
- Make him ask permission for extra helpings
- Arrange to run out of his preferred food so he has to fill up on something he likes less
- Avoid all high-fat, high-sugar "treat" food or use rigid guides about how much is allowed
- Limit menus to drab low-calorie food so he doesn't eat too much
- Expect him to eat the same food elsewhere that he does at home
- Make him eat certain foods or amounts before he can have dessert
- Closely supervise and be stingy with the butter dish or the salad dressing bottle
- Expect him to get by on only three meals a day
- Arrange to be home after school so you can supervise his eating

You aren't providing enough structure and limits if you

- Declare an open kitchen and don't have meals at all
- Offer unlimited amounts of high-sugar, high-fat "treat" food
- Fail to give clear expectations about the timing of snacks
- Fail to stock up on appealing and filling snack foods
- Fail to give clear expectations about his being home for dinner
- Do not make dinner at all
- Short-order cook for him or let him short-order cook for himself
- Let him have juice, milk, or other beverages—except water—whenever he wants them

but you can't fool your child. He will know you are restricting him, and as a consequence he will eat more, not less.

SUPPORT YOUR CHILD'S EATING COMPETENCE

Family meals are as important as ever. In some ways they are *more* important, because they give your mobile and outward-focused child reliable access to you and remind him he is part of a loving family. He may complain about giving up time with friends, but he will secretly appreciate your holding firm about family mealtimes. However, mealtime has to be pleasant. As Haley's case illustrated, struggles about eating can spoil family mealtimes.

Maintaining family meals helps you as well. It reminds *you* that you are important. You are as essential for your child during this stage as during every stage that has gone before and that will come after. While it is small consolation, your constancy has allowed him to take risks with your relationship by developing the obnoxious traits we have discussed!

Food Acceptance

Your child needs positive attitudes toward eating. He needs to know how to behave around food so he will, throughout life, take an interest in an ever-widening variety of food and continually increase the number of foods he enjoys.

What are those attitudes and behaviors? He will feel good about eating and about being at the table. He will be able to remain calm when he is offered new food and will be able to politely say "yes, please" or "no, thank you." He will know how to experiment with new food and learn to like it. He will be able to eat food he is not particularly fond of when there is nothing else available, simply to get himself fed. In short, he will be able to feel comfortable with the food that is in the world outside your home.

Good food acceptance skills for the school-age child are these: Come to the table readily, survey what is there, pick and choose from what is available *without making a fuss,* and be willing to experiment with new food. Experimenting for the school-age child looks the same as it did for the younger child: look, but not taste; taste, but not swallow; swallow, but not eat any more; not eat any more, but try it again another day. As before, your child will eat what tastes good to him and leave the rest. He may eat some of everything that is put before him, or just two or three food items to the exclusion of everything else. He may ignore vegetables for a full week—or for months. But like the younger child, the school-age child will eat a variety of food over time and will have a nutritionally adequate diet, even if his food intake doesn't look so well balanced on any one day. He will learn and grow—that is, as long as you offer regular and varied meals and don't try to get him to eat anything he doesn't want to eat.

Haley had poor food acceptance skills. She was sullen at the table, angry when she was offered new food, and she made a big issue of taking the smallest possible portion of whichever food her parents pushed. Why? Because she was being pressured to eat. More, she was being pressured to eat low-calorie food in the name of weight control. At mealtime, her mother reminded her of the lessons from the dietitian about the Food Guide Pyramid, particularly the one about required portion sizes of vegetables.

It is unrealistic and unkind to expect the school-age child to apply nutrition lessons to what and how much he eats. He can't yet do the abstract thinking required to make those applications. The school-age child is still a *child*. He is entitled to eat what his parents put in front of him. He needs his parents to make nutritional decisions so he doesn't have to worry about what to eat. He also doesn't have to worry about *how much* to eat. His body does that for him. His job is to eat as much or as little as he wants of the food his grown-ups provide.

Truth be told, it is unrealistic and unkind to expect *ourselves* to apply nutrition lessons to what and how much we eat as well. Certainly we apply nutrition and meal-planning principles to getting the meal on the table. However, once it is on the table, we can also pick and choose from what is available. Even if we planned it and cooked it, it may not taste as good as we anticipated. We don't have to eat it if we don't want it.

Special Requests

Increasingly, even your well-brought-up school-age child will

make requests for particular snack foods and will eventually
want to help plan some family meals. That is fine, provided he
has demonstrated his capability with food acceptance. If he
hasn't mastered food acceptance, he will simply be catering the
menu to his own limited likes and dislikes. It is a matter of
being able to take responsibility. A child gets to go to a friend's
house after school if he is willing to let you call the friend's
parents and determine that it is a safe environment. *And* if he
has previously demonstrated that he arrives home on time.
With responsibility comes privilege. A child with good food
acceptance skills gets to help plan the family menu.

Your child will continue to learn and grow with respect to
food acceptance. In fact, his industriousness and need to complete tasks will motivate him to begin experimenting with new
food and learning to like it. For instance, consider Lucas and
tabbouli. I had been preparing tabbouli since long before I was
married and had served it about once a month all during my
children's growing-up years. For the uninitiated, tabbouli is a
Middle-Eastern salad based primarily on cracked wheat and
parsley. One evening, my son Lucas, then about 11 years old,
announced, "I think it's time I tried this." I was startled to realize he hadn't been eating it—I hadn't noticed. The tabbouli,
however, had done its work. Over and over, it sat on the table,
saying, "Someday you will try this." He finally heard the call,
liked it, and has been eating it ever since.

Like Lucas, the gastronomically cautious child wakes up
one day in the school-age years, discovers he is missing out,
and applies himself to catching up. He applies himself, that is,
unless you have hounded him to eat or have given him too few
opportunities to be exposed to a variety of food.

Food Selection and Preparation
Your child will feel proud and accomplished when he can be
successful. That, in turn, depends on your giving him clear, limited, and achievable tasks—tasks that are not too difficult, not
too easy. Finding the balance is tricky. This discussion of food
selection and preparation will give you some concrete ideas of
what those clear, limited, and achievable tasks might be.

Provided he has good food acceptance skills, your school-age child can take modest responsibility for his own food selection and eating patterns. He can get his own snack right after school and choose it from foods you have provided. Your younger school-age child will still depend on you to be there to help prepare the snack and to keep him company while he eats. Your older school-age child will want to do more of the preparation himself, but will still respond when you sit down to talk while he eats. Eventually he will become independent with snacking, but you still must set limits by giving him an eat-your-snack-by-this-time rule so he doesn't spoil his dinner. Mastering that rule begins to teach him to be responsible about feeding himself.

You can share breakfast preparation with your child as he gets his own cereal and toast. You provide structure by seeing that the food is there and, very importantly, by eating breakfast with him. Take a few minutes in the morning to connect with him and his schedule. That's essential for providing backup and support.

Your school-age child may have been cooking with you since he was little. He can now become a genuine help in the kitchen. He will be able to read and understand recipes, follow directions, and apply cooking principles. However, invite him to cook *with* you; don't expect him to cook *instead* of you. Providing family food is still your responsibility, even if he helps with preparation.

Your school-age child can select some of the food he eats at school lunch and at friends' homes. Since he is out on his own, you don't get to say what he shall and shall not eat elsewhere. However, you can talk about it. It is important to give him license to experiment. An epicurean friend was shocked and appalled when her children returned from a visit eager to tell her about a new taste sensation they wanted to add to the family menu: boxed macaroni and cheese. Wisely, she kept her food politics to herself and supported their experimentation. We all have our food convictions and hang-ups. Rather than arbitrarily rejecting foods your child suggests, think his suggestion through and listen to his reasoning. You may learn something.

In fact, you may have to scrutinize your own comfort level.

Even if you can't bend, your child will benefit if you say, "We don't have that food, but it is all right with me if you eat it when you are at friends' houses." Consider the alternative, whether it is spoken or unspoken: "I don't approve of that food, and I don't think it is good for you. I forbid you to eat it, even when you are at your friend's house." What a bind for the child! Is he to refuse and create a fuss with the other family? Is he to eat and feel sneaky and bad about it?

Of course, if your child has an allergic reaction to a certain food, that is another story. In that case, the message is "Peanut butter makes you very ill. It's all right to tell Johnny and his mother you can't eat it. Tell them just a plain piece of bread will be fine." Or better still, ask a question that helps him take responsibility and do his own planning: "What are you going to do if Johnny and his mother offer you peanut butter?"

What does this have to do with overweight? Your child can't be good at eating the amount his body needs if he is afraid of food and unsure of his ability to manage eating situations.

Food Regulation

The child who is good at food regulation is able to tune in on his internal regulators and hunger, appetite, and fullness and eat the amount he needs to maintain consistent growth. If your school-age child has previously been good at food regulation, he will be capable now. The big condition, however, is that he will continue to be capable as long as you continue to do your feeding jobs and trusting him to do his eating jobs. Haley had lost her food regulation capability. Her parents had frequently crossed the lines of the division of responsibility and tried to limit the amounts she ate. As a consequence, she became food-preoccupied and sought opportunities to overeat. She also became angry and frequently overate just to spite her parents.

You and your child do not have to go that way. If he can depend on you to do your feeding jobs, his eating will be large-ly intuitive. Sometimes he will eat a great deal; other times not so much. Like other people young and old, he will regulate his food intake based on his internal cues of hunger, appetite, and fullness. He depends on you to put food on the table so he can go to the table hungry, pick and choose from what is available, and eat until he is satisfied. Then he will stop, knowing that another meal or snack is coming soon and he can do it all over again.

He will experiment with food regulation. At a party, he might eat a great deal of food. He might read a book about starvation and take a notion to try it out for himself. He might want to skip meals to find out what that is like. Your task in all this is to maintain the day-in, day-out of feeding. Maintain the structure of meals and snacks, and his experimentation will even itself out.

HELP YOUR CHILD TO KNOW WHAT HE KNOWS
One of your child's newly acquired intellectual capabilities is understanding his learning process. He knows how he knows what he knows. Your child knows how to regulate food intake and how to learn to like new food. However, his abilities are intuitive. Now he will benefit from beginning to bring his intuitive capabilities up to a conscious level so he can identify and understand them. Why is that important? Because increasingly, as he gets older, he will be with children who diet. To resist dieting, he needs to know that he has another, far superior way of regulating food intake.

To help him understand his process of food regulation, ask him a few questions. How does he know how much to eat? How does he know when to stop eating? How can he tell when he is hungry? When he is full? Does he ever eat so much that he feels *really* full? What happens next? Does he ever *not* get enough to eat and feel hungry? What happens next?

Share with him what you have observed about the way he regulates his food intake—that he eats more or less than other children do, that he does or doesn't seem to need snacks, that he has a sharp or more elastic end point. That is, either he gets full all of a sudden and won't eat another bite or he gets full gradually, slowing his eating down until he finally stops. You might observe that he eats a lot one time, not much another, but that his body knows overall how much he needs to eat.

To help him understand his process of food acceptance, ask

questions. What does he do when he is offered something new to eat? Does he remain calm? Can he politely turn it down? Those are food acceptance skills—if he can say no one time, he can say yes another time. Point out that his ability to remain calm and be tactful about refusing food allows him to go out with his friends or eat in other places. Is he interested in trying new food? Does he know how to try new food and learn to like it? Again, you can point out what you have observed about his food acceptance patterns—that it takes him a long time to learn to like new food—or not. Don't be critical—just point it out.

Remind him of the napkin trick: He can put a bite in his mouth and take it out again if he isn't ready to swallow it. As with the younger child, having an out will let him do and dare more. Use the napkin trick yourself. Keep a stack of paper napkins on the table to encourage it. You will find it easier to experiment with strange food if you don't have to swallow it. Like a new song, new food grows on you if you sample it over and over.

Teach your child that he needs structure and support in order to do a good job with his eating. Again, ask questions. How does he know that he will be fed? Does he plan ahead to make sure he gets fed when a meal will be late or he is out with friends? What happens to his appetite for lunch when a classmate brings cupcakes for mid-morning snack? Here is your chance to toot your own horn, if you don't make it obvious. Tell your child what you do to support him: Have regular family meals; maintain the structure of snacks; offer a variety of food; allow him to eat however much he wants—even if that means nothing at all—of any food he has been offered.

Ask your school-age child to do some problem-solving for himself. How does he feel in the afternoon when he rushes through lunch and doesn't eat much? How will he provide for himself when he goes directly from school to soccer and doesn't have time to go home for snack?

Beware of Traditional Nutrition Education

Traditional nutrition education teaches children food selection. It's not their job. The school-age child still depends on grown-ups to do *their* jobs of food selection and meal planning so he can do *his* job of eating the food he is offered. Developmentally, the school-age child has neither the intellectual capability nor the control over his environment to understand nutritional principles and to apply them to food selection.

A very typical nutrition lesson—in fact, one that is repeated annually from about the first grade on, is learning the Food Guide Pyramid. The pyramid teaches what and how much to eat. If a child takes the information to heart, he will learn to go by the rules—by expectations applied from the outside—and will ignore his internal regulators of hunger, appetite, and satisfaction. However, intellectually he is not equipped to follow the rules.

Your school-age child is in the *concrete operational* stage. That means he can think concretely about what he can see and touch. He can parrot such abstract concepts as "high in vitamin C," "low in fat," or "eat a variety of food," but they make no sense to him. He certainly cannot translate these concepts into food selection. He can learn lessons about the importance of fruits and vegetables, but he can't apply that information to food selection or menu planning.[8]

Even seemingly simple nutrition information will simply overwhelm and confuse school-age children and can lead them to apply the information in unintended ways. If children love and admire their teacher, they may become overzealous in applying nutrition lessons or even offhand comments about food. A mother I met on a speaking trip told of her 8-year-old anorexic daughter who had been sensitized to the "dangers" of dietary fat by her teacher. From then on, the little girl tried to eat *no* fat at all and eventually became so fixated on fat avoidance that she refused to eat anything unless she had first read the nutrition label.

Experts in nutrition education emphasize the importance of family involvement.[9] Essential to family involvement is avoiding any nutrition messages that cast aspersions on family food. During a radio call-in show, I talked with an angry father who told me his 9-year-old daughter began refusing family meals and losing weight when her teacher told the class that eating meat was bad. His little girl became obsessive about avoiding any food that came from animals, an obsession that was proving extremely difficult to resolve.

Both of these sets of parents volunteered that they knew there was more to the issue than simple food avoidance. Their daughters latched on to their teachers' messages to fill a need that went beyond managing their food. However, the message stands: arbitrary judgments about food can be destructive.

No self-respecting nutrition educator would give messages about avoiding groups of foods because they are simply incorrect. However, nutrition educators do continue to teach the Food Guide Pyramid. They don't realize the negative impact this teaching can have on eating attitudes and behavior. The message embedded in the pyramid, or any highly detailed set of guidelines on food selection, is that some foods are good and some are not-so-good. As I just said, those messages overwhelm and confuse children who don't have the intellectual maturity to understand them. Moreover, those messages criticize, directly or indirectly, family food choices. Such messages teach children not only that certain foods are bad, but that their parents are giving them what is not good for them.

Children need to be able to trust and depend on their parents to provide for them. Nutrition lessons must be taught in a way that supports the family. The key is avoiding lessons on food selection, which is a grown-up job. Instead, children can be helped to be curious about food and to feel comfortable with a variety of food. They can learn about broccoli at school and prepare it and maybe even taste it—if they want to. Then they can tell their parents about it, and maybe the parents will experiment with broccoli—or maybe they won't.

Children can learn about their own ethnic food traditions and tell their classmates about them—or teachers can invite parents to do the telling. Children can live with the discrepancy between the home world and the school world as long as neither is criticized or undermined. Children can do what is called *code-switching*—they can speak one language at home, another at school. They can do the same with food—they can eat one way at home, another at school.

However, have an answer ready in the event that your child comes home and says, "My teacher said I shouldn't eat that." That is your cue to say, "You don't have to worry about what to eat. I think about what is good for you when I plan meals, and for now, I will take care of that for you. Later on, you can learn how to do that for yourself. But not just yet."

Schools and Children's Weight

Today's schools are seen as being key in the campaign against child overweight. Schools are being encouraged to weigh and measure students, calculate BMI, and send those reports home to parents with more-or-less alarming messages about the importance of intervening with child overweight. Schools are being criticized for not providing enough physical education and for providing school lunches that somehow contribute to making children too fat. The American Academy of Pediatrics and other groups have strongly criticized vending-machine and other sales of soft drinks in school.[10]

I have discussed this topic in detail in appendix G, "Feeding and Parenting in the School Setting." In my view, making slimming children down the priority of the school over-all and the school nutrition and physical education programs in particular distorts the school's true mission. The school's responsibility with our children is nurturing them, helping them to learn to use the minds and bodies with which they have been gifted, and helping them be all they can be mentally, physically, emotionally, and socially. Giving children the message that there is something wrong with their bodies and teaching them to eat less and exercise more—when developmentally they can't even *comprehend* those messages—represents a *serious* and potentially destructive distortion.

Parenting considerations aside, school interventions to slim children down or to improve their health indicators simply *do not work*. Three highly funded programs targeting third- to fifth-grade children-the Child and Adolescent Trial for Cardiovascular Health (CATCH),[11] the Pathways study of American Indian children,[12] and the Kearney, Nebraska, study[13]—all failed to demonstrate changes in children's health indicators and body weights. All three studies *claimed* success on the basis of being able to modify the fat content of school lunches, increase physical activity in the school physical education programs, and teach children to give satisfactory responses to questions about nutrition and physical activity. However, the Kearney study, the only one to investigate changes outside of school, found that children's overall food intake and activity did not change.

What can schools do *instead* of such restrictive and coercive interventions?

- Optimize feeding and opportunities to be active to support children's natural growth processes.
- Follow the division of responsibility in feeding, providing filling, well-timed meals.
- Restrict children's access to food between times, including vending-machine sales of *any* foods.
- Provide safe places and encouragement for children's natural physical activity.
- Accept children just the way they are—fat, thin, or in-between—and teach them to make the most of what they have.

SCHOOL-AGE FEEDING PROBLEMS

The characteristics of the school-age child, in combination with our cultural attitudes about food and weight, set him up for feeding problems. He is capable and responsible. He acts like he doesn't need you anymore. He is out on his own. He thinks he knows it all. Little wonder that parents of many school-age children turn them loose with respect to their eating.

Home Alone

Many of today's parents don't know how important they continue to be for their school-age child. With parenting in general and food in particular, some children are left far too much on their own. Children rummage through the family kitchen, cook for themselves or for the family as a whole, or have a stash of money to spend at the convenience store or the fast-food restaurant. While I can understand today's stressed and overburdened parents making those choices, I do not condone them.

School-age children still need parenting. They need guidance and support, the knowledge that their parents are looking out for them, and the security of knowing that they *won't* be home alone, either literally or figuratively. Children turned loose too soon don't do well with providing for themselves. They become frightened and overwhelmed. Growing out of their fright, they often eat too much and gain too much weight.

Inability to Cope with the Outside Food World

Like Haley, children kept under too-tight control at home are likely to eat too much when they get access to food outside the home. A mother at an obesity conference complained that her 11-year-old daughter spent her allowance on soda, candy, snack cakes, and chips. She found the wrappers in her daughter's bedroom. I asked her, though I was certain of the answer, "What do you do about those foods at home?" "I don't allow them in the house," she responded. "I don't want her to get too fat." She made me think of the Pennsylvania study of the girls deprived of "forbidden" food described in chapter 2, "Feed and Parent in the Best Way."[14] Even when they were full, restricted girls who were given free access to high-calorie "treat" foods ate more and were fatter than girls who were allowed to eat them regularly.[15] It wasn't the foods that would make the girl in question too fat—it was the way she ate them. Since they were forbidden fruit, and since she was sneaking to get them, she ate a lot while the eating was good. The mother's unrealistic expectation—going without the tasty foods the other children were eating—put the girl in a serious bind. She simply couldn't be diligent enough to respect her mother's rules.

Because this concept is so difficult for parents and professionals alike, I will repeat the advice I gave you about "controlled substances" in chapter 4, "Help Without Harming: Food Selection." Don't throw away *all* controls, because too many high-sugar, high-fat snack foods can undermine the nutritional quality of the diet. But *do* find the middle ground. Offer snack cakes or cookies in unlimited amounts, along with a glass of milk, for an occasional snack. Offer an occasional soda for snacks or lunch, along with crackers and cheese. Include potato chips with the sandwiches for lunch—enough potato chips that there are some left over. Have dessert as regularly as you enjoy it, and manage it well—*only one serving* for a meal, and let him eat it before, during, or after the rest of the meal.

Children Diet

Societal weight standards filter down to children—through physicians, parents, teachers, extended family, and even casual bystanders—and give them the message that they are too fat and should therefore lose weight. From early on, large children develop patterns of restrictive eating and negative self-concept. Those patterns are likely to make them fatter, as well as making them feel bad about themselves.

Researchers at Pennsylvania State University followed relatively large girls (those whose BMI was at the 85th percentile or above) from ages 5 to 9 years. Those girls had clearly gotten the message that they were considered too fat. Compared with girls the same age whose weights were closer to the mean, the relatively large girls were more likely to feel bad about their bodies, to be concerned about weight, and to try not to eat as much as they were hungry for. Girls as young as age 5 years responded "yes" when asked questions like "Do you try to eat a little bit on purpose so you don't get fat?" Like the girls we met in the previous section, the relatively large girls ate significantly more than "normal-weight" girls (girls whose weights plotted closer to the mean) when they were given free access to high-calorie "treat" foods. The relatively large girls gained excessive amounts of weight as they got older—their weight gains accelerated.[16]

This research is extraordinarily concerning, not only from the point of view of children's weight gains per se, but also from the point of view of identifying a serious and pervasive iatrogenic condition. As I mentioned earlier, the word *iatrogenic* technically means physician-induced. In this case, I use it to mean *societally* induced. The problem wasn't the girls' high weight per se. The problem was the *societal perception* that they were too fat and the *societal expectation* that they should therefore eat less and get thinner. Because of this expectation, the girls became preoccupied with food and were prone to overeat when they got the chance. And they got even heavier. Their weight gains accelerated, which I have repeatedly emphasized is the *real* problem, not their relatively high weight.

Here is another bit of research evidence about relatively large girls that is even more concerning. Girls whose parents saw them as overweight, and whose parents restricted their access to food, felt bad about themselves overall and thought they weren't as smart as other children and not as physically capable.[17]

Little girls and boys are entitled to feel good about themselves, run and play, learn to use their bodies, focus their energy, and feel good about what they can do. The little girls on the cover are 7 and 9 years old, and they are doing just that. Even if those little girls had a weight problem, which they do not, we wouldn't want to hurt them or any other children by making them worry about eating less and losing weight. Teaching school-age children that they aren't good enough and saddling them with the impossible task of undereating and forcing down their body weight siphons off energy from what is truly important.

Dieting is not exclusive to large girls. Boys do it as well. So do small, thin girls and boys. Figure 6.4, "Why Do Children Diet?" summarizes some of the factors that precipitate dieting—and what you can do about it.

Parents Are Pressured

Parents, of course, suffer right along with their children. In today's weight-obsessed world, if you restrict, you create havoc with your child. If you do not restrict, you are suspected of being neglectful.

This attitude is expressed clearly by the Expert Committee Recommendations on Obesity Evaluation and Treatment. According to the committee report, parents who are not willing to go along with weight reduction efforts "express a lack of concern about the child's obesity or believe the obesity is inevitable and cannot be changed or are not interested in modification of activity or eating."[18]

However, according to the committee, parents are to engage in this virtually impossible task of trying to force their child's weight down (or maintain it at its current level) but not become

FIGURE 6.4 WHY DO CHILDREN DIET?

- Many times, children diet because they have been restricted from early on. As a consequence, they lack the ability to regulate food intake based on internal cues of hunger, appetite, and fullness. When they get out on their own, they grope for a way to manage. They turn to doing it in the only way they know how—by trying to eat certain amounts and types of food.

   What to do about it? Raise your child to be a competent eater. Get help restoring eating competence if it doesn't exist.
- Children assume that dieting is what it means to be grown up with respect to food. After all, their grown-ups diet, criticize their own bodies, and continually strive to be thinner.

   What to do about it? Don't restrict, don't diet, don't be critical of your own body.
- Children may diet because a coach or dance teacher or golf instructor tells them they will do better if they lose weight. This destructive advice makes a particularly strong impression on the task- and achievement-oriented school-age child.

   What to do about it? Tell your child—and the coach—that striving for weight loss is definitely *not* appropriate. Better still, have a serious talk with your child before he enters any activities, but particularly weight-focused activities like wrestling, gymnastics, and dancing. Make it clear to both your child and the coach that your child's participation is contingent on their *both* resisting pressures to diet.
- Children's friends diet. It's trendy.

preoccupied with the child's weight because such a preoccupation "may damage the child's self-esteem. If weight, diet or activity become areas of conflict, the relationship between the parent and child may deteriorate. When problems such as these occur, clinicians should refer the family to a therapist and should stop the weight control program *until the family can proceed without adverse psychologic or emotional effects*" (italics mine).[18]

At the risk of repeating myself, it is not possible to enroll your child in a "weight control program" without his experiencing "adverse psychologic or emotional effects." Going back to striving for weight loss after therapy won't make the effort any less malignant. This is like patching up soldiers and sending them back into battle. There is no way you can set the goal

FIGURE 6.4 WHY DO CHILDREN DIET? (CONTINUED)

> **What to do about it?** Raise your child to be a competent eater. Teach him about his internal regulators so he realizes he has a way of knowing how much to eat that is superior to dieting. Don't keep yourself on a diet, and don't be critical of your own body and strive to be thinner.
>
> - Children get chubby just before they go into the rapid growth of puberty. Rather than encouraging them to hang in there and see what happens, parents panic and collude with food deprivation.
>   **What to do about it?** Encourage your child to hang in there and see what happens. Encourage yourself. Remind yourself that if you are doing your feeding jobs and letting your child do his eating jobs, he will grow up to achieve the size and shape that is right for him. You do not have to feel responsible or make it happen.
> - Because their self-esteem dips, school-age children have much to learn and they feel overwhelmed. They seize on weight loss as the magic bullet for achieving self-esteem.
>   **What to do about it?** Be clear about your own struggle. It is hard to watch your child's pain. It is harder still to not try to fix it. Be ready to listen, ask helpful questions, don't be critical, and don't try to fix it. At most, help your child figure out his own solutions. Telling you about his troubles will help him. Your nonjudgmental listening gives both support and autonomy. It says to him, "I can understand your feeling that way. I am on your side, and I trust you to figure this out for yourself."

of reducing—or maintaining—your child's weight without getting into conflict.

If you do your feeding jobs and let your child eat and grow without interference, you are not being unconcerned, fatalistic, or uninterested. As I have said before, maintaining the division of responsibility day-in and day-out, 18-years-per-child, represents an enormous commitment that responsibly and appropriately supports your child's eating and growth.

Health Professionals Are Pressured

These attitudes about diagnosing and treating child overweight are hard on everyone. One of my reviewers, pediatrician Jim McGuire, spoke for many of his colleagues when he commented, "This is outrageous. We as professionals get the same guilt doled out to us. We are expected to treat obesity with restrictive programs that don't work. If we ignore obesity in the name of doing no harm, we are told we are not concerned and not doing our jobs."

FEED AND SUPPORT

As Dr. McGuire went on to observe, the feeding dynamics approach allows parents and processionals to actively *do* something, not just ignore the problem. What can you do to spare your child the kinds of struggles Haley experienced and Dr. McGuire prefers to avoid? You can feed and support him.

Do a good job of parenting with food as I have outlined in this book in general and in this chapter in particular. Establish the division of responsibility in feeding, even if you haven't been doing it all along. Let your child grow up to get the body that is right for him, and help him to feel positive and accepting of that body.

Find out how your child feels about his size and shape and the way his body is changing. Understand enough about normal growth and development to know that it is all transitory— anything can happen. Even at 9 to 11 years of age, your child has roughly a 50 percent chance of slimming down.

Even—or particularly—if he doesn't slim down, help your child come to terms with who he is so he can accept his size and shape as givens. How to do that? By helping him find activities he does well, activities that allow him to take pleasure in his body. By finding out what he is thinking. By providing a wise antidote to the craziness all around. Consider this typical example.

> "I'm too fat," lamented 11-year-old Rob.
> "Why do you say that?" asked his mother.
> "Because I have this roll of fat around my middle."
> "How do you feel about your body?" asked Rob's mother.
> "Well, pretty good. I am strong, and I can do a lot of things. I like to play soccer. I am good playing the backfield."

"What got you started worrying about being too fat?" asked Rob's father.

"My soccer coach said if I was thinner I could be a forward," said Rob sadly.

"Why is that?" asked his father, sensing he would hear something positive about Rob.

"He says I have good footwork and can see plays," Rob elaborated. "If I were faster, I could be a forward."

"Do you want to be a forward?" asked his mother. For his father, it was a foregone conclusion. Who *wouldn't* want to be a forward?

"Not really. I like being a sweeper. But he said I was fat." Rob's father was surprised. He didn't know Rob *liked* playing defense.

"What do *you* think?" his father, recovering quickly, was able to ask.

"I could be faster if I worked on it. But I *am* fat. I have this roll of fat around my stomach, and my legs are fat. The other day the doctor said I should eat healthy. But I knew he was saying I was too fat."

"How do you feel about that?" asked Rob's mother. She had heard the same thing, was disgusted with the doctor at the time, and was even more disgusted now. Rob's father stifled the urge to tear off immediately to give that doctor a piece of his mind.

"Well, I wish I weren't so fat. How do you feel about it?" asked Rob, somewhat fearfully.

"We think you are fine, just the way you are," agreed his parents.

"Gotto go," said Rob, and the conversation ended.

Rob was satisfied his parents were behind him. His parents were left hanging, wondering if he had gotten what he needed. Children do that. The parents' inherent message in the conversation was "Everybody's different. Some kids are thinner; some are fatter. You are the way you are." Rob was getting that message, but the more important one was "We *like* you the way you are." Rob's parents could say it—once. If they said it

over and over, he would feel they were giving him a
snow job.

I hope you identify with Rob's parents. Of course, for you
to be this cheerfully confident, you have to be relaxed about
your own size and shape. If you continually diet and try to
force your body into somebody else's size or shape, your child
will do the same. If you are not accepting about your own body,
you are likely to say, "Well, I guess it is time to cut down."

Following this conversation, Rob's parents worked behind
the scenes, like all good parents of school-age children. They
had a private word with the soccer coach and one with the doctor. The coach was appalled at his own insensitivity. The doctor
couldn't see what was wrong with what he said, despite their
explanation that Rob was fully aware that "eat healthy" was
code for "Don't eat so much; don't be so fat." They kept the
coach and found a new doctor.

THE SCHOOL-AGE CHILD WITH HIGH BMI

The story of Rob illustrates that the school-age child with high
weight or BMI is vulnerable. All too often, professionals,
weight-loss organizations, or casual advisers recommend food
restriction and weight loss. You must protect yourself and your
child from that interference. Even the large child is entitled to
depend on his parents to do their feeding jobs and then to be
trusted to do his eating—and growing—without interference.

Even the large child is entitled to like his body and must
not be made to worry about eating and weight. Even the large
child is entitled to go to the table hungry, eat until he is satisfied, and then stop, knowing another meal or snack is coming
and he can do it again. In feeding *any* child, the emphasis must
be on *providing*, not *depriving*. Anything else amounts to neglect.

Professionals Are Likely to Restrict

In most cases, a child's high BMI is taken at face value, diagnosed as overweight, and standard interventions are imposed.
That "overweight" diagnosis is often based on low and arbitrary cutoff points that misdiagnose between 5 and 15 percent
of children and overlook children whose weight gain is accel-

erating. Expert Committee Recommendations on Obesity Evaluation and Treatment label as *overweight* children whose BMI plots at or above the 95th percentile.[18] Children are labeled *at risk of overweight* when BMI plots between the 85th and 95th percentiles. As nearly as I can tell, that diagnosis is based on the faulty assumption that a child's weight will accelerate if it plots high. Why is this a misdiagnosis? One in 20 children normally grow at or above the 95th percentile; almost 1 in 7 normally grow above the 85th percentile. Those children are simply *relatively* large. They are not necessarily abnormal, nor is their growth any less stable than if they plot in the lower percentiles.

Standard treatment is based on deprivation and weight loss. According to the Expert Committee, the goal is forcing the child's weight down to the 85th percentile or below, either by getting the child to stop growing with respect to weight as he gets taller or by outright reducing his body weight.[18] Pro-weight-loss people consider the weight-leveling approach to be moderate and realistic. It is not. A child's natural state is *growth*; a child who isn't growing is essentially *losing.*

FIGURE 6.5 HOW HEALTH PROFESSIONALS CAN HELP WITHOUT HARMING WITH RESPECT TO CHILD OVERWEIGHT

- Review your child's growth history to identify whether his weight is high and stable or accelerating.
- Identify weight acceleration at any weight level, even if your child's high weight doesn't get above the standard cutoffs of the 85th or 95th percentile.
- If your child's weight is high and stable, assume his growth pattern is normal for him.
- Support you in accepting that high, stable weight pattern.
- Whatever your child's weight, give you accurate feeding information based on a stage-related division of responsibility.
- If your child's weight gain is accelerating, set aside an hour or so to help you identify what is disrupting his growth—or refer you to someone else who can take the time.
- If it emerges that you have complicated or long-standing issues with respect to feeding, refer you and your child for assessment and treatment.

While some professionals accept Expert Committee recommendations and strongly support weight-reduction efforts, most are trying to help without doing harm. Most processionals know full well that weight-loss efforts don't work, but they are nonetheless being exhorted to diagnose overweight and treat it. Surveys show that, like Haley's doctor and dietitian, most pediatricians, dietitians, and other health professionals attempt to soft-pedal their recommendations about weight reduction. They talk about "changes in eating patterns," "portion sizes," "limitations of specific foods," "low-fat diet," and "modest calorie restriction."[19] The problem is that health professionals don't realize these tactics are restrictive and therefore counterproductive. Since these approaches to food selection and weight management are so pervasive in our culture, that is not surprising.

What can health professionals do instead of restricting? They can do a more precise assessment of your child's weight, then give you information and support. Figure 6.5 gives more detail.

High Normal Weight or a Weight Problem?
As illustrated with Haley, to help a child and his parents with a weight problem, we must understand in detail the child's history with eating and weight. Then we are in a position to help. Simply applying the standard intervention is a disservice to children, and applying that "cure" more, harder, and under multiple professional supervision doesn't make it work any better.[4]

To understand your child's weight, jump ahead now to read chapter 10, "Understand Your Child's Growth." Understand the difference between high normal weight and weight acceleration. Know that your child is growing well if his weight consistently follows a particular percentile curve. Know the difference between a normal and an abnormal growth adjustment.

If your child's weight is high but stable, if you have been doing a good job of feeding, and if you are all pretty relaxed about his eating and weight, the task is to hold steady with feeding and parenting and keep doing what you are doing.

On the other hand, things are likely *not* going well if any of the following are true:

- Your child's growth veers abruptly upward or downward.
- You are making no progress toward having enjoyable, relaxed mealtimes.
- You worry a lot about your child's eating or growth.
- Your child seems immature, has trouble taking responsibility, or has significant problems with friends.
- Your child worries a lot about his weight and is extremely self-consciousness about his size and shape.
- Your child chronically sneaks to eat or sneaks to avoid eating.
- You can't seem to resolve your struggles about his eating.
- You feel the need to stay home to supervise his eating.

Start with a Careful Assessment
Any feeding problem that requires advice going beyond basic good parenting, positive feeding, and supporting normal growth and development is *treatment*. Doing treatment absolutely mandates doing a careful and detailed assessment to provide a clear understanding of the problem. I describe that assessment in appendix E, "Assessment of Feeding/Growth Problems."

For the child and family requiring treatment, restrained feeding is highly likely to be causing the problem. The standard interventions—restricting the amount of food the child eats, giving lists of what to eat or not eat, and recommending portion size in the name of reducing or maintaining the child's body weight—have likely all been unsuccessfully tried before.

Haley and her family provide a perfect example of that dynamic. Their previous "helpers" looked only at Haley's current weight and imposed food restriction. It was only when I looked at her *whole history* that it became apparent that more food restriction was likely to exacerbate her weight acceleration. Rather than encouraging her parents to restrict her still again, the assessment helped me to support them to find the middle ground with respect to feeding—the division of responsibility—and to support Haley as she developed her eating capabilities.

In my clinical work, I have encountered other families who have other stories of direct or inadvertent food restriction. Those stories became apparent only when I looked beneath the surface. I introduced Mary and showed you her growth charts in chapter 2, "Feed and Parent in the Best Way." From age 6 months until 10 years, Mary's mother restricted her relatively large daughter to slim her down. Then, in the midst of a family crisis, the mother stopped restricting, and over the next two years Mary's weight accelerated from the 50th to the 97th percentile. Overcontrolling Mary's eating, then totally leaving her to her own devices with respect to feeding herself had left Mary with neither internal nor external regulators. Mary's weight fluctuated over the next several years until, at age 19, she approached me for a diet. By this time she was binge-eating and vomiting to control her weight. Rather than more dieting, Mary needed careful and focused treatment to help her recover her sensitivity to her internal regulators. If I had seen Mary and her parents when she was 12 years old, I could have encouraged Mary's parents, as I did Haley's, to establish the division of responsibility in feeding to support Mary as she developed her eating capabilities.

Ten-year-old Salvador was so heavy he had to be in a wheel chair. He was the focus of health professionals, teachers, and treatment specialists who were frantic to restrict his food intake and force his weight down. Looking beneath the surface showed that his mother was alternately indulgent with food and unable to provide. She was overwhelmed by living with her alcoholic husband. Salvador gained weight rapidly from the time he was a toddler because he couldn't be sure he would be fed or provided for in other ways. Salvador was under enormous stress, and he didn't need further stress in the form of food deprivation. He needed good parenting, reliable feeding, and help rediscovering his internal regulators. With appropriate support, Salvador had a chance to develop his eating capabilities, to gain some self-respect with regard to his eating, and possibly to lose some weight.

It's not easy to hold steady with feeding on the one hand and let go on the other—to keep doing your jobs and then let your child grow up to get the body that is right for him. You will benefit from support, and finding supportive health professionals can make all the difference. The norms in our society are to be casual and unconcerned about feeding and preoccupied with weight. The pressure to impose food restriction and strive for weight loss is everywhere. As one of my readers, dietitian Carol Walsh, observes, "This is a strong statement—what you describe is the *opposite* of the division of responsibility."

She is right. In observing and maintaining the division of responsibility, you are parenting in ways that are decidedly contrary to the norms. That takes commitment and courage. The good you are doing may not be apparent, but the harm you will avoid will be considerable. To understand that harm, remember the story of Haley and other children who have been introduced in this book.

Doing a good job with feeding your school-age child means he will be ready to take on the challenges and rewards of being an adolescent. As you approach this most challenging and poignant of ages, you and your child will once again reap the harvest of your holding steady with feeding and parenting and trusting him to do his part—in all ways—with growing up.

NOTES

1. Rocandio, Ansotegui, and Arroyo, "Comparison of Dietary Intake."
2. Kern et al., "Postingestive Consequences."
3. Serdula et al., "Obese Children."
4. Epstein et al., "Treatment of Pediatric Obesity."
5. Fredricks and Eccles, "Children's Competence."
6. Wallace, Cunningham, and DelMonte, "Change and Stability."
7. Erikson, *Childhood and Society.*
8. Lytle et al, "Children's Interpretation of Nutrition Messages."
9. Lytle and Achterberg, "Changing the Diet."
10. Committee on School Health, "Soft Drinks in Schools."
11. Luepker et al., "Outcomes of a Field Trial."
12. Caballero et al., "Pathways."
13. Donnelly et al., "Nutrition and Physical Activity Program."
14. Birch, Fisher, and Davison, "Learning to Overeat."
15. Fisher and Birch, "Parents' Restrictive Feeding Practices."
16. Shunk and Birch, "Girls at Risk for Overweight."
17. Davison and Birch, "Weight Status."
18. Barlow and Dietz, "Obesity Evaluation and Treatment."
19. Barlow et al., "Treatment of Child and Adolescent Obesity."

UNDERSTAND AND PARENT YOUR ADOLESCENT

If all goes well, at the end of this period, your adolescent will be ready to make her way in the world. However, she will continue to depend on your backup and support.

Your Child's Growth and Development
- In early adolescence, the theme is autonomy. Your child focuses on peers and learning to make it in a teenage world.
- In later adolescence, the themes are intimacy and identity. Adolescents begin to form a picture of who they will be as adults.
- Adolescents find ways to be both close with others and separate.
- Boys and girls grapple with sexual identity as well as "finding themselves" in general.

How to Parent Your Adolescent
- Find the nebulous middle ground between being controlling on the one hand and throwing away all controls on the other.
- Assume that your child wants to please you and master what you find important.
- Give privileges and autonomy as your child becomes skilled and responsible.
- Talk and listen; consult and support to work out expectations and limits.

How to Parent Your Adolescent with Feeding
- Continue to have family meals; retain leadership with family food selection.
- Help your child to know what she knows about her intuitive eating capabilities.
- Give the expectation that your child will feed herself responsibly, including participating in family meals.
- Teach your child to plan family and independent meals as well as to learn to prepare food.

CHAPTER
7

OPTIMIZE FEEDING:
YOUR
ADOLESCENT

Your reward for doing a good balancing act during your child's school-age years is to go up to an even more challenging level. Like high-wire artists the Flying Wallendas, now you get to walk across the Astrodome! For parents, the theme of the adolescent years is "Oh, no, what do I do now?" But despite the bad press that adolescence receives, most adolescents, most of the time, are calm, predictable, and purposeful. Certainly, problems from depression to breaking the law are more common than they were earlier. About one adolescent in five has deep and sustained problems.[1]

While for some adolescents and parents, the time is simply awful, it isn't that adolescents suddenly become different people and turn on their parents. Families of troubled adolescents have been experiencing problems of interaction all along. Those problems just become impossible to ignore during this stage. Adolescents who turn to eating disorders, drugs or alcohol, promiscuity or delinquency do so in an attempt to solve or forget long-standing problems. The acting-out provides only temporary relief and in the long run adds to their difficulties with growing up.

Before we start, let me share a note about gender and this chapter. Until now, my strategy has been to alternate between using *he* and *she* from one chapter to the next when not referring to a specific child. That pattern would make this a "she" chapter. But because gender attitudes and behaviors diverge so much during adolescence, that won't work very well for this discussion. Therefore, in the name of keeping the book balanced, this will still be mostly a "she" chapter. However, I will include "he" paragraphs, sections, and examples to remind us all that we are talking about boys as well as girls.

ADOLESCENT GROWTH AND DEVELOPMENT

The adolescent grows rapidly toward being an adult intellectually, physically, emotionally, and functionally. The basic themes of adolescence are autonomy, intimacy, and identity. Early in adolescence, the major subtheme is autonomy, as a child focuses on peers and learning to make it in a teenage world. Later in adolescence, the subthemes are intimacy and identity. The adolescent finds out how to be both close with others and separate. Boys and girls grapple with sexual identity as well as "finding themselves" in general. They begin to form a picture of who they will be as adults.

If all goes well, at the end of adolescence your child will be ready to make her way in the world. At that point, you will be out of a job. Don't expect her to know it all. She couldn't possibly. Don't try to completely protect her. You couldn't possibly. Life is complex and challenging, messy and full of surprises and rewards. Instead, expect her to have the tools for learning from life—for figuring it out as she goes along. It's like learning a foreign language. If you study long and well, you learn enough words and communication skills so you can use the language to learn. If your child has basic capabilities, life will be challenging but not scary and overwhelming.

The adolescent finishes the job of learning to provide for herself that she started in her school-age years. You continue the process of doling out tasks and responsibility as she is able to manage them. The principles are the same: Challenge without overwhelming; provide support without controlling; give independence without abandoning.

Adjust Your Attitude

Your adolescent finishes getting ready to take adult responsibility with respect to eating. She learns to take care of herself. This is a priority for boys as well as for girls. Although attitudes are changing, the unconscious expectation is usually that managing food and being deliberate about eating are primarily women's and girl's issues. Girls are presumably concerned about eating; women take the lead with providing meals for families. The attitude is that boys are waited on, they are casual about eating, and they are even less likely than girls to learn food-management skills. It doesn't have to be that way. My sons are good cooks and make it a point to take care of themselves with respect to food. The same applies to my friends' sons—and to our daughters. Some of the boys took such an interest in food and cooking that they livened up family menus. So did some of the girls.

Although our lives and family patterns have changed enormously in the last 50 years, our attitudes about feeding ourselves are stuck somewhere in the 1950s. We expect to get serious about taking care of ourselves, including feeding ourselves, when we get married and *certainly* when we have children. That is a lot of time to go without self-nurturing. That attitude leaves almost all young people stranded in some sort of waiting room for life. Nowadays, many people remain single or childless for a long time—or indefinitely. They wait to establish relationships or they establish nontraditional relationships.

If your son decides to wait until some female comes along to take care of him, he may wait in vain. While managing food is still *seen* as being a woman's job, many women simply aren't *doing* that job. I could speculate on the reasons for that—women in the workforce, time pressures, changing roles among men and women, mothers not wanting to saddle their girls with traditional female roles. I am not going to get into gender politics, but I will say that feeding oneself is far too important to let it get stranded in a debate about gender roles.

I recently told a graduate student, "You are a family when you take care of yourself." Her face lit up, and she said, "Well, next week I am a family." She meant that next week she would finish her Ph.D. and could start taking care of herself. I enjoyed her humor and optimism, but I privately thought that was a bit late. She was at least 8 years out of high school. That's a long time to go without nurturing.

Teach your boy—and your girl—the attitude of *self*-nurturing: "I have taken care of you up until now. When you leave home, it is your responsibility—and your right—to take care of yourself."

Adolescent Eating Competence

Now to your job of getting your child ready to take that step. In chapter 5, "Optimize Feeding: Birth Through Preschool," I encouraged you to think about the future. When your child is approaching the time to leave home, I asked, What would you like her to be able to do with respect to her eating? If all has gone well with feeding her, by now she will have these eating attitudes and behaviors:

- Positive attitudes about eating. She will feel comfortable about eating and about her enjoyment of rewarding food.
- Good food acceptance skills. She will be interested in unfamiliar food and have ways of continually learning to like new foods.
- Good food regulation skills. She will be able to automatically eat the amount she needs and maintain body weight based on her sensations of hunger, appetite, and satisfaction.

She still has some learning to do. She needs to remember what she knows—her intuitive capabilities with food acceptance and eating the amounts she needs. She also needs to know what *you* know—how to go about managing food selection, meal planning, and food preparation.

It is still your job to manage the *what*, *when*, and *where* of feeding. That job includes providing regular and reliable family meals. Your teenager builds on her earlier eating competencies to progressively take more and more responsibility for her own food selection and for seeing to it that she gets fed. With your guidance and support, she finishes working her way through the list introduced in figure 5.1, "Children's Eating Capabilities" (page 137). We pick up in the overlap at the end of the school-age competencies, and complete the list:

11. Increasingly understand intuitive food regulation capabilities.
12. Increasingly understand and refine food acceptance skills.
13. *Independently* apply food selection and meal- and snack-planning principles outside the home—at restaurants, convenience stores, and snack bars.
14. Manage the schedule for feeding herself, including participating in family meals.
15. Plan family and independent meals.
16. Prepare food.

As an adolescent, your child works up to having enough skills with food selection, planning, shopping, and cooking to provide for herself after she leaves home. At that point, she will have the ability to feed herself regularly and reliably. Whether or not she *does* it is up to her. You will have done your job. Even if she feeds herself poorly for a few years, it is likely that at some point she will go back to feeding herself the way you fed her. Remember the wisdom of the prophets: "Train up a child in the way he should go: and when he is old, he will not depart from it" (Proverbs 22:6).

Teenage Children Know How to Eat and Grow

Provided you have done nothing to undermine his capabilities, your child still knows what he knew at birth: how much to eat in order to grow in the way nature intended. His ability to regulate, however, still requires that you maintain the division of responsibility in feeding. For the teenage child, that means you maintain the structure of meals. By now you have taught him to attend to structure with respect to snack times, and beyond your stocking the pantry and refrigerator, he controls the *what,*

when, and *where* of snacks. Rapidly growing teenage boys challenge structure, because they seem to be able to snack constantly and still tuck away a substantial meal. Often the issue
becomes maintaining structure on behalf of younger brothers
and sisters.

It is still legitimate to go by the eat-your-snack-by-this-time
rule. Adolescents who arrive home filled up from a big snack or
so famished they can hardly stand to wait for dinner have not
done a good job of seeing to it that they got fed earlier in the
afternoon.

You must still respect your child's prerogative of deciding
how much and *whether* he eats of what you provide. Your being
able to respect his right to decide still depends on *trust.* You
have to trust that he wants to eat, that he *will* eat the amount he
needs, and that he will grow appropriately *for him.*

TWO CHILDREN WHO WEREN'T TRUSTED

If you do not trust, and instead control what and how much
your child eats, your child will grow up devoid of internal controls. As a consequence, when she gets away from your external
control, she will come undone. She will have long since lost
track of her internal regulators of hunger, appetite, and satisfaction. On some level, she will be tired of being controlled and
will feel resentful about it. She will do one of two things: try to
impose *your* controls on herself, even though she feels negative
and ambivalent about those controls, or throw away *all* controls
and eat chaotically.

Maureen, Who Didn't Know How

Maureen depended on her parents to provide her with familiar
food and to tell her how much she could eat. They limited the
menu to foods she could readily accept and served the same 10
or 12 foods over and over again. They dished up her plate for
her and expected her to eat it all. They particularly reminded
her to finish her vegetables and milk. Sometimes they let her
have sweets, French fries, and other "forbidden" food, and
sometimes not.

That arrangement worked as long as Maureen was at home,

but when she got out on her own, it was a different story. She encountered unfamiliar and forbidden food in unlimited amounts, and she was overwhelmed. Her poor food regulation and food acceptance skills left her with few resources for managing her eating. She didn't know *what* to eat, because her parents had always managed that. Portion size was a problem, because her parents had managed that as well.

Maureen's solution was to organize for herself a monotonous diet of familiar foods, just as her parents had done for her. She controlled portion size by eating what she thought was the right amount—a bowl of cereal with milk for breakfast, a peanut butter and jelly sandwich with two slices of bread for lunch. Dinner was more of a challenge, but she solved both the *what* and *how much* problem by having one of the three or four Lean Cuisine frozen entrées that she liked. For snacks, she had apples.

Maureen's was an ingenious, if misguided, solution. Another child would have overeaten on all the goodies available to her; still another would have become bulimic, overeating and then purging to get rid of the excess. Some university students in fact binge and then purge routinely—without conflict or shame—as a way of regulating food intake. The problem was that her menus didn't add up to enough calories, and she was essentially starving herself. Her parents gave her more food than she was giving herself, but since she hadn't paid much attention, she didn't know that.

One of my reviewers concluded that Maureen was not too smart—why didn't she just eat more? He illustrated an important point. People who intuitively eat as much as they need simply have no *concept* of what it is like to be handicapped by external constraints—by outside expectations of *what* and *how much* to eat. Maureen was being driven by her hunger, but she was completely unable to trust her body's pleas for more food.

Instead of responding to her hunger cues, Maureen concluded that she was a compulsive eater. She was hungry all the time, thought about food constantly, was irritable and depressed, and lost interest in her schoolwork. She edited out the peanut butter and jelly sandwiches because she began binge-eating on them.

Instead, she had a second Lean Cuisine entrée. She began to fear she had an eating disorder and attended a lecture I gave at an eating disorders awareness week at the University of Wisconsin. She was startled when I talked about the symptoms of starvation, because the list described her perfectly.

Maureen didn't have an eating disorder; she was just *hungry*. She was not using her eating—or lack of it—for emotional reasons. She simply had such poor eating competence that she could not manage. She required counseling, though, because she was doing poorly emotionally and socially. Maureen had been a compliant child who grew up with overprotective parents. Rather than challenging how controlling they were, Maureen deferred to them. She ignored her own wishes in all things, including her food regulation cues. Maureen deferred to her friends as well and secretly felt they took advantage of her. As a consequence, Maureen remained a child even when she was old enough to leave home, and she knew it. She was ashamed of her inability to cope and felt helpless and overwhelmed at the prospect of providing for herself.

In treatment, Maureen learned to detect and trust her emotions as well as her hunger, appetite, and satisfaction. She developed the skills to provide for herself—with food and in other ways. She became confident, orderly, and positive about her eating. She learned to stick up for herself—tactfully—with her friends and became skillful at working things out with them.

Maureen's parents supported her, and their support helped enormously. Maureen loved them and didn't want to alienate them in the process of learning to meet her own needs. Her parents had the courage to examine themselves and their contribution to her problems. They took responsibility for the errors they had made in raising her, gave her support, and developed the realistic expectation that she could manage her own life. They were also able to see that in many ways they had been positive and faithful parents. They loved their daughter and had done their best for her.

Wesley, Who Was Forced to Eat

I introduced Wesley briefly in chapter 2, "Feed and Parent in the Best Way." Let me refresh your memory and tell you more details about him. Wesley ate until he was stuffed every time he ate. Even though he was an adult, that pattern went back to his earliest childhood. As he put it, his mother was a terrible cook, put huge amounts on his plate, then expected him to eat it all, reminding him he was lucky to get enough to eat. The only way he could choke down those huge portions of revolting food was to put himself on automatic pilot. He learned to disengage from his awareness of himself and the eating process and simply eat until the food was gone.

Wesley became hugely fat by the time he was three or four years old and stayed fat from then on. He despised his fatness and considered himself to be a glutton. In high school, he found excuses to avoid his mother's meals and dieted and lost weight. He went back to overeating when he went off to college, and regained his weight. That up-and-down pattern continued for several years. While he dieted, he felt moderate with his eating and lost weight. But when he reverted to stuffing himself again, he felt out of control and gained all the weight back and more besides. When he was in his forties, he made a particularly determined effort and forced his weight down to a near-average level. That time, he maintained it through rigid attention to food restriction and strict physical training. That lasted a year.

Then Wesley's daughter died. His grief and anguish took away his energy for food deprivation and forced activity, and he rapidly gained almost 100 pounds. He came to me for help, steeling himself still again to lose weight. He felt, in fact, that weight loss was the way out of his depression. He found the prospect absolutely daunting and dreaded starving himself still again. But he couldn't go on stuffing himself either. He felt awful physically, and he was ashamed of his eating.

I offered Wesley help of a different sort. I reassured him he could find someone else to help him if he was determined to diet, but dieting hadn't worked for him in the past and it was unlikely to work now. Instead, I could help him discover what held true for him—what it would be like for him to learn to eat in an orderly and positive fashion, depending on his internal regulators—and what would happen with his weight when he did. Skeptically, he decided to take me up on my offer.

Once he committed, Wesley worked hard. The results were astonishing. He learned to slow himself down and become aware of what went on inside of him while he ate. It was hard for him, because he got into so much anger and anxiety—all the feelings he had been stuffing down when he ate without awareness. But as he increasingly tolerated those feelings, they began to dissipate. He gained insight as to where the feelings came from. As he repeatedly ate in an orderly and tuned-in way, his internal regulators became apparent to him.

He was first aware of his appetite and was gratified to notice how he rejoiced in the flavors and textures of well-prepared, well-seasoned food. Wesley's wife was a good cook, but he had discouraged her from being creative because he felt good-tasting food sent his eating out of control. It helped when he became aware of his attitude that his wife was as controlling about his eating as his mother had been. That was coming from Wesley. His wife truly did not care how much or little Wesley ate of the food she had prepared.

At first, the excitement of such rewarding eating threatened to overwhelm him. He had a strong impulse to eat fast and stuff in as much as he could. But he contained his urgency and continued to eat in an orderly and tuned-in fashion. Then he came upon his feelings of satisfaction and a *true* willingness to stop eating. This wasn't the old dilemma he had experienced before—either eat moderately and feel deprived, or eat more and feel like a glutton. This was a new sense of truly being willing to stop because he had had enough. Eating rewarding food helped, because it gratified his need for pleasure.

After he discovered his stopping place, Wesley was able to refuse food offered to him—or pressed upon him—by other people. It made him angry to be coerced to eat, and he used his anger to remind himself to act on his own behalf.

SOCIAL AND EMOTIONAL COMPETENCE

Both Maureen and Wesley focused on their eating problems. Painful as it was, however, eating was the least of both their troubles. Neither of them felt comfortable and competent in the world. Maureen's struggles with eating accurately reflected her overall incompetence and anxiety. Wesley's eating reflected the way he felt inside. From the time he entered high school, he appeared to be successful in all ways. He achieved his success, however, at great emotional cost. Inside, he felt incompetent and anxious—like an imposter who was constantly on the verge of being exposed.

It was little wonder that they both turned to eating management as a way out of their dilemmas. We live in a society where achieving a particular appearance is used as a vehicle for solving emotional and social problems. Achieving slimness is a cultural preoccupation. The advertising industry and media are particularly virulent with messages and role-modeling about size and shape, and many of those advertising and role-modeling tactics are directed at adolescents.

Adolescents, in turn, are susceptible to taking in narrow and judgmental messages about body size and shape. Developmentally, they are working on being successful with their peer group in general and with intimate relationships in particular. In addition, they are preparing themselves to make it in the outside world. As a consequence, they are particularly vulnerable to messages that promote achieving a particular *look* in order to be successful. Conversely, failing to have that *look* is considered without question to be responsible for social difficulties and erosions in self-esteem. Thus many adolescents fall prey to drastic attempts to diet and lose weight.

There is no denying that for people of any age in our culture, it is easier to be thinner. However, everyone has something about themselves that they have to learn to manage and integrate in order to be successful in life. For some people, it is being heavier than average. Dealing with that reality requires emotional and social competence.

Defining Emotional and Social Competence

Let's start with the end in mind. What kind of *person* do you want your child to be by the end of adolescence? Rather than focusing your efforts on what you *can't* achieve—how your child's body turns out—why not focus on what you *can* achieve:

raising a socially and emotionally competent child. That competence includes good character, common sense, effective ways of
responding to feelings, a sense of responsibility, problem-solving skills, and the ability to get along with others.

To be socially and emotionally competent, an adolescent
needs positive and self-confident attitudes. She will be pretty
relaxed about life and its challenges. Certainly, she will feel
stressed and beleaguered at times, but she won't feel so anxious
and unprepared that life's challenges overwhelm her ability to
cope. She will be able to manage her level of stress and her
response to it and therefore think clearly and strategically
enough to be successful. She will be independent but not have
to be alone. She will know that she can fall back on you if she
has to, but she won't expect you to make her way smooth. She
will be prepared to make it on her own.

The competent adolescent will be interested in and flexible
about the people and situations in the world and, as a consequence, have good social skills. He will be able to learn and
gain comfort and familiarity, but also protect and preserve himself. Since he will be able to diplomatically defend himself
against the pressures of new situations, he will respect his own
tempo and reactions in adapting to new situations and be able
to proceed in a way that fits his comfort level.

The competent adolescent needs a certain level of emotional maturity. She will be able to consistently tune in on and trust
her own feelings and values in relationship to herself, other
people, and outside challenges. Rather than grabbing for solutions in response to her feelings and life's pressing necessities,
she will tolerate her upset, take her own needs into account,
and be honest, creative, and matter-of-fact in working things
out. She will be comfortable with feeling her feelings and sharing them with others because she knows that emotional self-
awareness is essential for making appropriate choices.

The competent adolescent will take responsibility for providing for himself and living up to his obligations to parents,
teachers, and other important people in his life. He will be able
to set and adhere to goals and gain satisfaction from achieving
those goals. He will take responsibility for managing the com-

plexity of his living situation, money, relationships, and multiple life issues. He will be able to maintain his self-regard and take care of himself in relationship to other people, being neither dependent on the one hand nor dictatorial on the other.

Finally, the competent adolescent will know what she knows. She will know that she has capabilities and resources with respect to her thinking, actions, and feelings. She knows, in short, that she has the tools to act on her own behalf, and she knows what those tools are.

RAISING A COMPETENT CHILD

How do you raise a child with such good character—with such social and emotional competence? Good character builds on your adolescent's relationship with you and her desire to please you. Maintaining values, taking responsibility, accepting the consequences of choices and actions, and standing up for what she believes all build on the solid grounding of her relationship with you. To preserve that solid grounding, you must be clear about what your adolescent can do to please you, but you must not make her choose between pleasing you and pleasing herself.

That statement sounds like a riddle, and in some ways it is. You must again find that nebulous place—the middle ground. You must *not* go to the easier-to-define but nonetheless destructive extremes of either being controlling on the one hand or throwing away all rules and expectations on the other.

The research is clear that the middle ground works best. Adolescents of parents who share control—neither give up all control nor insist on obedience—tend to be high achievers and are unlikely to be seriously disruptive and disobedient. In a classic and often confirmed study of 7,400 adolescents, psychologist Glen Elder saw parents' orientation to their children during adolescence as ranging from control over every aspect of the adolescent's life to no control at all. Although Elder saw control as falling into seven categories, parenting styles during adolescence essentially reflected the same three orientations introduced in chapter 5, "Optimize Feeding: Birth Through Preschool": *authoritative, authoritarian,* and *permissive.* Children of authoritative parents fared best.

Parents at the *authoritarian* extreme were autocratic. They laid down the law and didn't let their adolescents express their opinions or make decisions about any aspects of their own lives. Parents at the *permissive* extreme acted like anything was all right. These parents showed no interest in guiding their child's behavior and failed to lay out expectations. Permissive parents hid their impatience with their child's negative behavior until they could no longer stand it. Then they blew up, felt bad afterward, and then tried to make up for it. Parents in the middle—about half the parents—were judged to be *authoritative*, neither giving up all control nor insisting on obedience. Those parents talked with their children to arrive at realistic expectations, gave children responsibility for following through, and enforced the expectations when it was necessary. However, parenting style also reflected the family environment. Parents living in dangerous areas tended to monitor and control their adolescents more carefully to keep them safe.[2]

In research conducted since the 1962 Elder study, adolescents have never been found to benefit from families that are permissive to the point of irresponsibility or strict to the point of mistreatment.[3]

The Division of Responsibility in Parenting
Learning to do a good job of feeding can help you find that nebulous middle ground. Ellyn Satter's Division of Responsibility in Feeding is an authoritative approach to parenting. Parents find that applying the division of responsibility to the relatively concrete interactions of feeding teaches them to apply it in other areas as well.

In addition, feeding reflects the overall parent-child relationship. As such, its impact on your child's well-being extends far beyond feeding. In chapter 5, "Optimize Feeding: Birth Through Preschool" (page 132), I mentioned my research indicating that adults who are competent with eating are more self-aware, more trusting of themselves and other people, and more comfortable with other people. Their emotional maturity gives evidence of their having been treated respectfully, not only in the area of feeding but in all ways.

Figure 7.1 gives some ideas of what the principles of the division of responsibility look like when they are applied to parenting in general. In many cases, you will be able to anticipate your responsibilities and distinguish them from your child's responsibilities. You provide shelter, food, a quiet place to sleep and to study, an alarm clock, clean clothes. Your child manages herself and her time—she gets herself where she is expected, when she is expected, clean, rested, and with her homework done.

Other times, your child springs something on you. Let's say your 13-year-old son says, "Mom, can I go have dinner and hang out at the mall with my friends?" You have one of those "Oh, no, what do I do now?" moments. Your job is to decide whether he is capable of handling the situation he wants to put himself in. Here is the key to your dilemma: You don't have to know the right *answers.* You just have to ask productive *questions.*

(Mom, thinking. "Now what do I do? Is it all right to go to the mall—or not? How should *I* know?") Mom, out loud, buy-

---

FIGURE 7.1 WAYS TO APPLY THE DIVISION OF RESPONSIBILITY TO PARENTING YOUR ADOLESCENT

- Be respectful of your child.
- Trust your child to want to learn, grow, and be successful.
- Assume that your child wants to please you and to master what you find important.
- Be clear with your child about what you will and won't do.
- Once you have been clear, trust your child to make her own choices.
- Administer your tasks—provide food and shelter and control the family money and other resources, such as the family car.
- Clarify the nature of the tasks your child must master.
- Identify and provide the help your child needs in order to be successful and safe.
- Identify your own needs and rights and be clear and firm about maintaining them.
- Give privileges and autonomy as your child becomes skilled and responsible.
- Allow your child to experience the consequences of her behavior.

ing time, but also doing exactly the right thing: "Tell me more about your plans. How would you get there and get home, how long would you stay, who all wants to go?" Your child briefly answers—they will eat at the food court, he will spend his own money, they will walk around, poke around in the music store, maybe look at clothes. His friend's mom will drive, and the usual crowd is going. "So can I go?"

Mom, now having had a chance to think, says, "A lot goes on at a mall, and it's crowded. How do you plan to keep yourself safe there? How will you stay out of trouble? How will you avoid bothering other people?" Of course, Mom asks these questions one at a time and gives her son time to answer. At some point, she has an additional stipulation that would apply whether her child were a boy or a girl: "I think it's great to go with your friends to get ideas about clothes. However, I'm not ready to have you buy clothes on your own. Are you willing to just look and not buy?"

If your child discusses the issues willingly and is able to provide adequate answers, there is still the matter of *dinner*. This is not a *big* deal, because he could have an entirely worthless meal and still be all right nutritionally. However, it is a *precedent*. He will likely be eating at food courts and other fast-food establishments quite a lot in the next few years, and you can remind him to start thinking about providing for himself nutritionally. From our list of eating capabilities, his job at this stage is to "independently apply food selection and meal- and snack-planning principles" to just such eating situations.

If you have been applying the guidelines suggested in figure 4.7, "Family Meals in Restaurants" (page 115), he will likely have been more-or-less indoctrinated in doing the same. However, you can still ask some questions. "What about your milk? Those places don't have any fruits and vegetables. How are you going to get them?" Since he will no doubt be an *alert* child, he might tell you, "I can have a milkshake. I am planning to have tacos." Or he might say, "I can eat fruit for a snack when I get home." Those are all good answers. However, the *answer* is less important for him than the *question*—and the expectation that he will think about it.

Girls may plan to skip dinner altogether. Then the question is, "You will be hungry. How will you feed yourself?" She might say they will just grab something to eat on the run. That is not an adequate answer. The issue is standing up to her peers. She will ignore her own needs and fail to stand up to her friends if she becomes casual about feeding herself. If she isn't ready to do that, it could stand in the way of her being allowed to go.

But say you have received satisfactory answers, and your child gets to go to the mall. You might suggest that since this is the first time, the trip be limited to 2 hours. If your child can handle that, another time it can be longer. On the other hand, if your child isn't willing to discuss the issues, doesn't provide satisfactory answers, or hasn't demonstrated reliability in other areas, the trip will have to be postponed. Make it clear, however, exactly what it will take in order to get to go another time.

Children Want to Please Their Parents
What stops a child of this age and mobility from doing exactly what she wants to do? Her own desire for mastery and wanting to please her parents, just as with the feeding relationship. In addition, she won't have to resort to doing exactly what she wants to do if her parents make it possible to please them without her having to ignore her own needs and wishes.

The imaginary mother in the example above was able to hold the middle ground and take an *authoritative* approach with her son. She gave autonomy, helped him think through the new social opportunity, listened to his point of view, then made the decision based on their discussion. If all went well, she would have even been impressed by his thinking and able to say so. In the process, she treated him with respect. She trusted that he wanted to please her and at the same time wanted to learn and grow.

If, on the other hand, she had taken an *authoritarian* stance (a stance that her son invited with his blunt question), how would it have turned out differently? Say she said no. Or say she said no and then explained all the trouble her son would get into at the mall. He would have been left with two choices: to angrily comply on the one hand or to go anyway on the other, either by outright defying his mother or by sneaking out. He would have had to give up on pleasing his mother and getting her guidance in order to do what he wanted.

Now say the mother took a *permissive* approach. She just said yes. Like many parents who have questions like this sprung on them, she may have decided to swallow her misgivings and avoid conflict. Then her son would have gotten the privilege without earning it—without having to think things through or take responsibility for himself or his own behavior. The boy would know that his mother was knuckling under to him, and he would lose respect for her. He *could* please himself and do what he wanted. The problem was, he didn't *care* about pleasing his mother, and that left him without her backup and support. He likely would have felt—and acted—anxious and unsure, or blustered to cover his anxiety.

Dealing with the Big Time

Going to the mall is a relatively benign issue. Once you establish the pattern, however, you can apply it to issues that are far *less* benign, such as experimentation with alcohol, tobacco, and drugs. Whether they experiment or not, these substances are a fact of life for today's adolescents. According to the annual *Monitoring the Future* survey of nearly 50,000 8th-, 10th-, and 12th-graders in more than 400 U.S. schools, most children do try them. Eight in 10 high school seniors have drunk alcohol, two out of three have smoked at least one cigarette, and about half have tried at least one illegal drug, usually marijuana.[4]

Substance abuse is a big problem. It feels safest to keep our adolescents from using these substances, but that is an unrealistic expectation. Monitoring your child helps—knowing where she is, what she is doing, and with whom.[5] However, monitoring that becomes harsh and suspicious does more harm than good.[6]

Once again, the task is finding the middle ground—maintaining a positive relationship with your child, being clear about your point of view, talking things over,[6] arriving at an understanding of what is, and isn't, all right. The primary problem is *safety*. The adolescent's difficulty coordinating her impulses and behaviors with her moral values and better judgment can make her impetuous and therefore can put her in harm's way. Laying down the law won't help. She can as readily use her impulsiveness to get around you as around her inner constraints.

Teenagers take risks, but they do not have to take stupid, pointless risks. In fact, a teenager benefits from a thoughtful discussion about different levels of risk for a particular activity. Given such a discussion, she can decide just how much risk she wants to assume. Keep in mind, parenting a teenager with respect to risk-taking behavior demands the division of responsibility. Your job is to help her think through the hazards and lay out your limits and expectations. Her job is to decide how much hazard she is willing to assume.

Lay out the issue and then ask helpful, not manipulative, questions. "I don't want you to drink. You are too young and it is illegal. On the other hand, I can't stop you and I won't try. However, if you decide to drink and your drinking gets out of control, there *will* be consequences, and I will not rescue you from those consequences. I do not know whether those consequences will come from me or from some outside source, but those consequences will emerge. I do trust you to make good choices. To help you as much as I can, I have some questions for you." Here are some good questions to ask:

- How will you keep yourself safe?
- How will you stay out of trouble?
- I know you say a couple of beers won't hurt you. I say you will be impaired. We don't have to agree on that, but we do have to talk about the plans you have made for taking care of yourself if you drink. What are they?
- What if you get caught and are sent to jail? If your party gets raided, the police won't care whether you were drinking or not. They will arrest you.
- What about if you are with a group? What will you do to keep yourself safe if the group is being reckless?

Your child wants to please you. Conversations like this let her know that you back her up. They also make clear that you expect her to use good judgment, behave responsibly, and say no to her friends in order to take care of herself. If your child abuses alcohol, you have to be prepared to follow through. Stifle the impulse to protect her from the consequences of her own actions.

Perhaps it will help you to know that I became this clear only after going through these issues again and again with my own three children. It was a process of trial and error. My oldest child, my daughter Kjerstin, asked me whether or not she should go to a party at the park where there would be alcohol. I stammered, "I don't know what to tell you. I just don't want you to get hurt." Later on, she told me that had been a helpful answer. To her, it meant I was backing her up and trusted her to make the right choice. Parenting is like life. Once you figure it out, it is almost over.

All parents would like these issues to just *go away*, but that won't happen any time soon. To help yourself stay calm and think more clearly as you grapple with this difficult issue, remember one encouraging bit of research. Experimentation is not the same as getting hooked. Adolescents who experiment are generally those who are doing better socially and emotionally than either the abstainers or the frequent users.[7]

WHAT DOES THIS HAVE TO DO WITH EATING AND WEIGHT?

Allow me to be clear about what this seeming digression has to do with eating and weight. Physical self-esteem is closely related to self-esteem overall. Your child needs to feel comfortable with herself and capable of coping with her world in order to feel comfortable with her body. She also has to be willing to behave differently than her friends do.

In our weight-obsessed culture, having the right *weight* and the right *look* is seen as being essential to success. From that conviction, it is a small step to misusing eating and weight in an attempt to solve life's problems. Such misuse is likely to disrupt eating competence, destabilize weight, and impair the ability to deal directly with life.

For Maureen and Wesley, eating and weight were the *least*

of their problems. Their greater problems were accepting themselves and being able to feel comfortable in the world.

However, they attempted to *solve* their problems by managing their eating and weight. They clearly illustrated the consequences of childhood distortions in feeding and parenting.

Maureen's and Wesley's stories are also encouraging. It is unlikely that your errors have been as extreme as those of the parents in these accounts. Even if they were, it is still possible for your child to learn, grow, and recover her eating competence at *any* age.

It is also possible for you to learn, grow, correct your errors in parenting, and develop a more positive relationship with your child. Maureen's parents came through for her, even though they had made a lot of mistakes. She became a self-confident young woman who liked her body, took joy in her eating, and developed a new, more rewarding relationship with her parents. On the other hand, Wesley's relationship with his mother was broken—no retrieval was possible. The problems were too deep, they had gone on too long, and she was unwilling to take responsibility for her errors in parenting.

Having observed what can go *wrong*, let's focus now on how you can feed your child in such a way that things go *right*. We continue our discussion of normal growth and development and of stage-related feeding, now turning to the teenage child.

EARLY ADOLESCENCE: ROUGHLY 12 THROUGH 16 YEARS OLD

The young adolescent struggles with autonomy—with establishing herself as a separate person. She has to cope emotionally with the dilemma of being separate but being attached, of being let go by her parents, but not abandoned. In many ways, her struggle is the same as that of the toddler. She becomes exquisitely tuned in to issues of control and profoundly fearful—in her heart of hearts—of becoming so obnoxious that her parents give up on her. She will be sensitive to criticism, but at the same time, very critical. Before she can build her own self and ideas, she has to come to terms with what has gone before.

Everything about the young adolescent changes. Physical

changes make her feel uncertain and uneasy, particularly if she is out of sync with her age-mates. Puberty starts somewhere between ages 9 and 14, but possibly as early as 8 and as late as 16, with boys starting, on the average, 2 years later than girls. Increasing hormone levels cause, in sequence for boys, growth of testes, growth of the penis, first pubic hair, ejaculation, growth spurt, voice changes, beard development, and completing of pubic-hair growth. For girls, the sequence is beginning breast development, first pubic hair, widening of the hips, the growth spurt, menarche, and completion of breast and pubic-hair growth.

Hormonal changes give both boys and girls insistent sexual feelings and worries about appearance. Girls are concerned about the size and shape of their breasts; boys worry about their height and muscles and the size of their genitals. They all think about sex a lot, and some worry that they are sex-crazy. Boys can get an erection at any moment and worry about when it will happen. Girls worry that they will let their sexual interest show too much—or too little.

Once the growth process starts, every part of the body changes and the adolescent reaches close to adult size, shape, and proportion in 3 or 4 years. Appetite increases, and both boys and girls get heavier before they get tall. They all get bigger rapidly, and their shapes continually change. They can appear awkward and unbeautiful as their hands, feet, nose, lips, and ears get bigger before their heads and torsos. Sometimes an adolescent may have big ears that stick out; other times ears that are the right size for the rest of the head.

No wonder adolescents spend so much time looking in the mirror—keeping track of it all is an ongoing challenge, and those years of waiting to see how it all will turn out can seem to last forever. Few adolescents are satisfied with their physical appearance, even those whose genes give them bodies that are close to the cultural ideal.

The young adolescent becomes focused on friends at the same time as all the rules of socializing change in her new middle school or junior high. Peer pressure briefly becomes more important than anything else, then recedes in importance as she gets older. Parents are prone to blame other children for the trouble their child gets into. However, adolescents tend to associate with like-minded others, and together they get into escapades that none would consider alone.[8] The young adolescent becomes more self-conscious, and her positive and negative feelings about herself come and go. As mentioned earlier, self-esteem bottoms out at about age 12 and then gradually improves.[9,10]

The early adolescent develops intellectually. She becomes logical and imaginative and can tell the difference between what is hypothetical and what is real. Her egocentrism is a glaring exception. She believes she and her experiences are unique, that she is immune from danger, and that her parents can't possibly know how she feels. She acts as if she is on stage and the whole world her audience, paying attention to her as closely as she does to herself.

She is likely to have mood swings that shift from euphoric to despondent. It may be difficult for her to make decisions, and she can become extremely frustrated when she is confronted with a choice. She may shift between autonomy and dependence, one day insisting on being out in the world and doing things her own way, the next day coming back and wanting to be told what to do. One day she will be sensible; the next illogical and unreasonable. She will demand your advice, then reject it. Nothing seems to suit. This sounds more and more like the toddler's struggles, doesn't it?

Hard as it is to parent the young adolescent, I would rather *parent* one than *be* one. Indeed, the struggles that most of us have parenting during this stage have to do with our own history. Most of us feel we were not good at being teenagers. That's just as well, because those who were good at being teenagers often have difficulty getting beyond the people they were in high school.

The Parents' Role with Respect to Autonomy
As with the school-age child, you have to see through the smoke and mirrors in order to find your path with parenting. Your adolescent will act as if you are no longer relevant. You are an impediment, in fact, to her doing what she wants. Moreover,

the people she *really* values are her friends. She will also act as if she is ready, willing, and able to tackle any social, physical, or other opportunity presented to her. If only she could get you out of the way.

Totally bogus, but don't say so, and don't say *I* said so. She still needs you—needs you a lot. She just can't acknowledge that she needs you. Your task with your young adolescent is to give her liberty without abandoning her and to maintain structure and limits without policing her. It is a very tricky business, because now the structure and limits exist in your *relationship*. As with eating, what she does when she is out on her own is almost entirely under her influence. You hope that the values and capabilities you have raised her with will serve her well in the outside world. And they will.

Unlike with the toddler, you will not be physically present to see to it that your adolescent does and does not do what you want. In fact, you can't possibly tell her what to do or not do, because she knows far more about her world than you could possibly know. You simply have to know that you are important, that you still have your authority. Moreover, she has inner constraints: her desire to please you and the values and standards of behavior that she has learned from you.

You have a lot to build on. Despite all the struggles, most young people have considerable respect for their parents as individuals. They wish they and their parents could see eye to eye about some of their issues, but generally their disagreements are on finer points rather than on fundamental convictions. They *want* to talk with their parents, but they *tend* to talk more with their friends. Parents shut down conversations when they try to impose their own perspective, make judgments, and tell their child what to do. Friends listen sympathetically to blow-by-blow accounts, don't make judgments, and wait to be invited before they give advice.[11]

LATE ADOLESCENCE: ROUGHLY 17 THROUGH 19 YEARS OLD

During the last year or two of high school, the older adolescent gradually finds a balance in the contradiction of fitting herself into the world while establishing a sense of herself as a unique person who is stable and mature. Having for the most part resolved the autonomy issue, the older adolescent's struggle is with *identity* and *intimacy*.

By this time, your child's rapid growth spurt is at or near its end. She will be finding out what her size and shape are likely to be in her adult life and coming to terms with her physical capability and appearance. Her thinking ability matures and becomes more abstract. Rather than having to be concrete in her thinking, she can think in terms of possibilities and mentally run through scenarios. She can apply scientific principles to tasks and use abstract principles for guiding her behavior.

Now her growth is *internal*. If all goes well, she will spend a couple of years in limbo as she tolerates not knowing who she is and waits for herself to emerge. During that emerging process, she will arrive at her unique gender roles, vocational aspirations, and political values.

Your adolescent struggles with intimacy as well. While she begins breaking away from home and moving toward the future, she struggles with being loyal and connected to her roots—her parents and her culture, including her religious beliefs. Achieving and maintaining this balance is a fluid process that goes on throughout life. She discovers that closeness with people she loves can be maintained over geographical or philosophical distance. She finds ways to be emotionally connected with others without being bound to them, and ways to be separate from them without rejecting them. She must do this in all ways: sexually, morally, politically, and vocationally.

The Parents' Role with Respect to Intimacy and Identity

To support your child through this transition, remain true to yourself. Continue to be a force in your own right, being clear about your own needs, limits, and values. Tolerate your child's turmoil, but don't let her take it out on you or other family members. Prepare for your child to accept some of your values and goals but reject others. Give up your agenda for her and instead cultivate an attitude of *curiosity*.

Love and accept your child for being the exact person she

is, and expect her to do the same for herself. In chapter 9, "Teach Your Child: Be All You Can Be," we'll discuss accepting and supporting your child of *any* size or shape and helping her learn to love her body. Acceptance is a nebulous but nonetheless painful process that we all have to go through. That process is most evident for parents of children who have handicaps. Those parents say that parting from lost dreams comes up again and again at each milestone in the child's life. However, once attended to at the major juncture between child- and adulthood, each reprise feels more like an echo, without the original intensity. This observation may relate directly to you if you are raising a child with high body weight. In our culture, high body weight is a handicapping condition. However, unlike other handicaps, it is blamed on the sufferer—or the sufferer's parents.

If all has gone well with parenting your adolescent, you will have ways of talking openly with her and supporting her as she thinks through her own issues and makes her own plans. Soon she will be making all her own decisions, so give her the opportunity to try herself out. Now is the time for lightening up on constraints and letting her make her own decisions. The major limits at this stage are those that grow out of her relationship with you and with the broader culture. She is living in your home and using your property and therefore has to be considerate of your wishes and limits. Having lived there her whole life, she will think she owns the place. She is wrong. You paid for it. To live in your house, she has to be respectful of your rights and wishes.

As long as she lives in your house, it is legitimate for you to expect your child to participate in the sociability and responsibilities of the family. That means she joins in with family meals and occasional other social situations and helps with the chores around those meals. She also joins in with housekeeping, yard work, and other chores to keep the family going. It is not okay to for her to come home long enough to raid the refrigerator and then leave.

Maureen and Wesley Had Trouble with Identity
Ambiguity and conflict are an essential part of the adolescent's

achieving identity. Some adolescents can tolerate being in that limbo; others can't. If adolescents live with too much criticism or too few expectations that they will be mature and responsible for themselves, they find a way of prematurely resolving their dilemma.

Rather than struggling with her identity as an older adolescent, Maureen foreclosed on it. She accepted her parents' values and expectations, made them her own, and failed to forge her own unique identity. Rather than coming to terms with her need to be individual, Maureen's parents had accepted and even congratulated themselves on how easy and compliant she was—what an ideal child.

Wesley, on the other hand, submitted resentfully to his mother's dictates and then formed a *negative* identity. He set out to be the opposite of everything his mother had raised him to be. He worked hard in school, cultivated friends who could help him move up in the world, and aimed himself toward a profession in which he could be influential. His strategy worked. He got rich, had a great house, married a sophisticated woman, and had wealthy and powerful friends. All along the way, Wesley's mother was angry with him and ashamed of him for "getting above his raising." Under it all, Wesley still felt he belonged on the wrong side of the tracks.

PARENTING THE ADOLESCENT WITH RESPECT TO FOOD

The division of responsibility in feeding continues to apply until your child grows up and leaves home. You remain responsible for the *what, when,* and *where* of feeding; your child continues to be responsible for the *how much* and *whether* of eating.

In executing your responsibilities, family meals continue to be a priority. Even older adolescents do better in all things if they have family meals. In the face of multiple activities with competition for attention at dinnertime, you and your child may have to make difficult or inconvenient choices. Those difficult choices are well worthwhile. As we discussed in chapter 3, "Make Family Meals a Priority," adolescents who participate in family meals do better socially, emotionally, academically, and with respect to eating competence and normal growth and development. Family dinner grounds the adolescent because it means that family is there and functioning. As schedules evolve, take leadership in tinkering with mealtimes. How will the shopping get done? Who will do the cooking on any given night? Will it work to eat late in the evening, after practices or meetings? Will it work to eat early, before it all starts? Will you have to declare a dinnertime and have family be whoever is there? Even if an adolescent can't make it at times, she will benefit from knowing that family dinner is happening and that she can eat when she gets home. Perhaps it will work best, as one family found, to have their reliable family meal be breakfast. They had omelets and frittatas and once in a while a quiche. Like people in many cultures around the world, they even included salads and other vegetables.

Your adolescent can help shop for meals and get them on the table. However, even if he or she takes such a responsible role, family meals are still your primary responsibility. You, not your child, are in charge of nurturing. You may be more of an administrator and manager and less of a cook. Nonetheless, you are the one who sees to it that your family has meals on a regular basis.

Adolescents Take on More of the What, When, and Where
Earlier, your child learned to manage simple tasks of food selection within the limited menus at home and school, and at restaurants with your guidance. And he learned to take responsibility for his own snack times and choices. Now it is time to expand on all those capabilities.

When he is away from home, your adolescent will take on more and more responsibility for choosing his own food and providing for himself nutritionally. Again, I consider taking on that responsibility to be just as important for *boys* as for *girls*.

Now your child's intellectual development lets him understand the principles of menu planning and other nutritional principles. As a consequence, he can learn to manage the *context* of his eating: maintaining the structure of meals and snacks, identifying the components of a satisfying meal, planning meals to please others as well as himself, cooking food and keeping it clean and safe.

Your adolescent is in the *formal operational* stage. That means he can think abstractly and formulate and imagine alternate hypotheses. Such abstract concepts as "high in vitamin C" or "low in fat" or "eat a variety of food" make sense to him, and he can translate these concepts into food selection. He will be able to answer questions like "How will you get your vitamin C? What about your calcium?" Prior to this time, he could learn lessons about sources of nutrients and the importance of fruits, vegetables, and milk, but he couldn't apply that information to food selection.[12]

Keep in mind, you will be teaching your child to be unusual in his mastery of food management principles and skills. It isn't a bad idea to acknowledge that, even as you remain firm in your expectation that your child *will* do this. Otherwise, he will be handicapped. Ann Merritt, dietitian, educator, and one of my reviewers, commented, "I have met so many college-age and early-twenties people who are completely helpless in the kitchen. Even dietetics students in my food science classes didn't know the first thing about cooking. It was astounding!"

Given your older adolescent's ability to think abstractly, you can begin to teach him some of the principles presented in chapter 4, "Help Without Harming: Food Selection."

- How do you put together a breakfast or lunch that has staying power?
- How do you feed yourself after school and before activities?
- How do you see to it you get a vegetable or fruit when you eat lunch at the convenience store?
- What gaps did your lunch have, and how can you make up for those gaps the rest of the day?
- What do you consider when you plan a menu for the family?

If all goes well, your child will take an interest in menu planning and food preparation. In fact, if you have been cooking with him all along, that process will evolve. If you are careful not to be critical or pedantic, you can teach him a lot of food-management skills. Children appreciate parents' taking the lead with teaching life skills, and you will get a kick out of knowing enough to teach it. I strongly recommend that you teach your child these bottom-line principles:

- How to shop for and prepare three or four simple meals
- How to cook frozen vegetables
- How to open a can of fruit
- How to store food to keep it safe
- How to read labels to find adequate and filling prepack- aged meals

To help equip him for cooking simple meals, give your child a copy of appendix D, "Cooking in a Hurry." (You can also find this at www.EllynSatter.com.) Introduce him to *Secrets of Feeding a Healthy Family,* supplemented with a few of your family's favorite recipes. Show him the section in that book about grab- and-dump meals (page 118). I wrote *Secrets of Feeding a Healthy Family* too late to send it off with my own children, but it is a good primer for a young adult who is working to master food management. It presents valuable information on planning, shopping, cooking and sanitation. For more help learning—and teaching—the principles, get in touch with your local county extension office.

Relative to reading labels on prepackaged meals, teach your child to look for meals that have about 20 to 25 grams of pro- tein, 15 to 20 grams of fat, and 30 or more grams of carbohy- drate and a fruit or vegetable. That would be the equivalent of a meal with three ounces of meat, poultry, or fish, a sauce or some butter, and potatoes, rice, or other starchy food. To get that, he will likely have to look in at the Hungry Man dinners. Your daughter might have trouble with buying Hungry Man dinners, but Lean Cuisines and other meals marketed to women don't have enough calories to be filling and sustaining.

Your child will likely begin contributing ideas for foods that he would like to include on the family menu. Provided he has good food acceptance skills, take his suggestions seriously. But he has to tolerate unfamiliar food and learn to like new food before he can have the privilege of planning and preparing family meals.

There is more to contributing new food ideas than agreeing

on the family menu—being together and being separate at the same time are also involved. Parents from other countries struggle with separateness and togetherness in their dilemmas about assimilation versus cultural purity. The adolescent wants to bring home the broader culture in the form of food selection. Parents feel that this challenges their authority and criticizes their cultural values. Certainly, it is appropriate for parents to continue to take a leadership role with respect to food selection and maintaining the structure of meals and snacks. But now, being flexible and receptive about food selection offers a wonderful way to help and support the adolescent. Working through this concrete issue shows him ways both to be in the world and to remain connected with family. The adolescent's desire to experiment also presents a learning opportunity for parents: How can they be true to themselves without being so rigid that they create barriers between themselves and their child?

This dilemma is shared by parents whose children become vegetarian or beg for salads with the meat and potatoes or want Wonder bread with the lentil soup. Parents tend to take such requests as criticism of their ways. That may be true—adolescents *are* critical—but taking the criticism as an opening for discussion will create connection rather than barriers.

Understanding Intuitive Capabilities
In chapter 6, "Optimize Feeding: Your School-Age Child," I encouraged you to help your child to know what she knows—to bring her intuitive eating capabilities up to a conscious level. Now, her intellectual development lets you deepen that discussion. Why does she need to understand her intuitive capabilities? So she will know that she has the tools to manage her eating without having to resort to forcing down new foods or going by a diet to guide her in how much to eat. Consider this: If your child knows how to swim and *knows* she knows, she won't have to be afraid of the water. She won't have to wear a life preserver whenever she goes in over her head. Not only that, but she will be able to learn to do other things in the water, like canoe, or snorkel, or even scuba dive.

Knowing she can learn to like new food will make your

child more comfortable in the world. She can go to a friend's house or a foreign country and manage the food there. It will also allow her to accept her own reactions. Knowing, for instance, that she is very tuned in to taste and texture and has always taken great delight in delicious food will help her to accept and appreciate that about herself—even when she moans softly with the pleasure of eating. Knowing that tuned-in quality makes her slow to warm up to new food is the same. That is the way she is.

Knowing she is good at eating the amounts she needs will let your child eat less or more than her friends do. How deeply social expectations permeate even the amounts we eat! Boys feel self-conscious if they don't eat very much; girls feel self-conscious if they eat a lot. Your boy with a small appetite and your girl who enthusiastically eats large amounts deserve to know that they eat the amount they do because that is what they *need*. You can help by saying, "That's just the way you are; you have always been that way. If a baby does it, it must be right."

Because she knows about food regulation, your child will arrive at an intuitive understanding of and respect for her body's ability to weigh what it needs to weigh. However, at some point you need to tell her your philosophy about her weight. To keep yourself out of the "parents can't win" category, tell her what you did and why you did it. I have worked with people who are angry at their parents for putting them on diets when they were small—and others who blame their parents because they didn't try to restrict them and keep their weight down. You can tell your child that you maintained the division of responsibility in feeding and let her grow up to get the body that is right for her—and why you did it. Have her read chapter 1, "Help Without Harming."

THE ADOLESCENT WITH HIGH BMI

Adolescents with a high BMI often want to diet and lose weight. Putting your child on a diet or supporting her in her putting herself on a diet will make her fail and preserve her conviction that her true self is thinner. Remember, for the adolescent a major task is coming to terms with *identity*.

Maintaining the myth of some other, thinner self simply post-pones achieving that task. In our culture, many people diet their whole lives and go to their *graves* without ever coming to terms with their size and shape. You don't have to collude with that.

Most Professionals Will Restrict

Most people encourage adolescents with high body weight to diet and lose weight. This applies to health professionals, weight-loss organizations, parents, and even extended families. At times, the pressure to diet grows out of myths that even moderately elevated weight is a killer disease. At times, the idea is that children and adolescents who weigh a relatively large amount lack the ability to regulate food intake and must have it done for them or they will get heavier and heavier. At times, the pressure grows out of the adolescent's struggle for identity, compounded by distorted societal views about ideal size and shape. At times the issue is more benign—she is as tall as she is going to be, and she wants to find out if she can be thinner.

In figure 7.2 on page 250, I list my arguments against diet-ing. These arguments are intended to support you in resisting the pressure to send your child off for a weight loss regimen. The arguments are unlikely to have much impact on your ado-lescent. Adolescents believe that what happens to someone else won't happen to them.

No matter how it is labeled, any attempt at weight loss is a *diet*. Even weight-loss organizations that tout "nondiet" meth-ods encourage food restriction and striving for weight loss. They all amount to the same thing. When diets fail, the diet purveyors encourage adolescents to try again and try harder. Like their elders, children get caught in dieting and the pursuit of thinness.

Consider what would have happened with Maureen if she had found someone to put her on a diet. Under the best of cir-cumstances, she would have learned something about food selection and menu planning. She would have learned to force down vegetables and keep track of servings and portion sizes from food groups. But it would have been a big strain, and she

FIGURE 7.2 REASONS FOR YOUR ADOLESCENT *NOT* TO DIET

- Restricting her food intake can disrupt your child's energy balance—her ability to automatically eat the amount of food that is right for her.
- Weight-loss efforts can create the very problem they are intended to correct. Teenage children who diet are fatter, not thinner, by the time they graduate from high school.[13]
- Adults who started dieting when they were teenagers are often heavier than those who did not.[14]
- Adolescents who diet don't lose much weight, and they gain it back.[15]
- Adolescents who diet often don't get the nutrients they need and can become less healthy as a result.
- Adolescents who diet are cranky, hard to be around, and have a tendency to be depressed.
- Forcing unnaturally high levels of activity in the name of weight loss is depressing and can't be sustained.
- Dieting can make a child shorter than she would be otherwise.
- Trying to do the impossible is hard on anyone. The adolescent is particularly vulnerable to the upset that comes from chasing an impossible goal.
- Diets are often a Band-Aid solution to dealing with more difficult issues and developing social and emotional competence.
- Dieting and chasing weight loss postpones the time when your child comes to terms with the size and shape she is likely to be.

would have given it up and gone back to eating the old way. She wouldn't have learned anything.

Consider Wesley, who *did* put himself on a diet. Rather than eating enormous amounts, Wesley learned about "correct" portion sizes, and the "right" foods. While he dieted, he ate modestly. When he went off, he went back to stuffing himself. He didn't learn anything.

Do Good Parenting with Respect to Weight Issues
Even without pressure from health workers, parents, or family, in our weight-obsessed culture, sooner or later even the best-raised adolescent is likely to feel pressure to lose weight. She

will want to find out if she can be thinner.

Instead of going along with your adolescent's impulse to diet or "motivating" her to lose weight, why not help her grow up? Make sure that you are doing your jobs of feeding and parenting; then offer to help her find out what holds true for her. See to it that she knows how to *eat* and take care of herself with her eating. As I explain in chapter 9, "Teach Your Child: Be All You Can Be," expect her to learn to love and make the most of the body she *has*, not the one she *wishes* she had.

Then help your child to understand her own body and how it got to be the way it is. You might be able to do this yourself. Introduce her to the principles of size, shape, and energy balance that I teach you in this book. Talk about her history with respect to eating and growing. To make sure you understand growth principles, including the difference between *high normal* weight and weight *acceleration*, jump ahead now to read chapter 10, "Understand Your Child's Growth." Explain the principles to your adolescent, or let her read the chapter. You both need to know that your child is growing well if her weight consistently follows a particular percentile curve. If she has always grown that way, changing it will be very hard and likely won't work.

Adolescents can deal with complexity. While they may not like it, they can also accept unappealing—but freeing—reality and give up their fantasies. In the meantime, how competent is your child with her eating? Where does she need improvement? How competent is she with her activity? Where does she need improvement? Is she willing to increase her competence with respect to eating and activity and make improvements— permanently? What will happen with her weight if she does?

Find a Professional to Help Find Out What Holds True
For an adolescent, it is likely to be easier to examine those issues in detail with a professional than with a parent. If you can find one, a professional who understands the issues as I have outlined them in *Your Child's Weight: Helping Without Harming* can be wonderfully helpful to your adolescent. That person would be able to consider your child's whole picture

with respect to eating, activity, and weight issues and help her find out what holds true for her. You could raise all these issues yourself, but an outside person will do a more complete review and will be in a better position to tell your adolescent things she doesn't want to hear.

Those professionals exist. In my workshops "Feeding with Love and Good Sense" and "Treating the Dieting Casualty," I have trained many health professionals in supporting positive, internally regulated eating. Other experienced professionals are aware of the harm and futility of continually striving for weight loss and take other approaches. What is common to all is that they identify themselves as working toward *health at any size* rather than toward weight loss.

Allow me to demonstrate the process by telling you about Tyler. As he neared the end of high school, Tyler started to think along the lines of weight loss. He was strong and heavily built, and he wondered if he could be thinner. Tyler had a solid foundation for asking that question. His parents accepted his size and shape and fed him well. He fed himself reasonably well and had pretty good health habits. He continued to participate in family meals, and he played on one of the high school sports teams.

But Tyler wondered if he was too fat and had even run a few short-term experiments with his eating and weight to see if he could get thinner. He discovered that after a week or so of skipping snacks, he lost 10 pounds. But he gained the weight right back when he started eating snacks again.

Tyler's parents found a dietitian who set up a working relationship with their son. Together, she and Tyler looked at his size and shape history; evaluated his food selection, eating, and activity; and identified where he had room for improvement. Tyler had grown consistently and had always had a relatively heavy build. Changing that was unlikely. His activity level was already high, so increasing that would have been a stretch. His meals were moderate, so there wasn't much room for change. The one place there may have been room for change was with his snacks. He ate a lot of high-fat, high-sugar snacks that he wolfed down in a hurry.

He wasn't particularly attached to those foods and thought

he could skip his snacks. However, the dietitian told him that was unrealistic. He ate his snacks because he needed the energy to keep him going. They were working on something he could *live* with, not just jump on for a while and then fall off. She gave him some appealing ideas for other easy, filling, more nutritious snacks.

The dietitian told Tyler that he might drop a few pounds if he switched over to lower-calorie snacks—and stayed switched—or he might not. He would be getting more nutrients, but his meals already gave him all the nutrients he needed. He seemed to be a good regulator, and he might just get hungry and eat something different. He was still growing and putting on muscle, so he *would* get hungry. His body seemed to weigh what it wanted to weigh, and that might not change.

Then the dietitian asked Tyler some questions about taking care of himself when he went off to college. How was he going to get fed? What was he going to do for activity? Not only were those important considerations in general, but they applied to the current discussion. His weight was stable when he ate well and maintained consistent activity. Continuing to eat well and be active would be key to maintaining stable weight when he went off to college.

The dietitian wasn't holding out much hope for weight loss, but Tyler didn't give up. He wanted to know if he could go on the Atkins diet just to drop a few pounds. Instead of answering, she asked, "What do you think would happen?" Reluctantly, Tyler applied the lessons he had learned from her and from his own experiments. His weight would go down, and then it would go right back up again when he went off the diet. The dietitian agreed and said that if he wanted to get his weight down and keep it down, his changes would have to be *permanent*. He would always have to be careful to eat less than he was hungry for and exercise more than he really felt like. It would be a big change, because now his eating and activity were pretty automatic for him. But it was up to him what he decided to do.

Tyler had mixed feelings about his work with the dietitian. He learned a lot about himself and about what to do to take

care of himself, and he guessed that was good. But he also
wasn't happy to know how hard and complicated it would be
for him to weigh less.

After that, it was up to Tyler. He could make up his own
mind about what he wanted to do.

The Adolescent Whose Weight Gain Has Accelerated

Your direction is considerably more involved if your child's
issues are established or complicated. That is likely to be the
case if any one of the following is true:

- Your child's weight has diverged significantly and rapidly
  up or down from her normal growth curve.
- Her eating competency is low.
- You have ongoing struggles about her eating.
- She is chronically and significantly upset and anxious about
  her eating and weight.
- You and she can't find solutions to her issues on your own.

For you and your child, working your way out of these issues
will require an intervention that is both detailed and long-lasting
enough to enable real change to take place. You need *treatment*.

Your Child's Weight can give you general guidelines for what
you are working toward with respect to feeding and parenting.
However, correcting the distortions in your relationship may
require more focused guidance and support than you can find
in *any* book. Look for a family therapist who is good at helping
adolescents and their parents. It would be best if that professional is knowledgeable about feeding and weight issues as I
have addressed them in *Your Child's Weight*. However, be fore-
warned that the attitudes toward eating and weight held by
many mental health professionals are about the same as those
of the general population. Many mental health professionals see
weight loss as an essential first step in resolving emotional
problems. The best you may be able to hope for is a mental
health professional who will regard your child as "normal."
Then you can get help addressing your issues from the point of
view of establishing and maintaining good parenting, and your

child can get help addressing her issues from the perspective of gaining emotional and social competence.

Once you work your way out of those social and emotional issues, you can find help with feeding. Find a dietitian or other health professional who understands appropriate feeding such as I have described it in *Your Child's Weight*. Get her help and support to resolve the feeding and eating issues.

In presenting your child for such scrutiny, you invite scrutiny of yourself—of your history of parenting your child. While it takes courage and commitment to engage in such a process, you stand to gain as much or more than your child does. A careful assessment and treatment plan offers you a priceless opportunity to correct your errors in parenting, restore a more positive and satisfying relationship with your child, and build a foundation for a long life with her.

It is possible that reading this chapter or this book has been painful for you. You, like many parents, may have recognized your errors with feeding and parenting. Don't be too hard on yourself. You acted as you did for specific reasons, many of which have been addressed here. Your reading this book gives evidence that you love your child and are willing to go to some trouble on her behalf. Taking responsibility for your part in creating her problem and finding better ways of parenting go a long way toward helping find a solution. Your child had—and has—a contribution to make as well and, with your help, can develop more positive ways of dealing with herself, her eating, other people, and her life circumstances.

By the end of adolescence, your child will be ready to go out into the world. You will have done what you can for her. She can always fall back on you, but for the most part, now it is up to her. By whatever path she takes, the task for your child is to come to terms with herself, to love and appreciate herself just the way she is, to take responsibility for her own choices, and to do the best that *she* can.

NOTES
1. Powers, Hauser, and Kilner, "Adolescent Mental Health."
2. Elder, "Structural Variations in the Childrearing Relationship."

3. Demo and Acock, "Family Structure, Family Process."

4. Johnston, O'Malley, and Bachman, *Monitoring the Future.*

5. Rogers, "Sexual Risk-Taking Behaviors."

6. Stattin and Kerr, "Parental Monitoring."

7. Shedler and Block, "Adolescent Drug Use."

8. Adelson, "Friendship and the Peer Group."

9. Simmons, Rosenberg, and Rosenberg, "Disturbance in the Self-Image at Adolescence."

10. Fredricks and Eccles, "Children's Competence and Value Beliefs."

11. Buhrmester and Furman, "Development of Companionship and Intimacy."

12. Lytle et al., "Children's Interpretation of Nutrition Messages."

13. Stice et al., "Naturalistic Weight-Reduction Efforts."

14. Ikeda et al., "Self-Reported Dieting Experiences of Women."

15. Epstein et al., "Treatment of Pediatric Obesity."

ELLYN SATTER'S DIVISION OF RESPONSIBILITY FOR PHYSICAL ACTIVITY

Parents provide *structure, safety,* and *opportunities.* Children choose *how much* and *whether* to move and the *manner* of moving.

The Division of Responsibility for Infants:
• The parent is responsible for *safe opportunities.*
• The child is responsible for *moving.*
The parent provides the infant with a variety of positions, clothing, sights, and sounds. Then the parent remains present and lets the infant experiment with moving.

The Division of Responsibility for Toddlers Through Adolescents
• The parent is responsible for *structure, safety,* and *opportunities.*
• The child is responsible for *how much* and *whether.*

Supporting a child's physical activity is good parenting. Parents' jobs include the following:
• Develop judgment about normal commotion.
• Provide safe places for activity the child enjoys.
• Find fun and rewarding family activities.
• Provide opportunities to experiment with group activities such as sports.
• Set limits on television but not on reading, writing, artwork, or other sedentary activities.
• Remove the television and computer from the child's bedroom.
• Make children responsible for dealing with their own boredom.

Fundamental to parents' jobs is trusting children to decide *how much* to move, the *way* to move, and *whether* to be active.
• Children will be active.
• Each child is more or less active depending on constitutional endowment.
• Each child is more or less skilled, graceful, energetic, or aggressive, depending on constitutional endowment.
• Children's physical capabilities will grow and develop.
• Children will experiment with activities that are in concert with their growth and development.
• They will find activities that are right for them.

CHAPTER
8

PARENT IN THE BEST WAY:
PHYSICAL ACTIVITY

Your job is to support your child's natural inclinations to move so he can get the body that is right for him. Your job is *not* to get your child to be active as a way of preventing or curing overweight. Children are born loving their bodies, curious about them, inclined to move, and driven to be as physically competent as they can possibly be. The goal of good parenting with respect to physical activity is to preserve your child's positive attitudes about his body and his joy in moving it. Joyful activity is sustainable.

Managing your child's physical activity will no more guarantee keeping your child slim than managing his eating. To parent well with physical activity, you must identify and give up your size-and-shape agenda. Otherwise you will fall prey to the current attitudes that say, "Well, diet doesn't seem to work to slim children down, but surely activity will." Such attitudes turn parents into personal trainers rather than parents, encouraging, cheerleading, nagging, and even coercing children to *move* in the name of slimness.

With physical activity as with all the other issues we have discussed in *Your Child's Weight,* to act on behalf of your child, you will have to resist interference and pressures to change or control your child's weight. The pressure is all around. An August 2004 article in *National Geographic* showed a 9-year-old boy on a treadmill, trying get rid of what was perceived as his excess fat. (Is there nowhere to escape this weight mania?) The child had apparently been put on an exercise regimen in hopes of wearing him down to be more svelte. He was also taking tae kwon do, "but still weighs 134 pounds. 'It's been a struggle,'" sighs his mother.

The boy's mother was on the right track with the tae kwon do. It could let him have fun as well as help him experience his body as strong and capable. But participating because he *had* to, for the purpose of slimming him down, would take all the fun and reward out of it. Children at this age explore and play and try out their bodies and learn about life. Why would anybody condemn a 9-year-old to a routine that is so dead boring and demoralizing that all but the most determined adults use a treadmill to store unused clothing?

Agendas hurt children. Your child will naturally be as active as is right for him, and he will naturally seek out what he enjoys—he will find the forms and levels of activity that are right for him. Children are more or less active, more or less strong and coordinated, more or less aggressive, more or less graceful—the list goes on. There are some activities your child is good at and some that are right for him. He will find those activities—unless he loses his good feelings about moving.

SUPPORTING ACTIVITY DEMANDS A DIVISION OF RESPONSIBILITY

Opposite the first page in this chapter is Ellyn Satter's Division of Responsibility for Physical Activity. You will note that there are clear parallels with Ellyn Satter's Division of Responsibility in Feeding. I modeled the activity guidelines directly on the feeding guidelines. Both *divisions* advocate supporting without controlling, giving autonomy without abandoning. Both help you find that tricky balance that is the essence of good parenting. Both support your child's growth and development in a stage-related fashion.

The Division of Responsibility for Infants

You are responsible for providing safe opportunities for your baby to move. He is responsible for *moving*.

Even your young baby is active. He actively explores his body. He moves around while he sleeps, waves his arms and legs and moves his head, arches his back, squirms, stiffens himself to stand up. Once he discovers his hands and feet, he holds them up and studies them for long periods. He plays with his voice by talking and yelling and plays with his saliva by letting it drool on his lips and sucking it back in again.

Here are some ways you support your infant's activity:

- Pay attention to him.
- Conduct little baby conversations with him.
- Hold him rather than keeping him in the infant seat (when you aren't driving).
- Keep him company while he is awake.
- Put him on his tummy to play rather than always keeping him on his back.
- Vary his clothing and sometimes take his clothing off.
- Give him something to look at and follow with his eyes.

All of the activities on this list, and many others you will think of, let your baby experience and develop his body as well as support his mental development. Don't keep up a steady barrage of activity and stimulation. Like us, your baby needs time when he engages with you and times when he is left to his own devices. Go by what he tells you. He will look at you when he is ready to talk or play, look away while he calms himself down. If you wait while he gets calm, he will look back and be ready to play again.

Rather than hauling your baby around in an infant seat, hold him as you carry him from place to place. He needs the body contact to feel close to you and to make his brain develop. Hold him while you talk with other people—he will take part.

Hold him while you wait in line—he will liven things up. Certainly, at times putting him in an infant seat is the only way you will be able to safely get your tasks done. At times he gets tired of being handled and wants to be put down. Go by what he tells you.

The current advice is to put your baby to sleep on his back to prevent SIDS (sudden infant death syndrome). However, when your baby is awake and you are around, it is important to put him on his tummy. He will move more as he lifts his head and tries to raise himself on his arms and legs. That lifting and raising will allow him to roll over and crawl sooner.

Babies love being allowed to have their clothes off. Observe your baby's puzzlement and delight as he kicks and squirms in a whole different way. Being without clothes feels unfamiliar to him, and he experiments with the sensations—air on his skin rather than covered up, cool rather than warm, free movement rather than restricted by clothing.

The Division of Responsibility for Toddlers Through Adolescents

For older children, you are responsible for providing *structure*, *safety*, and *opportunities* to move. Your child is responsible for deciding *how much* and *whether* to move.

Toddlers, preschoolers, and young school-age children can't help moving. Early play is mastery play, and children work to master new skills. They work on keeping their balance as they kick, run, hop, fall, throw, swing, jump, slide, leap, dodge, gallop, and catch. Rather than the sports activities we adults organize for them, young school-age children most enjoy cooperative games they make up themselves. Those are games that have lots of action, such as kickball, dodgeball, king-of-the-mountain, hide-and-seek, and kick-the-can. Since young children's priority is keeping the game going, they take care to choose up evenly balanced sides and negotiate do-overs.

Prior to late school-age or early adolescence, your child has innate limitations in his ability to be successful with organized sports. He may or may not be able to watch a moving ball and intuitively predict where that ball is likely to go. His attention is overly inclusive, meaning that he has trouble discriminating the key action in the midst of a lot of activity. His reaction time is slow, and his tolerance for prolonged, high-endurance activity is limited. His lung capacity is not yet fully developed, and his body is not efficient about getting rid of excess body heat.

In late school-age or early adolescence, children cross a proficiency barrier. With respect to tracking, attention, discrimination, reaction time, and endurance, they physically approach adult ability to learn and perform. Their drive for task achievement makes them interested in developing skills, learning the rules of the game, and developing strategy.

Whether or not your child chooses to participate in sports, the growing-up years have everything to do with his developing sustainable activity throughout life. Primarily, what contributes to your child's participation in sustainable activity are attitudes such as these:

- Your child has a positive attitude toward his body and his capabilities.
- He is interested and *wants* to move.
- He finds movement rewarding.
- He is reasonably strong and coordinated and able to move his body.

THINK IN TERMS OF *CAPABILITY*, NOT SIZE AND SHAPE
Physical capabilities are strength, agility, coordination, stamina, endurance, quickness, flexibility, speed—the list goes on. As with eating, some capabilities are inborn; others are learned and developed. Slimness is not a physical capability. It is an *attribute*.

Until he learns otherwise, if your young child thinks about his body at *all*, he will *not* think in terms of how it *looks*. He will think of what it can *do*. More likely, he will just *move* and in the process discover what he finds rewarding. Keeping the emphasis on *function* rather than on *appearance* will support your child in being active and feeling good about his body throughout his growing-up years. Moving his body and experiencing it as strong and capable lets him feel good about his body at *any* size and shape.

As usual, children in their intuitive wisdom are ahead of the innovative thinkers. A June 2004 *New York Times* article describes a "transformative" approach to fitness in which trainers offer customers not toning and slimming but *functional fitness*.[1] The goal of working out is preparing the body to perform daily activities—walking, bending, lifting, climbing stairs—without pain, injury, or discomfort. In short, it is training for *life,* not *events*. The idea is that one's body can be useful and that striving for fitness can be in the name of living fully!

Large Children Can Be Fit and Healthy

The research is clear: With respect to health and a long life, it is better to be fit and fat than thin and unfit.[2] Moreover, fat people can be active, fit, and healthy. Stephen Blair, a well-known fitness researcher at the Cooper Institute in Houston, uses himself to make the point about size, shape, and health before he launches into his lectures about his data. "I thought when I started running I would be slim and muscular," he observes. "But look at me. I run five or six miles a day. I weigh what I did when I started." Dr. Blair is short and stocky and has a layer of fat on his body. He is the living illustration of his research.

The bottom line with physical activity is preserving your child's good feelings about his body and his inclination to move. Until or unless they are taught, children with high BMI don't think they are physically incapable. Three-year-old Benjamin thought he had found heaven when his father first arranged for him to be at Head Start. Benjamin ran and played and climbed and swung. He was so busy playing that it was a chore to persuade him to sit down to lunch with the other children.

Benjamin taught everyone about size, shape, and physical capability. He was so fat that when he first started attending, the administrator worried about his physical safety. She sent a teacher to ride the bus with him, fearing that he simply could not manage it on his own. Benjamin surprised her—and a lot of other people as well. He *moved*. He *gloried* in movement. All he needed was the opportunity.

Don't Make the Wrong Assumptions

Protect yourself against the common assumption that people are fat because they are not very active and that if they become more active, they will get slim. Instead, go with the assumption that people have natural inborn tendencies pertaining to activity, body type, and energy intake. The first assumption will have you pushing physical activity in an attempt to keep your child slim. The second will let you do a good job of parenting and then trust the evolution of your child's size and shape to normal growth and development.

From the first, children are different from one another with respect to energy need, body type, and activity level. In a classic study done at Harvard University, nutritionist Jean Mayer and his then-graduate student H. E. Rose set out to understand normal processes of energy regulation as it related to size and shape. They observed the food intake, activity, size, and shape of 30 infants, 4 to 6 months old. Researchers weighed and measured what the babies ate and monitored their activity by strapping tiny pedometers to their wrists and ankles. The results were clear: The least active babies ate the least and were the fattest. The most active infants ate the most and were the leanest.[3]

The point is that from birth, children *are* the way they *are.* They have *constitutional* inclinations regarding activity, food intake, size, and shape; and if we try to change those inclinations, we will be destructive.

Recent studies illustrate the same variations. Tufts University researchers found that 8- to 12-year-old girls with a "high activity temperament" moved more and were slimmer.[4] Unlike Mayer, who concluded that placid, chubby children simply represented a variant of normal, the Tufts authors concluded that the less active, less slim children were somehow abnormal. As they put it, "a constitutional predilection for movement" may aid in the avoidance of obesity. Instead of natural variations in activity, size, and shape, the authors thought they were identifying a cause-and-effect relationship.

Researchers at Boston University followed children for 8 years, from roughly 4 to 12 years of age. They found that children at the higher levels of activity showed lower increases in

BMI and body fatness. Those in the lower levels of activity showed greater increases. Those researchers concluded that their results "add strong support for the hypothesis that higher levels of physical activity during childhood lead to the acquisition of less body fat by the time of early adolescence."[5] On the other hand, it is equally possible they were identifying natural differences among children's natural activity levels, size, and shape.

How the data are interpreted all depends on spin. Considered another way, both sets of researchers demonstrated what the Rose and Mayer study did: There are natural variations in body type and activity. Had they studied the children's food intake, they would likely have found, as Rose and Mayer did and as have other researchers that have studied food intake and weight, that the heaviest children ate the least, the lightest the most.[6]

Expect Your Child to Make Good Use of the Body He *Has*
Every child is limited—or empowered—by the body he was born with. Some sports will be a good fit for your child; others are simply out of the question. If your child wants to participate in sports, there is one that is right for his body.

My accountant, Justin, 6 feet tall and on the slender side, commented that he is prepared for his slender, short 6-year-old. "I was always small, and I expect he will be the same," he observed. "In fact, I didn't get my full growth until I was out of high school." Justin didn't seem to think he had missed out on anything, although football was the big sport at his school, and he decided that at 130 pounds and 5 foot 6 inches tall he wasn't up for bouncing off when he tried to tackle and being crunched when he was on the receiving end. Instead, he wrestled in the 130-pound category. The only time he seemed a bit wistful was when he commented that he would have liked to have played soccer, a sport that wasn't available in the rural community where he grew up.

When I last saw him, Justin was nursing an arm he had broken water-skiing. Justin enjoys moving his body because he has not been overprotected. I expect his son will be the same. Too often, parents see a child who is unusual with respect to size and shape as being vulnerable. Rather than accepting the child's natural rowdiness or encouraging him to take reasonable physical risks, parents protect him and in the process teach him that he is fragile and incapable.

My 25-year-old patient Carson saw himself that way. He tried to walk and ride a bike, but he got all upset when he started to puff. He worried that he was hurting himself. It helped Carson to have a sports medicine evaluation so he could identify his body's capability and realize that he wasn't hurting himself when he worked hard enough to breath heavily and sweat.

I won't even tell you whether Carson was fat or thin. Anybody can be overprotected and learn to perceive himself as fragile. People of size just pay the price in the form of weight criticism and the judgment that they are slothful.

Don't Criticize Your Child's Weight

Your child will be most active if he is spontaneous and uninhibited about moving. That, in turn, depends on positive physical self-esteem. Weight criticism backfires—it makes children less active, not more. When their grown-ups criticize their weight, children see their bodies as being less capable. From there, they become self-conscious, embarrassed about their bodies, and inclined to hold back on moving.

The destructiveness of weight criticism on physical self-esteem starts early. Research at Pennsylvania State showed that very young girls didn't feel as good about their bodies when parents were concerned about weight. The damage was even greater when parents restricted the girls' food intake. The association between concern about overweight and lower physical self-esteem was particularly marked for fathers. Parenthetically, lowered self-concept extended to intellect as well as overall self-esteem. Girls whose parents saw them as overweight and whose parents restricted their access to food, thought they weren't as smart as other children and felt bad about themselves overall.[7] As I have said before, children do not compartmentalize their attitudes about themselves. If they are seen as flawed in *one* way, they experience themselves as flawed in *all* ways.

Regardless of weight, children with low physical self-esteem appear to be less active than children whose physical self-esteem is higher. Children whose weight is criticized become self-conscious and inhibited in their movement. A Columbia University study showed that weight criticism lowered fifth- through eighth-grade children's leisure-time activity and sports enjoyment. Overweight children commonly reported being "embarrassed doing physical activity and playing sports." Children's coping skills diluted the association but did not neutralize it.[8]

Children criticize each other and establish pecking orders with respect to sports achievement. The more talented roll over the less talented. There is little you can do about that. You can, however, do much about your *own* criticism and that of other adults. Weight criticism is often indirect, offhand, or clothed in euphemisms that are intended to disguise true feelings. Children are not fooled. A child knows you don't approve of his weight when you ask *him* how he feels about it, when you tell him he should eat certain foods to "be healthy," hint that being more active will tone him up, or even *feel* that there is something wrong with his weight. Children are exquisitely tuned in to feelings and attitudes and can read us even when we don't want to be read. The bottom line is *attitude* and *intent*. If your *attitude* is that there is something wrong with your child and your *intent* is get him thinner, you are being critical.

For more about preserving and supporting your child's positive attitude about his body, read appendix H, "Development of Physical Self-Esteem."

Activity Fine-Tunes Food Regulation

Adults often make the association between food intake and activity by saying that exercise allows them to eat all they want without gaining weight—they can eat more and get away with it. Activity *will* support your child in eating all he wants, but the mechanism is far more positive and sophisticated than simply allowing him to overeat and wear it off. Throughout *Your Child's Weight*, we have discussed automatic processes of food regulation based on hunger, appetite, and satisfaction. When those processes work well, your child is able to go to the table hungry, eat until he is satisfied, and then stop, knowing another meal or snack is coming and he can do it again. He will *automatically* eat the amount he needs to grow well, and as an adult he will be able to maintain a stable weight.

Here is the important part: Given a certain minimum level of activity, the amount your child *wants* and the amount he *needs* will be the same. That is in sharp contrast to the experience of many adults, who feel deprived when they eat what they feel they *need* and gluttonous when they eat as much as they *want.* In addition, getting a certain minimal level of activity makes those internal regulators more prominent, making it easier to detect hunger and fullness and to eat the amount that the body needs. Be careful not to decode this as the standard message that your child should exercise to lose or maintain his weight—the point is that physical activity enhances your child's natural ability to regulate his food intake.

In a 50-year-old but by no means outdated study, Harvard nutritionist Jean Mayer, who was introduced earlier in this chapter, set out to examine regulatory processes as they related to activity. The study focused on adult males, but the results are applicable to children and women as well. In contrast to today's research, which attempts to control or manipulate regulatory processes, Mayer's research was designed to study *natural* regulatory processes. Mayer chose a jute factory in Bengal, India, for his study setting. The factory was a self-contained environment. Everyone ate the same type of food, and the workers engaged in widely varying levels of physical activity. The most sedentary men were stall holders and supervisors, who sat most of the time. The most active men were the load carriers, coalmen, and blacksmiths, who kept the fires going and moved huge, heavy loads. The moderately active men between the two extremes were the clerks and mechanics, who moved around during their day's activities, walked to work, or played sports.

With the exception of the people in the sedentary range, the more active the men became, the more they ate. The active men's weights remained stable. They were able to automatically balance their energy intake with output and maintain a consistent body weight. In contrast, the people in the sedentary ranges, the ones who sat most of the time, ate more than they needed and gained weight.[9] The group replicated in humans well-established observations in animals: The way to fatten an experimental rat or mouse is to immobilize it. Back in the old days when we liked fat meat, farmers would restrict the activity of cows or pigs in order to fatten them.

The moral of the story is the same as with all the other issues we discuss in this chapter. The goal of good parenting with respect to physical activity is to preserve your child's positive attitudes about his body and his joy in moving. Interfering with your child's physical activity can undermine his food regulation and make him fatter than nature intended.

SUPPORT, DON'T PUSH, ACTIVITY

As the division of responsibility for physical activity points out, your child will grow and develop with respect to movement. If all goes well, he will develop to the limits of his physical ability. He will arrive at his school-age and high school years ready to participate and to have as much fun as he wants in whatever activities are available. He will be prepared to enter his adult years having found activities that are right for him and that he will take pleasure in pursuing later in life.

Stow Your Agenda

Ellyn Satter Institute consultant Pam Estes helped write Ellyn Satter's Division of Responsibility for Physical Activity. She feels particularly strongly about the part that says to "trust children to decide *how much* to move, the *way* to move, and *whether* to be active." Pam is a slender and active woman who loves walking and yoga and participates in an annual mini-marathon. Her husband, Jim, enjoys teaching tae kwon do and running races. Jim dreamed that their son Adam would run and bike with him and play sports so that Jim could cheer him on. Jim loved sports as a boy, and he wanted to give Adam all the support for physical activity that he himself had not received. Pam's dad coached her brother in every sport, and she looked forward to being a "soccer mom."

Wouldn't you know, Adam loved the computer! He rode

his bike to get where he wanted to go, played Little League to please his parents, and thought running for the fun of it was rather curious. Jim and Pam couldn't figure it out, and they kept pushing and encouraging. Adam went along as best he could, but what he really liked was the computer.

During a tae kwon do class, Pam could see that Adam was starting to feel bad about himself. She talked to Jim about it, and together they realized the error of their ways. They gave up on their dreams of having a sports-enthusiast son and came to accept and support the son they *had*. Both Jim and Pam were tested in their resolve when Adam went through a period of preadolescent chubbiness, but they both held firm with accepting and supporting him. He slimmed down as he got taller, and he is now of average weight, off to college, pursuing environmental studies.

After a series of e-mails and phone calls in which they aired out their feelings about the issue, Pam, Jim, and Adam gave me permission to share their experience because they felt it would be helpful to other families. As they wound up their discussion, Adam e-mailed *his* observation: "I think Ellen should include that once you guys left me alone I did my own choices of physical activity! I walk (I would hike if Indianapolis had trails near us!), I kayak (not recently but I plan too!), and I jog (I have been running when I take Rocket [the apartment dog] out. . . . She keeps pace with me, which is nice, since I am much slower than her)."

Pam and Jim learned what we all have to learn at some point in order to be good parents: Love the child you *have*, not the one you *thought* you would have.

Don't Be Overprotective

For whatever reason, sometimes children get stuck and need help to be able to grow and develop with respect to movement. Many times, a bit of encouragement is all that is needed. A friend said he was a klutzy kid who needed encouragement from his parents to play games with the other children. He could get so he could keep up, they reassured him. He could learn to throw and catch a ball and score a basket. His father took some time to help him master throwing and kicking, and they reassured him he didn't have to be the best. The idea was to have fun. Children who move into a new neighborhood feel self-conscious if they can't do the same activities the other children do. Parents can help a child learn to ride bike, skateboard, or jump rope so he can join in with the other children.

Being too protective can undermine a child's capability. The father in one of my chubby-child families sympathized when his 6-year-old daughter came home crying about being teased on the playground. "Who needs that?" he asked. "We'll just play a game ourselves." The father had been a chubby boy, and his daughter's experience brought back painful memories for him. His own parents didn't want to be bothered. They sneered, "Well, if you weren't so fat, you wouldn't have that problem!" Another parent, also of a 6-year-old girl, did better. She heard her daughter out, helped her to think of ways to deal with the teasing, and encouraged her to go back out to play with her friends. She could insist on her turn, even if she *was* fat!

Given the backward way that children have of getting their needs met, the well-intended father was undermining his daughter's social and physical capability. What little girl wouldn't rather have her father's undivided attention than learn to make it with her friends? If whining worked so well and was so rewarding, why tough it out with the other kids? What this father missed was that he was a better parent than his own parents had been. He loved and accepted his daughter and looked out for her. Given his backing, she could be a lot more resilient than he had been.

Develop Your Tolerance for Normal Commotion

Moving is what children do. With young children, the task is not to *get* them moving but to learn to *live* with all the movement while you preserve and protect your own civil rights.

Develop your tolerance and judgment about a child's normal level of activity and risk taking. Visit child care centers, preschools, and school playgrounds. Talk with experienced parents. Know some tricks of the trade. Boys—and many girls—love rough-and-tumble play. In the course of it, they deal with others in ways that to the uneducated eye seem downright anti-social. Consider this example: After a few moments of observing three other boys building a sand castle, 5-year-old Jimmy smiles, climbs on a tricycle, and plows the structure apart. The builders take off in hot pursuit, yelling menacingly, "Come back here, you!" Soon Jimmy stops his tricycle and the others pounce on him. The four of them tumble around in the grass amid shouts of glee, wrestling, and punching.[10]

How can you tell whether all the yelling, wrestling, and punching is fighting or playing? If the one on the bottom is smiling, it is rough-and-tumble play. It is rare for anyone to get hurt, and then it is only by accident. When my sons were small, it seems they had only to brush against each other to end up rolling over and over on the floor. Tolerate this sort of thing, but you don't have to tolerate it under your feet when you are reading or in the middle of your living room. Children can learn to do their rough and loud playing where they don't bother others.

Don't forget your sense of humor. Using its own brand of stating-the-obvious humor, a December 27, 2000, article in the satirical newspaper *The Onion* outlined the challenge of living with children. Under the headline "More U.S. Children Being Diagnosed with Youthful Tendency Disorder," the article described how "day after day, after arriving home from pre-school, Caitlin would retreat into a bizarre fantasy world. Sometimes, she would pretend to be people and things she was not. Other times, without warning, she would burst into non-sensical song. Some days, she would run directionless through the back yard of the Sernas' comfortable Redlands home, laughing and shrieking as she chased imaginary objects."[11]

After months of sessions with a psychologist, the Sernas were given the "heartbreaking news that Caitlin was among a growing legion of U.S. children suffering from Youthful Tendency Disorder (YTD), a poorly understood neurological condition. YTD is characterized by a variety of senseless, unproductive physical and mental exercises, often lasting hours at a time. In the thrall of YTD, sufferers run, jump, climb, twirl, shout, dance, do cartwheels and enter unreal, unexplainable stages of 'make believe.'"

The point is clear. We have to let children be children.

Provide Safe Places for Activity Your Child Enjoys

This is two-part advice: *Safe places* is one part; *activity your child enjoys* is the other. To begin with the second part, follow your child's lead. As children gain control of their muscles and movement, they practice continually. They climb trees and fences, they run through open fields and along busy streets, they find ways to play with almost anything they can get their hands on. As they get older, they range farther and master a greater variety of activities as they explore, ride bikes, climb, swim, skateboard, ski, ride scooters.

Children need help keeping safe, and they are more active if they *feel* safe. In most communities, families need help keeping their children safe and giving them a place to play. To move around freely, children need to feel safe. Consider the old story of the playground with the fence. Children using a playground bordered by busy streets clustered toward the center of the space and were inhibited in their movements. After a fence was installed, they ran and played freely all over the playground, right up to the fence. Not having to worry about boundaries freed them to do more.

The key concept in keeping children safe is *injury control*. You can't watch a child all the time, but you *can* help keep him safe with forethought and supervision. You practice injury control when you put up child safety gates to keep a young toddler off stairs and childproof a play area by putting away breakables and tall objects that a child can pull over on himself. You do injury control when you put medicines and cleaning products on high shelves and make sure that open windows have child safety barriers. You also practice injury control when you survey your environment with a child's eye, moving or removing hazards to a running, climbing, swinging child, such as a woodpile at the base of an attractive climbing tree.

Communities practice injury control and help keep children active and safe with strict traffic enforcement, crossing guards, and requirements for bicycle helmets and bicycle reflectors. Communities also help keep children safe and active by providing safe playground areas and putting soft surfaces under playground equipment rather than cement or asphalt.

As children get older, they benefit from thinking about injury control for themselves. Teenagers in particular take risks, but they do not have to take stupid, pointless risks. In fact, a teenager benefits from a thoughtful discussion about different levels of risk for a given activity. After such a discussion, he can decide just how much risk he wants to assume. Keep in mind, parenting a teenager with respect to risk-taking behavior demands the division of responsibility. As I said in chapter 7, "Optimize Feeding: Your Adolescent," your job is to help him think through the hazards. His job is to decide how much hazard he is willing to assume.

Find Fun and Rewarding Family Activities

What activities do you enjoy? Cruising the mall, window shopping, and visiting with friends? Walking the dog? Camping? Playing Frisbee? Riding a bike? Going to the beach? Playing ball? Going to the gym or the Y? Building or tearing down? Gardening? Dancing? As far as your child is concerned, the best part of any activity is *you*. Edie Applegate, who worked with lots of children at Rockford Clinic in Illinois, says children's eyes always lit up when she asked them, "Would you like your parents to play with you?" That response from your child is reward enough. If you have fun with your child, it is likely he will grow up to enjoy many of the activities you do.

When your child is little, the term "family activity" has to be used rather loosely, at least as far as you are concerned. I see young families shuffling through the woods, parents mostly standing around as the toddlers and preschoolers examine everything they see. I see parents being spotters next to slides and endlessly pushing swings. I see them patiently throwing balls while their child swings and misses, swings and misses. I see them sitting on front steps while children ride their tricycles up and down, round and round. The reward for parents is in being with their child and participating in their growth and discovery. If children are outside, they are likely to be active. The trick for parents is finding ways to be outside with them.

At times, "family activity" means parents are active and children are not. Children ride in bike seats and carts behind bikes, in strollers, and in backpacks. Even if they are passive participants, children are exposed to the activity and to a love of being outdoors. It isn't long before a school-age child begins to ride his own bike and walk far enough so the whole family can take walks and hikes. Then, one day, children kick in and you can't keep up with them! Parenting can be a thankless business.

Provide Opportunities to Experiment with Group Activities Such as Sports

Prior to about age 8 to 10 years old, children are simply not developmentally ready to play sports. While many children start to play soccer when they are 5 or 6 years old, at that age they are more running back and forth chasing a ball than playing soccer. They swarm around the ball, moving up and down the field tightly grouped around the kicker as if they were a flock of birds. The coach stands at the edge of the field, yelling, "Spread out! Spread out!" They can't spread out. Developmentally, young children are simply not capable of thinking in terms of position, strategy, and moving the ball from one person to the next and thereby down the field. You can't train a child beyond his developmental limitations. Accepting those limitations is essential. Criticizing a child for failing to do the impossible takes away his good feelings about the sport and about himself.

I remember watching the swarming—and yelling—scenario when my son Lucas was 6 years old. "Do you remember that?" I asked him? "How did you feel about it?" "I remember him yelling, but I didn't pay much attention," Lucas responded. Interesting—and relieving. I imagine if his father or I had gotten after him about his performance, it would have been a different matter.

Which brings us to your ego involvement as a parent. If a child is to try things out, you must keep your ego out of it. If your good feelings about yourself depend on your child's being a star, you are in trouble, and so is your child. One of the most difficult eating disorders cases I ever worked with was a university runner who got caught in trying to force her weight down in a desperate attempt to run faster. She was in such bad shape nutritionally that she knew she had to give up dieting and possibly even give up her sport. However, she was getting pressure from home. Her father kept her trophies in a special room and spent hours each day admiring them and remembering her victories.

You can dream about raising a great soccer star or swimming medal winner, but keep your dreams to yourself! Most of us raise competent children who enjoy moving, and that is just great! While Lucas and his teammates eventually learned to *spread out* and he became a good soccer player, as an adult, he enjoys puttering with bikes and playing pickup hockey games with the neighborhood kids.

Set Limits on Television Watching

To find today's equivalent of those Bengalese sedentary workers, we could look in the vicinity of television sets. Population studies find that the more television children watch, the heavier they tend to be. An analysis of the 1988 to 1994 National Health and Nutrition Examination Survey found that one-quarter of U.S. children ages 8 through 16 watched 4 or more hours of television each day. Furthermore, boys and girls who watched 4 or more hours of television each day had greater body fat and had a higher weight-to-height ratio than those who watched less than 2 hours per day.[12] California adolescents who watched more than 2 hours of television a day were twice as likely to be overweight at follow-up as adolescents who watched less than 2 hours.[13] Time spent watching television is increased when families eat meals in front of the television set and when children have television sets in their bedrooms.[14]

There is, of course, a logic to the association between television and body weight, especially if we extrapolate from the Bengalese study. Children who watch too much television may not have the opportunity to get themselves out of the sedentary range of physical activity and may eat more than they actually need. There may also be more to it than that. Studies in a Memphis metabolic laboratory of 8- to 12-year-old children showed that children watching television fell into a trancelike state. Their metabolic rate dropped to roughly 15 percent lower than when they were awake but at rest. Extrapolated over the course of a day, the average decrease in expenditure was 211 calories.[15]

Studies that have attempted to increase children's activities in the name of weight management have indirectly demonstrated television watching to be significant in children's activity—or lack of it. The greatest impact on children's overall activity level was produced by restricting sedentary activity, not by encouraging or even rewarding children for being more active. In fact, children deprived of television appeared to increase their activity level and energy expenditure, even when they turned to other sedentary pursuits.[16]

The association between television and weight is not an open-and-shut case. Some studies of children, television watching, and weight find no association. Moreover, it's not clear whether television watching is more likely to be related to weight gain than other relatively sedentary activities are, like reading, coloring, playing video games, and working on the computer.

Lacking such answers, what it comes down to is good parenting. Restricting television is good parenting. Discouraging television viewing for children younger than 2 years is good parenting.[17] Encouraging more interactive pursuits, such as talking, playing, singing, and reading together is good parenting. Encouraging more *creative* pursuits, such as reading, writing, and artwork, is good parenting.

Children who are glued to the tube are not doing their jobs of exploring their world. Other sedentary activities are better for children than television watching is. Rather than being mesmerized, as they are when they are watching television, children engaged in other activities, even sedentary ones, are actively involved with their world.

Remove the Television and Computer from Your Child's Room
Do not allow your child to have a television or computer in his bedroom. I realize this is an audacious statement, particularly when it comes to the computer. However, the American

Academy of Pediatrics backs me up.[17] The issue is supervision—and isolation. Children who have a television in their room watch more. You can't supervise what your child watches if the television is in his room. You can't sit down and watch with him or have him nearby while you work. Therein lies the problem with the computer.

The computer brings the whole world to your child's bedroom. That world may not be nice. Clio Bushland, my very important right-hand-woman, knows whereof she speaks on this issue. As part of her family therapy graduate training, Clio worked at Briarpatch, a crisis facility for teenagers. Clio tells stories of teenagers doing homework who accidentally log on to pornography sites that won't let them out. She worked with a girl who struck up an acquaintance on the Internet and was raped when she met the man who had represented himself as another teenager. She talks about the no-holds-barred social anarchy and brutality that is often a part of instant messaging. People can be horribly wounding via e-mail and may say things they wouldn't dream of saying face-to-face or even on the telephone.

How does it help to have the computer in the common family space? Clio points out a new Internet acronym: POS. It stands for Parent Over Shoulder. A child who happens onto a porn site will be all-too-aware of the possibility of his parents' walking into the room. He won't be as tempted to look around and instead will ask for help getting out. He will be less likely to be brutal and inflammatory in his messages to friends if he runs the risk of his parents' seeing those messages. His Internet mailbox will be potentially open for public view, and therefore he will be less inclined to set up intense Internet relationships. That is not to say that it is legitimate to read your child's e-mail. But you can certainly see what is coming in—especially frequently—and ask about it.

What does this have to do with weight? With television the connection is more clear: more television, less activity, higher risk of excess weight gain. With the computer the connection is a bit of a stretch. It has to do with good parenting to support *emotional* competence. A child closeted with a computer misses out on a lot of interaction with other people and therefore opportunities to learn social skills. The emotionally competent child has more resources, is therefore more likely to move his body, and is less likely to use food for emotional reasons.

Make Your Child Responsible for Dealing with His Own Boredom

Today's parents work hard, have difficulty finding time for their children, feel bad about it, and try to make it up to them by being overindulgent and by trying to entertain them. My parents and their age-mates worked hard, had little time for children, expected us to entertain ourselves, and didn't feel one bit apologetic about it. My parents had an easier time being parents. While I enjoyed the exceedingly rare times my parents played with me, I did not feel deprived. In fact, I enjoyed my freedom to do what I wanted.

Don't be your child's entertainment committee. In response to my recommendation to limit television to 1 or 2 hours a day, Adrianna, a young mother of my acquaintance, said, "Oh, Ellyn, get real! I couldn't possibly do that!" Adrianna's 5-year-old son, Jules, is a highly active and demanding child who gives Adrianna time to herself only when he is sitting in front of the tube.

Jules needs to learn to play by himself and give his mother a break. Of course, Adrianna is the one to deliver—and enforce—the expectation. Turning off the television need not—in fact, *must* not—mean that you will fill your child's time. In some ways, this is like maintaining the structure of meals and snacks. Certainly, you will take an interest, be companionable, and set aside regular times to play. However, once you have done that, it is up to your child to decide what he will do with the rest of his time. I see today's young parents wearing themselves out trying to entertain their children and keep them from ever being bored. Don't do that. Let your child be bored. If he gets bored enough, he will think up something creative and wonderful to do.

Your child does want to be with you, but that doesn't mean he has to have your undivided attention all of the time. Toddlers have a pattern of ranging out and coming back, showing you what they are up to, than going off and playing again.

In fact, studies show that toddlers check back in an average of seven times an hour, for an average contact time of 30 seconds to a minute. Admire whatever your toddler wants to show you, call it by name, demonstrate something new about it, and send him on his way.

Preschoolers are capable of independent play for more sustained periods of time, and if they have been allowed to have time to themselves they play elaborate pretend games with scripts for everyone. However, preschoolers still want to be where the grown-ups are. Keep your child's toys close to where you are working, take a moment to watch (but not interrupt) while he plays, and let him join in with your activities. Those are all ways of sharing enjoyable time with your child without your having to be an entertainment committee.

School-age children love playing with their parents, but they also spend most of their time playing with their friends. They need you to supervise, to take them places, and to occasionally provide them with tools and resources for play. They aren't quite as fond of *working* with their parents, but the activity is still there and so is the time spent together. School-age children can be a good help, and they feel good if they contribute to the family.

Take walks with your teenager. It's a good time to talk—if you don't try to get it to happen. Take bike rides, play Frisbee, rake the yard, wash the windows, clean out the garage. Don't be too ready to give your teenager rides or access to the car. If you think things through, he can probably manage many of the trips on his own.

A PROGRAM TO GIVE PHYSICALLY INCAPABLE CHILDREN A BOOST

The theme of this chapter has been normal growth and development with respect to physical activity. You have learned the importance of supporting your child's natural inclinations to move and his enjoyment in movement. To give you a more concrete picture of how important that is, I am going to tell you about a school physical education program for children whose growth and development were impaired to the point that they were inhibited in movement and took little joy from physical activity.

Stoughton, Wisconsin, seventh- and eighth-grade physical education teacher Bob Hanssen and school counselor Nancy Crassweller wanted to do something to give less physically capable children a chance. Often those children dislike physical education classes. They may be dismissed by other children, and they often act awkward and uncomfortable when they are in the physical education class, and many avoid the class whenever they can. At times, children dislike physical education class so much that they avoid school altogether—they make it a point to be sick or absent from school on physical education day.

Hanssen and Crassweller's sense of mission mirrored that of University of Wisconsin Sports Medicine and Pediatric Fitness Clinic physician Aaron Carrell, who had been looking for ways to help children with high BMI become more active. Underwritten by the University of Wisconsin Children's Hospital, a collaboration was formed to provide physical education classes and do clinical trials—Hanssen and Crassweller to provide the classes, Carrell to test children's fitness levels before and after the school term.

While children of all sizes and shapes can feel negative about physical activity, the grant defined the target audience: children with high BMI. Hanssen and Crassweller named their class Fit*4*Life and started looking for students identified by school health screening as having high BMI. (Incidentally, I do not like that screening. I think it holds children up to scrutiny in a setting where they are entitled to feel safe, and it singles them out for the scorn of their classmates.)

Hanssen and Crassweller were sensitive to the children's dilemmas. Despite getting funding for being a child overweight intervention, their primary goal for the children was *not* weight reduction. Instead, their goals were letting the children have a good time moving their bodies, experiencing their bodies as capable, and developing more-positive attitudes about activity and about themselves.

Both Hanssen and Crassweller are tuned in to the social and emotional challenges of middle school students. Initially they feared that the intervention would single out and further stigmatize that group of students and that the kids would avoid their special class like the plague. To make their class as accessible as possible, they were careful to find a setting that was out of sight and out of earshot of the other classes. The instructors started with the children right where they were, not making them feel they should be able to do more or be better. Then they made some accommodations. In Fit*4*Life, changing clothes for class, following the rules for games, and being skilled simply didn't matter.

The Pecking Order

What did matter was *effort*. Hanssen and Crassweller's purpose was to empower the kids to have fun and keep moving. Their expectation was that the children would participate. Although they both were so positive, the kids didn't make their work easy for them. Some children in their classes felt the need to establish a pecking order. Children who had always been at the bottom wanted to be on top, and at times they harassed others to get there. Hanssen and Crassweller had to deal with that negativity fast, before it undermined the class.

Crassweller's skill as a counselor proved essential in addressing this problem. Rather than getting after the children or making rules to snuff out the harassing, Crassweller took a compassionate approach. As a school counselor, she knew that combative, belligerent kids generally have something bugging them. They have strong negative feelings that they can't deal with or something going on in their lives that is bothering them. If they talk about it, they are less likely to act it out or take it out on other kids.

Crassweller has a knack for finding ways to help kids be comfortable talking with her. She tried having private sessions in her office, and they wouldn't talk. She tried having small "support group" discussions, and that didn't work either. One day she simply joined in the games, and that worked. The kids talked. Their confidences tended to be hit-and-run. Children would spend a few minutes playing near her, sharing their frustration with friends, schoolwork, or family. Then off they would go and somebody else would mosey over and talk. Crassweller was surprised at how quickly the kids got to the bottom of things in those brief chats—far more quickly than most ever did in her office.

Later in the semester, after they had gained some physical confidence, children were able to acknowledge how hard it had been at first to participate. One student had been particularly challenging to start with. As she biked with him later in the year, Crassweller commented to him that he had biked for the full 30 minutes and even made it up a hill. At first, he could bike only a couple of blocks. The student was quiet for a few seconds, then delivered a well-thought-out oration explaining himself. "Yes, at first I didn't like this class because I felt awkward and wasn't sure I could do the activities. But now that I find I can do it, I find it somewhat satisfying to move around."

Reluctant to Move

The kids had little confidence in their bodies and needed a lot of reassurance to participate in the class. Their anxiety *looked* like contrariness, and they made excuses: I can't walk, I can't run, I can't ride a bike. Some of the kids *didn't* know how to ride a bike, and they had to learn. Some of the kids came across as downright lazy and reluctant to move, but Hanssen saw through it. "They didn't have a clue about movement," he observed. "They couldn't fathom what their bodies were capable of."

Hanssen depended on the University of Wisconsin testing to reassure both himself and the kids that they were capable. The results from the exercise testing done by Carrell and his team indicated that the children were physically all right and that they weren't going to be hurt by the activity. The tests gave the children a real workout, they scored well, and they were told that during the testing. The testing helped them begin to discover that they *could* be physically capable.

For the children, learning they were capable was something they had to do with their *bodies*. They couldn't do it with their *heads*. The challenge was giving the children the experience of rewarding movement despite their reluctance. They were wary and firmly convinced that they *couldn't* be active. Hanssen and Crassweller didn't want to force them, because forcing would be shaming and would turn the kids off.

Instead, the instructors delivered realistic expectations.

They showed the children what they had to learn and let them rise to the occasion. Furthermore, they presumed the children would do well. Rather than accepting the children's assumption that they were somehow fragile or incapable, Hanssen and Crassweller expected them to be strong and able to hold their own. Hanssen encouraged them: "Come on, you can do it!" He didn't get excited when they got winded or tired, and he didn't buy into their attitude that they were somehow fragile or incapable. "It's all right," he would say. "Let's go!" "There were moments when they were drama kings and queens," observed Crassweller. "They had spectacular ways of saying, 'I can't do it. I can't *breathe*.'" She would remind them, "You are breathing hard, but I am, too. That's normal. You can do it!"

Keeping Kids Safe and Having Fun

The children gradually participated more fully as they came to trust that they weren't going to be shamed, criticized, or asked to perform in ways that they couldn't. Hanssen was careful to keep the activities doable, fun, and rewarding. He has a genius for making up and adapting games with the goal of keeping everyone moving, participating, and having a good time. He would stand on the sidelines and watch them play and ask himself, "How can we change that so everybody gets to play?"

The adaptation started with choosing sides. Sometimes Hanssen chose sides, and sometimes the kids did. However, he said he never let them choose down to the last person—the kids picked a couple and then he stepped in and divided up the rest so the teams could be evenly matched. As he put it, "There is nothing worse than being the last one picked!" They made up their own version of speedball, in which they could kick, carry, or throw the ball. Any form of getting the ball across a line drawn on the field was a touchdown. Hanssen laughed that except for trying to get the ball through the hoop, their basketball game only vaguely resembled the regular game. The kids didn't have to dribble. They could run with the ball, and if they got tagged, they had to give the ball up. But if they dribbled, they couldn't be tagged. There were no "out of bounds"—they retrieved the ball and kept on playing. Scores were low, and nobody worried about it. The object was to keep moving. When somebody stood around, Hanssen encouraged, "Come on! We are all playing."

The Program Worked

The Fit*4*Life program was wonderfully successful. The kids asked for the class to be repeated, and now the class is three days a week. As far as Hanssen and Crassweller are concerned, the important results are in the children's *attitudes*—attitudes about themselves, about physical activity, and about their bodies. The kids have a good time moving their bodies, and they learn that they *can* have a good time being active. They learn that they are physically capable, and they take pride in their achievements. They use their bodies in ways they were designed for and in the process increase their physical self-esteem. Some of the kids who have participated in the program have been so empowered that they have joined regular intramural and interscholastic sports teams.

Hanssen and Crassweller have lots of stories of individual children and their positive changes, and they both felt great about what their kids accomplished. In short, the kids loved it, and they came out feeling more confident of their bodies and their abilities to move.

Parents were pleased about the class as well. One mother observed that her son looked forward to physical education day rather than trying to get out of going to school. Another observed that her daughter's moods had improved and that she seemed generally much happier.

What about the medical results? The children's physical capabilities improved a *lot*. Endurance on exercise testing, a measure of cardiovascular fitness, increased. Their body composition changed—they developed more muscle. Insulin sensitivity improved, decreasing the risk for diabetes. What about body weight? On the average, there was little change. Weight loss wasn't one of the goals of intervention, which was probably essential to the program's success. It didn't have the agenda—and the stigma—that goes along with defining children as flawed and trying to correct those "flaws."

Why the Negativity?

For the moment, I will leave off telling the story of the Fit*4*Life class to contemplate some of the issues raised by the children. As I said at the beginning of this chapter, children are born loving their bodies, curious about them, inclined to move, and driven to be as physically competent as they can possibly be. What had happened over the years to the children who ended up in Crassweller and Hanssen's class? Why had they so thoroughly lost their physical self-esteem—their positive feelings about their bodies and their inclination to move? What do we as adults do to deprive children of positive physical self-esteem?

The standard answer, that their overweight was the culprit, is not sufficient. Many large children feel good about their bodies and enjoy moving them. Blaming the children's body size leads to the inevitable conclusion that children have to become slim in order to feel good about activity. That was clearly not the case with the children in the Fit*4*Life class.

Given our discussion earlier in this chapter on growth and development with activity, I have more questions than answers. From the time they were small, to what extent had the children missed out on opportunities to move and to like and accept their bodies? Were their parents able to tolerate commotion, or did they feel the need to keep their children quiet? Were parents able to let children take reasonable physical risks, or did they see the children as fragile? Parents have their own dilemmas and pressures in their lives that influence their ability to be supportive of children's activity.

Did the children have safe places to play or other children who could teach them to play? Were these children so uncomfortable with other children that they learned to avoid rather than learning to hold their own and work things out with others? Did they live in safe neighborhoods so they could get outside, or did they have to stay indoors because the area was dangerous? Rather than playing outside or being expected to pursue more creative pursuits, were the children allowed to watch a lot of television? Communities may or may not be able to provide environments that allow children to be active.

Were parents and other important people in the children's

lives accepting of their weight, or critical? In our era of thoroughgoing concern about child overweight, to what extent are we teaching large children that they are flawed and thereby depriving them of physical self-esteem?

Given these and other factors, to what extent did the Fit*4*Life students have delays in their normal growth and development as it related to activity? With respect to their attitudes and behaviors around movement, they acted like younger children. Young school-age children most enjoy cooperative games they make up themselves, they are invested in keeping the games going, and they make up the rules as they go along. Once they have those opportunities, children grow and develop further with respect to activity. In late school-age or early adolescence, children become interested enough and proficient enough to learn the rules and develop skills for organized sports.

Hanssen picked up on his students' stage of development, not their *age,* and played with them in ways that they found rewarding.

Children Can Regain Physical Self-Esteem

For whatever reason, the children in that first Fit*4*Life class had lost their positive feelings about their bodies and their inclination to move. Hanssen and Crassweller helped them to get those positive feelings back. As far as Hanssen and Crassweller were concerned, that was the major success of the program. For their Fit*4*Life children, physical activity became fun and rewarding, rather that something to be feared and avoided.

Hanssen tells a story about biking and one of their "drama queens." We'll call her Trudy. Toward the end of the school year, Hanssen decided the kids could handle the major grades and challenging curves at the local bike track. The kids were enthusiastic about attacking the hills. Each one in turn biked up the steep hill and disappeared into the course. The class time went fast, and soon it was time to go. There was one boy left on the track. "Come on, let's go!" Hanssen encouraged.

"Trudy's still up here," the boy responded. Hanssen climbed up, and there in a dip in the track lay Trudy, flat on her back, spread-eagled, covered with dirt. Beside her lay her bike, the front wheel bent in two.

"Trudy, what happened?" he asked her.

"Well, I was trying for some major air," Trudy responded. "I went over the jump, but I went off crooked. So I turned the front wheel to straighten out. And you know, it doesn't turn when you're in the air, does it? So I came down crooked." Hanssen picked up her bike, and together they trudged back to the truck. Trudy *may* have limped a bit, but it was a limp she was proud of.

"I was a football coach for 20 years," observed Hanssen, "and I enjoyed working with some very talented athletes. But working with these kids and their parents gave me more good feelings than I ever expected."

One of their boys said it all. "This is the first time I have ever been able to feel like a normal kid and do all the things the other kids can do."

NOTES

1. Leopold, "Functional Fitness."
2. Wei et al., "Low Cardiorespiratory Fitness and Mortality."
3. Rose and Mayer, "Activity, Calorie Intake, Fat Storage."
4. Anderson et al., "Temperament, Nonresting Energy Expenditure, Body Composition."
5. Moore et al., "Early Physical Activity."
6. Rocandio, Ansotegui, and Arroyo, "Comparison of Dietary Intake."
7. Davison and Lipps Birch, "Weight Status."
8. Faith et al., "Weight Criticism During Physical Activity."
9. Mayer, Roy, and Mitra, "Caloric Intake, Body Weight, and Physical Work."
10. Maccoby, *Social Development.*
11. "More U.S. Children Being Diagnosed with Youthful Tendency Disorder," *Onion* 36, no. 34 (2000).
12. Anderson et al., "Physical Activity and Television Watching."
13. Kaur et al., "Duration of Television Watching."
14. Saelens et al., "Home Environment Influences on Children's Television Watching."
15. Klesges, Shelton, and Klesges, "Effects of Television on Metabolic Rate."
16. Epstein et al., "Effects of Decreasing Sedentary Behaviors."
17. Committee on Public Education, "Children, Adolescents, and Television."

CHILDREN, WEIGHT, AND SELF-ESTEEM

- Your tasks are to feed well, parent well, provide opportunities to be active, and accept your child's natural size and shape.

- Help your child feel good about herself and be emotionally and physically healthy at any size that she turns out to be.

- Do good parenting: Children given both love and limits are likely to become successful, happy with themselves, and generous with others.

- In order for you to be accepting of your child, you may have to deal with your inner bigot.

- Children whose parents are preoccupied with keeping them thin do not appreciate their parents' efforts, nor do they feel good about themselves.

- As with any other characteristic that makes your child different, accept her feelings and support her in solving her own problems.

- Deal with your own feelings, and help your child to cope with hers. If you feel apologetic or treat your child as fragile, she will grow up to blame you and be a whiner.

- Children feel bad about themselves if we feel sorry for them and expect them to feel bad about themselves.

- Acceptance of one's own body—size and shape, capabilities, opportunities—is a task that we all have to do—ideally by the end of the teen years.

CHAPTER 9

TEACH YOUR CHILD:
BE ALL
YOU CAN BE

By now you are clear about your responsibilities and limits in helping as much as you can to let your child get the body that is right for her. If you have made it this far in *Your Child's Weight*, you know that your tasks are to feed well, parent well, provide opportunities to be active, and accept your child's natural size and shape. Conversely, you have come to terms with the fact that it is destructive to restrain your child's food intake, coerce her to be active, or try to get her to lose weight by *any* means.

Deciding to stow your agenda about your child's size and shape is a great gift to both of you. It opens the door to your parenting her well and feeling good about her. You are entitled to love your child just the way she is—short or tall, fat or thin, freckles, warts, and all. Ironically, if you can be *truly* accepting of your child's size and shape, and help her to be accepting as well, it is likely that she will grow up to be thinner than she otherwise would be. Large body size is a risk factor for dieting, which increases the likelihood that your child's weight will accelerate—it will increase at a faster rate than is normal for her.

Now we can turn our attention to accepting and supporting your child of *any* size or shape, raising her to feel good about herself, and supporting her in loving her body. Even if your child is slim or of average weight, this chapter applies to you and to your child. Our truly demented, thinness-preoccupied and fat-phobic culture puts pressure on everyone. For even the thinnest person, the specter of fatness—for self or child—lurks, creating tension and crazed behavior. To free yourself and your child, be prepared to love her and do a good job of parenting, no matter what.

Asking you to accept your child of size—or potential size— is considerable and may be extraordinarily difficult. However, as with all issues related to our children, it is your opportunity to grow. First you have to deal with yourself and get rid of your own prejudice. To do that you will have to swim against the tide of naïveté, truisms, and bigotry that say that if a child is at all fat there is something wrong with her—and probably with her parents—and that her parents should do whatever is neces- sary to correct that defect. While you *are* responsible for doing a good job of parenting and providing your child with the struc- ture and support she needs, getting caught in chasing an agenda will be destructive and painful for all of you.

You have to hold steady with your child when she comes in feeling bad that the other children have teased her about her size. Empathize, help her to figure out what to do, and send her right back out there to take her licks the same as any other child. You have to advocate for her and other children of size in the school system, identify hurtful and discriminatory behavior, and insist on more evenhanded attitudes and treatment. To do all that, you have to look at the overall culture and, like the boy in "The Emperor's New Clothes," you have to say, "It's all a lie!" You have to be able to see that the common intelligence about size and shape in general and child obesity in particular isn't intelligent at all. Having achieved that, you can struggle through to your *own* wisdom, hang in there with it, and prepare for the long haul in maintaining a moderate stand.

Don't get caught up in the weight-loss hysteria. You may—

in fact you *will*—be pressured to try to control or modify your child's weight. Don't. You can't tell until she is an adult how her body will turn out. Trying to make your child slim is likely to make her fatter. It will condemn her to a lifelong struggle with eating and weight and make her subject to periods of overeating and weight gain throughout her life.

Rather than trying to change your child's natural body, it's much better to put your efforts into parenting her well and supporting her in feeling good about herself. Help her develop in ways that really matter: good character, common sense, effective ways of responding to feelings, problem-solving skills, and the ability to get along with others. Children who are relatively fat, like children with other characteristics that make them distinct, need better-than-average life skills in order to succeed.

As a parent, you may be feeling, as one of my children observed when he was struggling to find his way through high school social quagmires, "I am really getting sick of these growth experiences." I don't blame you.

ACCEPT YOUR LARGE CHILD

Children can cope with their fatness if their parents can. Any of us would spare our child pain if we could. The bald-faced truth, however, is that life is hard. Everybody's got something, and everybody has to cope. About all we can do for our children is love and support them, teach them to manage as well as they can, and portion out the world in doses they can handle.

As important as it is, it's not easy to be accepting. Our culture is lipophobic—it is permeated with the extreme and irrational fear of fatness. In the face of that lipophobia, even the most ordinary and modest amounts of fatness are considered excessive. As many of my patients who have struggled with weight their whole lives have told me, "I look back at my photographs as a child, and I wasn't fat. I wasn't thin, but there wasn't anything the matter with me. I just wish I could be that slim again." Their parents overreacted, restricted their food intake, and in the end made them fatter than nature intended them to be.

These patients' parents weren't bad or awful. They did

what they did because they wanted to help their children—to keep them from being fat and having to deal with what they considered to be a dreadful fate. Often the parents restricted on the advice of health professionals, which made the inclination to limit their children's intake all the more compelling. For these patients' parents, as for society as a whole, fatness is viewed as a profoundly negative condition. It is perceived as being so bad, in fact, that even the most negative cures are preferable.

Consider the extraordinarily energy-consuming and life-limiting implications of becoming a zealot in the pursuit of thinness. Consider *dying*, as is evidenced by the number of overweight people who are willing to risk life-threatening surgery in order to lose weight. Consider how early people learn these attitudes: Friendship-preference studies find that children choose pictures of children of size *last* among children having other characteristics that make them distinct—physical limitations, race, handicapping conditions. Indeed, attitudinally and socially, having a relatively high level of body fat is potentially a handicapping condition. However, unlike other handicapping conditions, it is blamed on the sufferer.

For anyone who has ever loved—or been—a large child, such statements are like a dagger to the heart. The father of one of my young patients cried when he considered the prospect of his daughter's growing up fat. He had been a child of size himself and had been on the receiving end of a lot of teasing. "I love her so much," he said. "I would just like to spare her if I could." That father was missing the fact that his daughter had better parents than he did. His parents hadn't given him much help or guidance. They let him blunder along on his own and then criticized him severely when he made mistakes. They harped on what he *was* and *did* in general and his weight in particular. As a consequence, he not only felt bad about his *weight*, he felt bad about *himself*.

There are worse things than being a child of size. It is worse to be regarded as defective by your parents and have all issues in parenting focused around weight reduction. Before I figured out how to set up my office consultations more humanely, more than one set of parents furiously swept their humiliated child into my office and demanded, "Get my child thin! I will not have a fat child!" It is worse to be sent to fat camp with the express purpose of being slimmed down to be more acceptable to parents and peers. It is worse to be publicly deprived of treats that other children are freely allowed. It is worse to worry about getting enough to eat, to feel compelled to sneak and hide food, and to be shamed and criticized for wanting it. It is worse to be paraded for all the world to see on the *Maury Povich Show,* held up to disgrace and ridicule like a member of some new-age electronic freak show.

Let Yourself Nurture

Our lipophobic culture is hard on parents as well. It expects parents to deprive their children. Think of it—how unnatural can you get? The parent's job is to *nurture.* It's what we *do.* The child's job is to *be* nurtured. It's what *they* do. It's not natural for parents to make children go hungry. No parent wants to give up being a loving and trusting provider and instead become a police officer.

I have serialized the story of Leane. In chapter 2, "Feed and Parent in the Best Way," I told you the early part of her story. From birth, Leane's parents hadn't let her eat as much as she wanted because she was big and they feared that letting her eat would make her fat throughout her life. Rather than going by her signals of hunger and fullness and getting on the same wavelength with her in their feeding, they struggled. For *years* they struggled—managing, avoiding, policing the kitchen, and enduring whining and tantrums about food. They weren't bad parents—they were doing what they thought was right for her. In chapter 5, "Optimize Feeding: Birth Through Preschool," I used Leane's story to illustrate how seriously food restriction distorts normal growth and development. Here I will tell you the part of the story that has to do with loving and accepting a child.

When Leane was 6 years old, I helped her parents apply Ellyn Satter's Division of Responsibility in Feeding. Leane's eating changed dramatically. For a few scary and difficult weeks, Leane ate a *lot* at every meal and snack. Then she reverted to eating like a normal six-year-old: She ate a lot sometimes, not so much others, a square meal one time, a sketchy one another. Between times, she generally forgot about eating. Feeding became *so* much easier, and Leane's parents were grateful for that. What they were *stunned* about, however, was the change in their relationship with Leane and in the way they *felt* about her. For them, feeding had to get better before they realized the extent to which their weight concerns and struggles about food had tainted their whole relationship.

Leane's mother cried as she told me about how profoundly different things were for all of them. "Finally, after all of this time, I understand what you mean by the feeding relationship. I read your books almost two years ago, and you just can't comprehend what that means. 'Oh sure, my relationship is positive'—you think that way. Now for the first time, mealtime isn't stressful and is actually enjoyable. Each time, I'm conscious of practicing and trying to enforce the rules, but it's not that big burden hanging over me—that dread. When we started, I couldn't even look at her at the table. Now, easing up on the restriction—not having that big responsibility—has freed me up to just enjoy her—to look at her and appreciate her in a different way and not have food be the end-all. I can give her the freedom to be her own little person. She has so many great qualities, and I have just ignored them. What a waste! If she grows up to be fat—if that is her fate—then so be it. She will grow up knowing we love her and treasure her for being just who she is."

Like Leane's parents, you may find it difficult to feed and parent well and let your child weigh what she will. It's not easy to give up the dream of having a slim child, especially if you have been a child of size yourself. What is, after all, the *right* choice? As with other issues in parenting, in answering that question, I find it most instructive to look, not to the *method*, not to the *logic* of what is best or right, but to the way the children themselves react and respond to what we do.

Consider Your Child's Point of View
Children whose parents have dedicated their efforts to keeping

them thin do not appreciate those efforts, nor do they feel good about themselves. Even when parents' efforts have produced normal-weight or slim children, those children feel hurt, bullied, and ashamed. Jacolyn, a 15-year-old girl whose father marched her into my office saying "Get my child thin!" did not feel he was acting in her best interest. Jacolyn felt rejected. She picked up on his anger and disdain and responded by being sullen, oppositional, and resistant in *all* ways. Despite being very bright, she barely survived academically. She went out of her way to look poorly groomed. She hung out with kids who expected little of themselves and little of her. After all, how much did she have to offer?

Mary Ray Worley, now an adult carrying over 300 pounds on her 5-foot 1-inch frame, does not appreciate her parents' efforts to keep her thin. In fact, Mary feels strongly that all those years of restriction and struggles around eating made her heavier than she otherwise would be—*lots* heavier. Mary says, "Not only were all my problems attributed to my weight, but all of my family's problems seemed to have been attributed to my weight as well. I was most definitely the family lightening rod! My mother always talked—proudly—about restricting my food intake even when I was a baby." Mary first went to Weight Watchers at age 12 at the insistence of her parents and continued battling with her weight until she was an adult.

When she was in her thirties, Mary finally said *enough.* Being so focused on weight loss was giving her tunnel vision and taking away her energy and enthusiasm for *life.* She decided to define the problem in a way it could be solved. She let me help her become competent with her eating. She found a size-accepting fitness club where they helped her learn to manage her size and move her body in challenging and rewarding ways. She joined a support group to help her feel better about her body and about herself. Now she is happier than she has ever been before.

"Tell them to not not offer the same food to their fat children as their slim ones," recommended Ashley, an average-weight but bulimic 19-year-old who had spent years on the receiving end of her parents' food restriction. As my reviewers reminded me, Ashley's sentence structure was not the greatest. However, her meaning was clear. Her parents had offered cookies and chips to her brothers and sister, but not to her. As she recalled, "I felt hurt that they wouldn't give it to me and ashamed of myself for wanting it. It would have been so much better for them to offer it to me and let me turn it down." Truth be told, she *still* felt hurt.

I thought of that piece of advice when I read a recent newspaper article about child obesity intervention in schools. Some schools were maintaining a "do not sell candy" list for overweight children. Think of the shame that a child on such as list experiences! She is labeled a glutton for all the school to see and deprived of what the other children are freely offered. What in the world were schools doing selling candy to children in the first place? Actually, making candy freely available to *any* children is a disservice to them. It spoils their meals, rots their teeth, and lets them fill up on less nutritionally desirable food. Moreover, selling candy to children to make money for school events or programs exploits children.

Be Prepared for the Long Haul
Leane's parents found a resolution for the immediate problem with her eating and weight. Leane was getting too fat, but it wasn't because they were overfeeding her. It was because they were *underfeeding* her. They learned to feed her well, and she learned to eat well. However, she remained heavy, and despite their best efforts, she may still grow up to be relatively fat. It is important for them to remember that applying those best efforts will help her to be *no fatter* than nature intended her to be. More important, it will help her to feel good about herself and to be emotionally and physically healthy at any size that she turns out to be. Now their dilemma is the same as the one faced by other parents of constitutionally large children—they have to continue to hold steady with feeding and parenting through all the years to come.

In case you have started your reading of *Your Child's Weight* with this chapter, let me hasten to reassure you that I did not encourage them—and I am not encouraging you—to do laissez-faire parenting. I do not recommend throwing open the refrigerator door or giving unlimited access to the television remote control. In fact, I recommend that you spend years and years getting meals and snacks on the table, saying *no* to grazing and sipping between times, supervising screen time, hanging around playgrounds, and shuffling along on walks. In short, I recommend you do the kind of good parenting that you would do with any child, not just the one who has a potential weight problem. That is *definitely* not easy, but it is possible, and you can continue it for the long haul. Trying to restrict your child's food intake, force activity, and slim her down can be maintained only for a short time.

However, if it takes fear of excess weight to get you going, who am I to complain? Parenting in the name of weight management is not necessarily bad, as long as you don't judge your success on slimming your child down. The success is in the process itself—your doing a good job of parenting and your child's feeling loved and supported. Weight management gets people in gear. A lot of adults begin to make reliable meals, take regular walks, and take good care of themselves in general only when they go on a weight-reduction regimen. That's not all bad.

The problem comes in when you veer from one extreme to the other in taking care of yourself. Many people diet and are oh-so-careful to eat well and be active. When they stop, they go to the other extreme of being inconsistent and inattentive about eating and avoiding activity. If that is your pattern, like my patients, you will benefit from finding the gray area—the middle ground between the two extremes. In the middle ground, you can feed yourself well and find a way of being active that is rewarding and sustainable.

If it is just you, it is your business whether you blow hot and cold on taking care of yourself. Such a pattern will make you fatter in the long run, but so be it. For your child, however, you have to do better. Your child depends on you to take care of her. Children thrive on consistency and being provided for, day in and day out. They do poorly with inconsistency.

DO A GOOD JOB OF PARENTING
Today's parents do not know how important they are to their

children. At every step, the way you parent is the most important consideration of all. Your child will have to learn to cope
with whatever nature and her environment throw at her. Her
success or failure in coping to a large extent depends on your
parenting. That doesn't mean you can spare your child pain. It
means you can help her learn to handle life's challenges and
rise above them.

Your child feels good about herself and becomes competent,
not because you tell her over and over again that she is wonderful and praise her for every little thing that she does, but because
you do a good job of parenting. Children who grow up with parents who give them both love and limits are most likely to
become successful, happy with themselves, and generous with
others. Children whose parents are overly strict are likely to be
obedient but unhappy or angry and rebellious. Those whose parents are overly lenient and have provided insufficient guidelines
are likely to lack self-control, have unrealistic expectations of
themselves and others, and feel bad as a result.[1,2] As discussed in
chapter 5, "Optimize Feeding: Birth Through Preschool," and
chapter 7,"Optimize Feeding: Your Adolescent," the three types
of parenting are *authoritative, authoritarian,* and *permissive.*
Feeding follows the same three patterns. Authoritarian parents
say "Eat it or else." Permissive parents say "What would you
like? When would you like it?" Authoritative parents observe the
division of responsibility in feeding.

Authoritative parenting is not easy. It takes more time,
energy, judgment, and nerve than either being dictatorial or
being permissive. Authoritative parenting requires leadership.
To parent authoritatively, you have to make judgments about
appropriate behavior, set limits, take a stand, tolerate your
child's anger, and manage her aggression. Authoritative feeding
takes more knowledge, understanding, and energy than does
simply laying down the law about eating on the one hand or
letting children graze for food on the other.

Authoritative parenting also takes more nerve. At a certain
point, you have done your job of feeding—or parenting—and
have to trust your child to take herself the rest of the way.

As I have said more than once before, children grow best—

most consistently—when they have been parented authoritatively. Children are excellent regulators. They are able to tune in on their internal cues of hunger, appetite, and satisfaction and eat the amount they need to grow the way nature intended. However, in order to do that, children depend on adults to provide structure and support. To do a good job with food regulation, children need the structure and reassurance of regular meals and snacks, they need their grown-ups to make the decisions about food that will be available at those times, and they need people they trust sharing those meals with them. Children whose emotional needs are not met—who are chronically frightened, upset, angry, anxious, or lonely—have difficulty tuning in on how hungry or how full they really are. They may lose interest in eating, or they may eat too much in order to try to feel better inside or grow up fast.

Maintain a Positive and Accepting Attitude
Your attitude toward your child is absolutely critical and can make an enormous difference in the way she feels about herself throughout life. In her book *Eating Disorders: Obesity, Anorexia Nervosa, and the Person Within*, child psychiatrist Hilde Bruch reflected on her decades of work with patients, including people of size. She observed that she had become acquainted with two different types of people who identified themselves as being obese. First, there were those who felt good about themselves. They were busy and involved with their lives; they had families, lovers, friends, and rewarding jobs and generally saw their weight as only one of many characteristics. They sought Bruch's help with the same run-of-the-mill life issues as any other psychotherapy patient. In contrast, the other group of people, who were no fatter than the first, saw their fatness as being the be-all and end-all about them. Fatness was their presenting problem, and they were absolutely convinced that until they could get thinner they quite simply could not get any better. They could not find a mate, have a family, have friends, or succeed in life.

Bruch observed that the difference between the two groups of people was the attitude of the parents. In the first group, the healthy ones, parents did not make a big issue of the child's weight. Certainly, they recognized that the child was relatively fat and may have even made modest efforts to change it. However, they let go of the efforts when they found them ineffective or counterproductive. Fundamentally, they valued their child as a whole person and saw their child's size and shape as being only one of many characteristics. They laid out their mastery expectations just as they would for any other child and presumed their child would do well.

The attitude of the other group of parents was that the child simply could not do, be, or become worthwhile until she was thinner. Their only mastery expectation was that the child lose weight. And Bruch observed with considerable chagrin that "the greater the number of helpers, the worse the outcome for the individuals in terms of their self-esteem and ability to be successful in life."

To be like the first group of parents, you may have to deal with your inner bigot. In case you haven't guessed, that's the part of you that really *does* look down on people of size. A very lean athletic photographer stumbled across his inner bigot as he listened to my comments to a reporter about children's variations in size and shape. As he took his photos, he confessed, "I know you are right. But my 12-year-old daughter is chubby, and it is *very* difficult for me to accept it." Take heart—admitting your feelings is half the battle. We all recognize feelings we wish we didn't have. I tell my patients that once negative feelings are acknowledged, like radioactive substances, they have a half-life. Over time they decay and become less toxic. Unacknowledged feelings, however, stick around forever and cause you no end of trouble when you are trying to behave yourself.

Be Honest with Your Child About Her Size and Shape
Five-year-old Logan came home from school with the dreaded question. "Am I fat?" he asked his mother. Logan was big—his BMI was at about the 97th percentile, and he had a double chin and a roll of fat around his middle. But he was growing consistently, and his parents were doing an excellent job ensuring that

that continued to be the case.* They had regular meals and scheduled sit-down snacks. They kept a firm hand on the television remote control and regularly gave Logan opportunities to run and play. Logan, in fact, was an active child and could keep up with the other children in vigorous play. "You would think he would run some of that off," said his parents wistfully.

Despite Logan's electrifying inquiry, his mother kept her cool—to a point. "Why do you ask?" she responded. "We were weighed today in school, and they said my BMI was too high," he said. "And the other kids teased me—they said I was fat." At first, Logan's mother was just *mad.* How could they do that to him? She made a mental note to go to the school and have a few well-chosen words with the principal. But first things first—she had a question to answer. She got a grip as much as she could on her own upset and did the best she could to be kind and supportive. "Well, no, you aren't too fat," she said. "You are just stocky. You have always been that way." It wasn't perfect, but it was a good first try. To give her full credit, she avoided saying "Well, we'll just get you thin, and then they won't say that." That would have been hurtful and ridiculous. Hurtful because essentially she would have been saying "You *are* fat, and that is bad. You are not all right the way you are." Ridiculous because there was no way she could deliver on an intention to "get you thin," and trying would only have caused them all a world of hurt.

What would have been a better answer? Try this: "Why yes, you are sort of fat. Why do they tease you about that?" There is no mild or harmless term that will get you around this question. *Chubby* is a word that children know full well to mean "fat." *Stocky, chunky, solid,* or even *buff* are words often used by parents and other sympathetic adults to describe the relatively fat child. Those words are appropriate only when used to describe a physically dense child with a lot of muscle mass and bone. For a child who is heavy but not fat, the answer would be, "You are heavier than other children, but you are not fat.

---

* Logan had about a 60 percent chance of slimming down, but his parents weren't counting on it. He also had a 40 percent chance of staying right where he was with respect to his size and shape.

You have a lot of muscle and bone."

When you climb down from your alarm at the possibility of answering a child "Well, yes, you are fat," consider the issues. Logan was looking for information and help. In giving information, his mother was able to neutralize a message that is often used in a derogatory way. He wasn't expecting his mother to make a value judgment or to protect him from the slings and arrows of the playground. He just wanted to know. How would it have been different if he had asked, "Do I have freckles?" She could easily have said, "Well, yes, you do. Why do you ask?" For that, she wouldn't feel responsible. For weight, she would. You know how she feels.

But if you, like Logan's mother, are doing all you *responsibly* and *realistically* can to help your child maintain the body that is right for her, then you need to settle down. Stow your guilt and get on with parenting. Guilt simply gets in the way. You don't have the child you thought you would have or perhaps hoped to have. Your feelings are *your* problem, not your child's. Deal with them, and help your child to cope with hers. If you feel apologetic or treat your child as fragile, she will grow up to blame you and be a whiner.

Maintain Your Mastery Expectations

You can help your child of size by being honest and accepting about her body. As with any other child with any other characteristic that makes her different, accept her feelings and support her in solving her own problems. Help her find physical activities at which she can be successful. Recognize her capabilities. Be firm and fair, and follow through with parenting. But don't feel sorry for her or protect her. I realize we are talking about your own sweet child, but if you feel sorry for her, she will learn to work it for attention or to get around you.

Children of size can be as physically and emotionally tough and capable of holding their own with their peers as other children. When you ask your child "Why do they tease you about that?" you can find out what it means to *her*. It is a *real* question. You know the answer from *your* point of view, but children look at things differently. Your child might say, "Because everybody teases everybody" or "Because that's all they can think of to tease me about" or "Because I tease them."

That would give you the opportunity to ask, "How do you feel when they tease you?" She might feel bad, or she might like the attention, or she might say she doesn't feel one way or the other about it. If she doesn't like it, you might ask, "What do the other children do when they get teased?" Keep asking for examples until she comes up with one that is empowering for her. More than likely, that will be the end of the conversation, if you even make it that far. Children have a way of telling us about the most alarming things, getting us all worked up, then losing interest in the discussion before we have figured out a resolution. Take heart. Wherever the conversation stops, your child will have gotten what she needs—to know that you back her up. It is trusting and affirming to say, "I know you can handle this." Certainly, schools are responsible for managing bullying and hazing. Schools must take a stand that physical violence is *not* allowed. Schools must have clear nondiscrimination policies about all characteristics that put children outside the norm. However, no school can protect a child from teasing.

Children tease. If they can't target physical characteristics, they taunt with names, clothing, schoolwork—the list goes on. My well-liked, average-sized son Lucas's friends cheerfully taunted him by calling him "Lucas the pukas." Like children who are successful in dealing with teasing, he blew it off. Some children give a sassy retort. Or both. One little girl responded to the taunt "You are so *big!*" by saying "and *beautiful!*"

Another child was the target of the school bully who threatened, "I have a brown belt in Karate, and I am going to hit you in your big fat stomach!" She looked him right in the eye and said, "Oh, yeah! Well, I would like to see you try it." Like all bullies everywhere, he sidled off to find a different victim. I am not sure I recommend the threat of mayhem as a way to solve playground problems, but children have surprising solutions that work for them.

Deal with Social Attitudes
While your child of size can learn to deal with other children,

she does need you to run interference with other adults. Adults tend to feel sorry for children of size—or critical of them and of their parents—and are convinced that those children have to get thinner to be better. We are dealing with the Pygmalion effect. What is that? The Pygmalion effect is when something that is initially false is made to be true because of one's expectations. We have a faulty vision of a child, and the child conforms to that vision. Perfectly acceptable children learn to feel bad about themselves if we feel sorry for them and expect them to feel bad about themselves. Children do better in school when their teachers have been led to believe that they are smart and talented, whether or not they really are. Children do worse when we expect them to *have* or *be* trouble. With respect to weight issues, we have a societal Pygmalion effect. Our whole society teaches children of size that they *should* feel bad about themselves for being big and that they can *feel* and *be* better only when they are thinner. And they believe that and act as if they are inferior.

Consider quality-of-life research, which is prominent right now in medical circles. Essentially the studies say that people of size have a lower quality of life. A paper-and-pencil test measures a person's *perception* of his or her physical functioning, role limitations owing to physical problems, role limitations resulting from emotional problems, vitality, bodily pain, social functioning, mental health, and general health perceptions. Adults and adolescents with what is generally defined as high BMI frequently score low on their perceptions of quality of life.[3,4]

Generally, the gist of the medical research is "ain't it awful?" Here is still another way that people of size suffer because of their size, and why don't they slim down so they don't have to suffer? To paraphrase Susan Wooley, University of Cincinnati professor and long-time size-acceptance pioneer, if suffering could slim us down, we wouldn't have any fat people. Losing weight is not the answer. Stepping outside the current logic *is*.

Unless she is taught to do so, it does not follow that a relatively large or fat child will grow up to have a lower level of physical functioning and overall health, more physical or emotional problems, less vitality, more bodily pain, greater limitations in social functioning, or poorer mental health than a child of average weight. If she does, it is nothing more or less than the Pygmalion effect. Our expectations did it to her.

SUPPORT YOUR CHILD'S PHYSICAL SELF-ESTEEM
Any child can—and is entitled to—feel good about her body. Any child can see herself as strong, capable, durable, and even beautiful—if she thinks about it at all. Acceptance of one's own body—size and shape, capabilities, opportunities—is a task that begins at birth, accelerates during the school years, and is ideally accomplished in the late teen years. Physical self-acceptance is based on a clear perception of reality—seeing one's own body as it really is—beauty spots, warts, and all. In our culture, people go to their *graves* with that task undone.

You may be more accustomed to hearing about *body image,* which seems to mean feelings and attitudes about one's own body. I prefer the term *physical self-esteem* because it is more descriptive. In our culture, physical self-esteem is most often an aesthetic consideration—how do we look? Are we beautiful, toned, and sexy—or not? Less frequently we think of physical self-esteem in the *functional* sense. Do we have a strong, durable, flexible, or resilient body? Does it get us where we want to go?

Our cultural attitudes and behaviors make achieving physical self-esteem a challenging task. Aesthetic standards are impossibly narrow. Size and shape are seen as being within a person's control, and practically nobody is pleased about how they look. Sports stars are genetically at the extremes of size, shape, strength, and coordination, and they use drugs to build themselves up further. Super models and stars rue the microscopic rolls of fat around their midsections and subject themselves to grueling workouts and plastic surgery to get some parts trimmed down and others plumped up. Advertising and magazine publishers routinely airbrush their photos or mix and match body parts to bring their already beautiful subjects to an impossible ideal.

You will be pleased to know that there are a few who buck the tide. For instance, Jamie Lee Curtis will pose for the glamour shots only if the true Jamie gets equal time. For her, the issue has to do with overcoming the feelings of inadequacy she developed growing up with her famous parents, Tony Curtis and Janet Leigh. Even the beautiful and famous Curtis has struggled to achieve peace with her flaws. Not too long ago, actress Kate Winslet made a big fuss at *Gentlemen's Quarterly* magazine for airbrushing her cover photo to make her look thinner. The digital changes were made without her permission. Winslet has repeatedly taken stands defending the appearance of fuller-figured women. Emme, the full-figured fashion model, has made size acceptance a mission. "We live in a society that is based upon the attainment of unrealistic beauty. I want women to know their self-esteem is not contingent upon their dress size," says Emme.

Physical Self-Acceptance Is a Mastery Expectation

Your child's task is to develop physical self-esteem. If all goes well, as she grows she will come to terms with what nature has provided her, be realistic and accepting of her size and shape, feel good about her body, and find activities that are a good fit for her capabilities and interests. Your task as parent is to expect and support her development of physical self-esteem. It's a mastery expectation, the same as the eating competence mastery expectations discussed earlier in this book. The mastery expectation says or demonstrates through behavior, "Here is what you need to do. I know you can do this."

Your task is to maintain your mastery expectations with respect to physical self-acceptance just as you do with every other issue. Consider the mother who said to her appalled daughter, "No, you are not getting fat. You are getting hips, and you are getting breasts. You are developing a woman's body. You are not a little girl anymore." That mother was saying, "This is the way your body is going to be, so accept it."

Consider the father who said to his son, "It is hard to tell when you will grow or *if* you will. In the meantime, you may as well plan on staying small. What are you good at?" He was saying, "I love and accept you the way you are. You can do the same."

Consider the parents who said to their daughter, "Yes, you are fatter than the other kids. That is the way it goes. People come in all sizes. Some are big, and some are small." They, too, were saying, "I love and accept you the way you are. You can do the same."

On the other hand, consider the slender mother who brought her tall, powerfully built, well-proportioned adolescent daughter to my office seeking a weight-reduction diet. The daughter was willing. She compared herself with her mother and thought there was something the matter with her beautiful body. Consider the father who brought his handsome, relatively short, slender, nicely built son into my office wanting a diet to buff him up—both father and son wanted the boy to be big and heavy enough to be a hockey star. Both sets of parents were failing to deliver mastery expectations and were essentially saying to their children, "You are not all right the way you are. You have to be different before I will feel good about you and before you are entitled to feel good about yourself."

Jennifer Motl, dietitian, columnist, and one of my readers, wanted to know how I dealt with those parents' and children's expectations. In a word, poorly. Instead of helping them evaluate their expectations in the light of normal growth and development, I temporized. I tried to do the impossible—avoid taking a stand, but still do no harm. Given another chance, I would review each child's growth chart *from birth*. If the child's growth was consistent, I would explain the significance of that consistency and warn both parents and children about the distorted eating attitudes and behaviors and unstable growth that were likely to grow out of trying to change natural size and shape. If growth was *inconsistent*, I would encourage them to have a more detailed assessment to identify factors that were undermining normal growth. I describe such an assessment in appendix E, "Assessment of Feeding/Growth Problems."

Some regions of the country are more extreme than others with respect to the pressure put on size and shape—for children and for adults. If you live in a high-school-football-mad or appearance-mad or fitness-mad community, my sympathies. You are going to have to march to your own drummer.

The bottom line, of course, is that you have to deal with your own attitudes in order to be helpful to your child. The parents who gave their children appropriate mastery expectations had done the same for themselves. They had learned to accept themselves the way they were.

Development of Physical Self-Esteem

As in other areas of their lives, children develop physical self-esteem step-by-step as they grow up. What they discover about themselves when they are little provides the foundation for their learning at each stage of development. If all goes well, as they grow and mature, their attitudes and capabilities with respect to physical self-esteem become more and more empowered—and empowering. Appendix H, "Development of Physical Self-Esteem" discusses in detail these stages of maturation. Here, we will sum up.

Infants, toddlers, and preschoolers accept their bodies as they are, are curious about them, and try them out. They run and climb, look and name, and examine similarities and differences between themselves, other children, and adults. School-aged children want to know what their bodies can *do*. They try out their strength, speed, and coordination and experiment with various activities to find out what works for them. Early adolescence challenges physical self-regard as children strike out on their own from parents, focus on peers, and learn to hold their own outside the home. They get more concerned about size, shape, and physical attractiveness as they evaluate themselves and others, often in the midst of rapid bodily changes that leave them wondering what nature will do for—or to—them.

Later in adolescence, teenagers begin taking on adult identity and learning the skills necessary to do well in the adult world. At this point, they begin coming to terms with who they are in all ways and with their bodies in particular. Size, shape, and build influence and often dictate life direction. Will he be a football player or a jockey? Will she be a ballerina or a firefighter? Coming to terms with what one can or can't be and do is essential for living a happy life.

An integral part of the development of adolescent physical

self-esteem is sexual maturation and development of self-regard relative to sexuality. Stated or not, this issue is most concerning to parents with respect to their child's size, shape, and physical appearance.

Size and Sexual Attractiveness

Parents have difficulty holding steady with their children of size—or potential size—because they love them and don't want them to be hurt. Those concerns are particularly troubling in the area of sexuality. Whether we acknowledge it or not, lurking in the back of our minds as we raise children who are unusual in any way is the concern about whether they will be successful with intimate relationships. What might be in store for your large child sexually as she gets older?

Begin by laying to rest the worry that your child will be sexually handicapped if she is fat. Part of that worry may come from your high school memory of the friendless overweight child, seemingly socially isolated because of her unattractiveness. Think about it. Wasn't that child also limited socially and emotionally? Wasn't she a little strange, hard to get along with, in need of constant reassurance, or just plain unpleasant? Those qualities didn't come from her *weight;* they came from her *personality.* Even worse was the overweight girl who let the boys have their way with her as a way of feeling included. Think about it. Didn't that girl have a lot of other strikes against her as well—not much backing from home, negative feelings about herself, little sense that others would take an interest in her for whatever reason?

Now think about the children of size who were liked, included, felt good about themselves, were fun and good company and who could hold their own with the other children. The difference was *attitude,* not *size.* As Carol Johnson points out in her excellent book *Self-Esteem Comes in All Sizes,* "People only make an issue of my weight when I do." People who truly consider themselves to be sexy *are* sexy. Keep in mind when I talk about sexual attractiveness, I am thinking about it in the broadest sense—enjoying being with and looking at another person simply because they are sexually attractive, enjoying having these feelings directed at you.

Being sexy is not reserved for the 3 percent who fit into the category of the tall, slender, broad-shouldered folks with exaggerated upper body development who appear on magazine covers and in ads. Those are the people we may fantasize about, but do we really make those attributes primary when we seek out friendships and relationships? Maybe at first. But even if the package is great, if the person lacks positive human qualities, the attraction doesn't last long.

Twenty-five-year-old Chris had finally figured that out, and she said to her at-risk-of-being-ex boyfriend, "So you think I am too fat? It seems to me that is *your* problem, not mine." Chris was a bit—maybe quite a bit—over the line from average. She was lovely—voluptuous and elegant. She was naturally graceful. After years of struggling with her eating and weight, she had worked hard to learn to eat in a joyful and self-trusting way. She had learned to let herself enjoy moving her body and found activities that felt good to her. She had gradually learned to feel better about herself in general and about her weight in particular. She had begun letting herself dress in a way that emphasized her attractiveness. She had overcome her conviction that she was too fat and therefore ugly, and she wasn't going to let her boyfriend, no matter how much she loved him, take that away from her.

"I am puzzled by the way you feel here in the U.S. about weight," said the beautiful Gloria, who had recently moved from Chile. "In my country, I was considered attractive. Here I am considered fat and ugly. I met my American husband when he was in Chile, and he thought I was beautiful. Now he tells me I should lose weight." Gloria's body was like Oprah Winfrey's at her heaviest. Gloria didn't need my help losing weight—she needed help combating the size-related bigotry she found when she moved here. She also needed my help getting to the point where, like Chris, she could tell her husband that his attitude about her weight was *his* problem, not hers. As for Oprah—why does she need to be so preoccupied with losing weight?

In my experience, dating partners, significant others, and

spouses make an issue of weight when they are invited to. "Do I look too fat?" he says, looking for reassurance and a boost for his ego. "I hate the way I look," she says, looking first at him and then over her shoulder into the mirror. Not a fair question—for either of them. Others cannot possibly reassure us enough to maintain our good feelings about ourselves. When we become adults, we have to learn to maintain our *own* positive self-regard.

DRAW YOUR OWN CONCLUSIONS ABOUT SIZE AND SHAPE

You will have to swim against the tide of public opinion to maintain the middle ground in parenting your child of size or potential size. The world will expect you to put your child on a diet. The world "knows" that obesity is dangerous and reprehensible in all ways—medically, emotionally, socially. The world makes the judgment that if a child remains heavy, it is the parents' fault. It is little wonder that parents resort to putting their children on diets just to protect themselves against the beastliness of it all! But let's see if we can take out some of the sting and help you keep the courage of your convictions.

Excess Weight Is *Not* a Killer Disease

In my view, the health consequences of obesity in general and child obesity in particular have been greatly exaggerated. I do not make this statement lightly. I have done my research and have thoroughly supported this astonishing statement in appendix I, "Health Risks of Child Overweight." Why are my conclusions different? When I read the literature, I carefully consider studies that are not generally included in literature reviews. I also look in detail at the most commonly quoted studies and examine the study itself. I don't just accept the conclusions and caveats of the authors.

Questioning the truisms is not easy, and encouraging others to do the same is not popular. As one of the physicians at a recent presentation complained, "The scientific data was interpreted very differently than I have seen in past reviews of the material by actual medical experts in the fields of obesity, diabetes, and cardiology." Well, that is exactly the point. The "actual medical experts" have accepted at face value the truism that overweight and obesity are medically extremely dangerous. I read the same data and find, at *most,* medical concern, but certainly not catastrophe.

Panic about health consequences of obesity greatly increases the pressure to do the impossible—get children to lose weight. In my view, it does no harm to decrease the panic and anxiety about overweight. In fact, sustaining the panic makes it all the harder to arrive at reasonable solutions. I am fully cognizant of the responsibility to *do no harm.*

Certainly, we have a *problem.* Children on the average *are* getting fatter than nature intended them to be. Taking responsible action in the face of a problem will lead you to make your priority good parenting in general and good parenting with respect to feeding and activity in particular. We do *not* have a catastrophe. Taking emergency action in the face of a catastrophe would lead you to reach for drastic solutions that are potentially more damaging than the condition itself.

You don't have to take my word for it. I have given you the references. Do your own reading and thinking. It is a *lot* of work and takes enough of a research background to sort it out. Read the *whole* article and consider the way the research is conducted and the way statistics are set up and reported. Consider how the authors' conclusions and recommendations are arrived at and whether those conclusions are supported by the data.

Be Prepared for Bigotry

Beware the unquestioned convictions—the ones that are so commonly held as to be truisms. A widely held unquestioned conviction is that individuals have a choice about their body size and shape. The conviction is that children get too fat because they eat too much and exercise too little and that their parents are failing in their responsibility to do something about it. To be blunt, the thinking is that people of size "bring it on themselves," that children of size are gluttonous and slothful and their parents are neglectful.

Let me treat you to a few of the pronouncements that are delivered with absolute and unquestioned conviction:

"Children are fat because they eat so many potato chips and drink so much soda." "It's all the fast-food joints—children are allowed to eat at McDonald's all the time."* "It's the portion sizes—if the portions sizes weren't so big, people wouldn't eat so much." "They eat (their parents feed them) all the wrong things—they never eat a vegetable." "Parents just let those children sit around and watch television all the time—why don't they get them moving?"

These are truisms—commonly held beliefs. Like other truisms, they represent *opinion* rather than actual *fact*. Research shows that infants who grow up to be fat as adolescents ate no more or no differently throughout their growing-up years than did children who grow up to be average weight or below. They were no more likely to be breast- or formula-fed, to be started early on solid foods, to drink high-fat milk, or to eat high-fat, high-sugar snack foods.[5]

Today's eating patterns are not the greatest, and most families *do* have room for improvement with respect to maintaining the structure of family meals. Marketers *do* depend on supersizing in order to entice us to purchase their products.† The pronouncements of the know-it-alls from the previous paragraph don't apply just to children of size and their families. Almost all families depend on McDonald's, use chips and soda, have trouble getting vegetables on the table, and are challenged by the television remote control. The flaw is in thinking that those patterns are more prominent among families of children of size. Not true. Other families do all the same things, and their children remain slim.

My clinical work shows me that there is a whole lot more to the issue of unstable body weight than those sweeping and ill-

---

* With apologies to McDonald's, which is actually a reasonable place to go for a periodic family meal. Keep in mind there is a world of difference between sitting down with your family and enjoying your hamburgers and French fries and whipping through the drive-through and throwing a bag of food into the backseat.

† But why are we so easily sold? Because we restrict ourselves, that's why. If so many of us weren't dieting, we wouldn't depend so much on supersized packaging to help us break our diets.

informed generalizations would lead us to believe. "I can't figure
out why my daughter is so chubby," observed a mother who was
doing some design work for me. "She doesn't eat nearly as much
as her sister, who is slim. Not only that, but she is very active.
She is on the swim team and is on the go from morning until
night." That mother and daughter were not unusual—there are
lots of children like that, and lots of mothers who draw the same
conclusions. Some people are just easy keepers—they don't eat
much, and they are active, and they maintain a relatively high
body weight. For the time being anyway, her daughter just happens to have a relatively chubby body type.

I often get treated to the moralistic judgments right after I
have spent an hour—or several hours—trying to sensitize an
audience to the complexity of the issue of children and weight.
Often those judgments are delivered by people favored by
nature to be thin but who attribute their thinness, nonetheless,
to their own virtue and self-control. A friend calls that attitude
"born on third and thinks he hit a triple." While I have my
share of aggressive urges and unkind fantasies, I have come to
realize that some people simply have oak between the ears. No
amount of data and logic will convince such lipophobic folks
that fatness is not the scourge of epidemic proportions that we
have been led to believe. No amount of protesting that high
BMI is primarily a genetic condition will protect people of
size—young and old—from bigotry. There is nothing you can
do to change their minds. So tune it out, make up your own
mind, and help your child to do the same.

Challenge Assumptions About Weight

People of size often feel guilty about their weight and ashamed
of their eating. Many have accepted society's judgment that
they overeat and that they are digging their graves with their
knives and forks. In reality, people of size eat no more than thin
people. In fact, on the average, they eat less. As I have said
before and substantiate in appendix C, "Children and Food
Regulation: The Research," children who are fat—or who
become fat later in life—eat no more or differently than children
who remain slim. In fact, they eat less. People of size at times

eat chaotically, but rather than being a cause of the weight, the chaotic eating is far more likely to be a consequence of the *weight-reduction dieting* that they pursue in the name of becoming thin.

Many people of size accept society's judgment that they are slothful. They generally feel physically incapable and are convinced they can't get better until they get thinner. In reality, research shows that people of size move around just as much when you factor in the amount of energy and strength it takes to move more weight. The bodies of people of size have not only more fat, but also more muscle and bone. That muscle, like muscle that isn't padded by fat, can be trained to have greater strength, flexibility, grace, coordination, and endurance. If you don't believe me, think of the last time you watched a fat toddler running, climbing, crawling, bending. She didn't know she was limited by her fat—and she wasn't!

Parents and health professionals worry that overweight children will grow up to be overweight adults with a limited life expectancy. A careful examination of the evidence simply does not support that conviction. Moreover, the tendency for large children is to slimming as they grow up. For that matter, the tendency for small children is to getting larger. As they grow, most children diverge toward the mean with respect to body weight. The fat baby has no greater risk of remaining fat than does the thin one. The same holds true for the toddler and preschooler. It isn't until a child is 9 years old or older that the likelihood of her shifting to a different growth percentile becomes less than the likelihood of her staying the same. A child's growth divergence is likely normal if it is slow and smooth and takes place over an extended time. A child's growth divergence is likely *not* to be normal if it is sudden or abrupt and takes place over a relatively short time. For more help telling the difference between normal and distorted growth, read chapter 10, "Understand Your Child's Growth."

SUPPORT SCHOOLS IN HELPING WITHOUT HARMING
Today's educational policy is "leave no child behind." The endeavor pushes teachers to pack all they can into the little

minds in their charge so children can pass tests so the schools can continue to get funding. I prefer the slogan of Zero to Three, an advocacy organization for infants and toddlers, "To grow a child's mind, nurture a baby's heart." To think straight, learn well, and be successful—to *not* be left behind—all children need love and nurturing. They need to be well fed, supported in being physically active, and respected for being just who they are-size and shape, skin color, socioeconomic class, intellectual and physical capability.

Today's schools are being given the job of slimming children down. Because of the obesity "crisis," they are being rallied to weigh and measure children, to send home BMI measurements and overweight diagnoses, limit calories in school lunches, and teach children nutrition and exercise in the name of slimming.

Such interventions don't help, and they do harm. They single children out, shame them, and nonverbally pin targets on them to make them the object of other children's scorn. Those interventions harm schools as well. Schools *educate*, they do not do *treatment*. The school's job is to understand each child's capabilities, characteristics, and limitations and help children to be all they can be. It is *not* the school's job to try to resolve childhood weight issues. Like intellect and learning style, a child's size and shape must be regarded as a given and the school's role as helping the child to make the most of what nature has provided.

Teachers who are encouraged to be weight-preoccupied have difficulty liking their students. My son's first-grade teacher had a thing about fatness. Patrick, one of her students, was fat. As he ran across the playground, she said disgustedly to me, "What is the matter with those parents that they let him be so fat? You should see his lunch! I tell him, 'Don't eat those cookies and chips!' I say to him, 'You should be walking home from school.'" It didn't occur to her that even as we spoke we could see Patrick running and climbing and being as physically aggressive as any of her other students. It didn't occur to her that her thin students brought lunches that were every bit as reprehensible as Patrick's and got rides home from school. She was a good teacher, and the children learned, but her distaste for Patrick was destructive.

What Can Schools Do Instead?

As in the family, schools can take an active and healthy role in parenting with respect to food and activity. For a summary of some of the major principles regarding schools' involvement with these aspects of children's lives, see appendix G, "Feeding and Parenting in the School Setting." You know about good parenting with respect to feeding from reading chapter 2, "Feed and Parent in the Best Way." You know about good parenting with respect to activity from reading chapter 8, "Parent in the Best Way: Physical Activity." The same principles apply to schools.

Schools can parent well with respect to feeding by offering school breakfast. They can make school lunch an important part of the program day. They can schedule lunch around noon and give children enough time to eat. They can restrict access to snacks between times so children go to lunch hungry and ready to eat. They can reassure children they will get enough to eat and be considerate without catering with food selection.

School physical education classes can offer children safe and positive ways to learn and grow with respect to physical activity. Rather than learning to compete, children can learn activities that will give them pleasure throughout life.

While schools can never get rid of teasing, schools can include size acceptance in school antidiscrimination policies and offer consciousness-raising about discriminatory attitudes and behaviors. For more about maintaining the division of responsibility in nutrition education, read *Secrets of Feeding a Healthy Family,* chapter 10, "Raising a Healthy Eater in Your Community."

FIND THE MIDDLE GROUND

As with everything else in our lives, finding the middle ground is extraordinarily difficult. It is far easier to go to the extremes of being rigid and restrictive on the one hand or simply to do nothing on the other. If in doubt, think of your child as being of average weight. Think of your child as being able to regulate her food intake well and grow in the way nature intended. Then think of what you must do to responsibly parent that child. Every child does best with love and limits. Your child will eat and grow best when you provide them.

How do you provide that love and those limits? By following Ellyn Satter's Division of Responsibility in Feeding, of course!

NOTES

1. Baumrind, "Current Patterns of Parental Authority."
2. Elder, "Structural Variations in the Childrearing Relationship."
3. Lean, Han, and Seidell, "Impairment of Health and Quality of Life."
4. Schwimmer, Burwinkle, and Varni, "Health-Related Quality of Life."
5. Crawford and Shapiro, "How Obesity Develops."

UNDERSTAND THE STORY
THE GROWTH CHARTS TELL

Growth charts tell a story about a child's life and circumstances. Growth plotted over time on standard
growth charts provides a snapshot of the child's
physical, nutritional, emotional, and developmental
well-being. Growth charts reassure us that all is going
well and alert us early when there are problems.

- Normal growth can be consistently at the mean.
- Normal growth can be low and slow.
- The problem is not low growth per se, but abnormal
  growth deceleration.
- Normal growth can be high and fast.
- The problem is not high growth per se, but abnormal
  growth acceleration.
- Normal growth divergence is generally slow and
  gradual.
- Abnormal growth divergence is generally sudden
  and abrupt.
- A single measurement tells little about growth, even
  when it is plotted on the growth chart.
- Most children's growth diverges toward the mean—
  unless we spoil it by becoming controlling.
- Compare the child with himself; arbitrary cutoffs for
  overweight or failure-to-thrive distort feeding and
  growth.

CHAPTER
10

UNDERSTAND YOUR
CHILD'S GROWTH

Read this chapter when you
have the *need*. Your health professional will weigh and measure
your child and tell you how his height and weight plot on the
growth percentile curves. To correctly interpret that information,
you need to understand growth charts. Your child's school may
send home notice that his BMI is above the 85th or the 95th
percentile and that he is therefore overweight. A single growth
measurement, even a BMI measurement, doesn't tell you *anything*
useful. Your health professional may tell you your child is "overweight" or even "underweight." Or your child may decide that
his weight is all wrong and want to try to lose weight. To accurately interpret such judgments and to help your child understand his normal growth process, you need to know how to use
growth charts.

Growth charts provide vital information and give the best single indicator of a child's progress and well-being. Growth plotted
over time on standard growth charts provides a snapshot of the
child's physical, nutritional, emotional, and developmental health.

323

Growth charts tell a story about the child's life and circumstances. I find that teasing apart that story is an exciting and engrossing process, one that makes me feel like I am being a detective.

To protect yourself and your child from interference and to make sure real growth problems aren't overlooked, you have to understand growth charts. Some health professionals who work with young children simply do not understand growth chart principles and therefore misuse them. Some use them to *prescribe* rather than *describe* growth. Many set up arbitrary cutoffs and say that a child growing above or below a certain percentile is growing abnormally. Some tell parents to *get* their child to grow on a particular percentile. Some go to the other extreme and pooh-pooh growth charts and tell parents not to worry about their child's growth. Most fail to appreciate how essential it is to evaluate *feeding dynamics* as a part of understanding growth. They evaluate based on medical and nutritional issues but fail to take into consideration the influence the feeding relationship exerts on growth.

You were introduced to growth charts elsewhere in *Your Child's Weight* when I used them to illustrate the profound impact feeding errors can have on a child's growth. Now I will turn the sequence around and use growth charts the way I do clinically. We will begin with the growth charts and then tease apart the story they tell us. However, to solve the puzzles and unearth the stories, we first examine the principles of the growth charts themselves.

UNDERSTANDING GROWTH CHARTS

Most of your child's growth is determined by genetics. Your child has a natural way of growing that is right for him, and he knows how much he needs to eat to grow that way. To put a finer point on it, your child has a strong genetic predisposition to grow in a certain way. That predisposition is supported by, and is in exquisite balance with, his individual need for more or less energy and his natural individual inclination to be more or less active. If you maintain Ellyn Satter's Division of Responsibility in Feeding and Ellyn Satter's Division of Responsibility for Activity, including trusting your child to do his part with eating and moving, you generally don't need to worry about normal growth—it happens.

Your child's body shape and size are determined mostly by heredity: the size and shape of his mother and father. Growing out of this genetic predisposition are countless possibilities for normal shapes and sizes.

Assessing children's growth is a fluid and constantly changing process. Clinicians use growth charts such as the ones in the figures in this and other chapters to monitor children's continual changes in height (or *stature,* in the language of the growth charts) and weight. These charts were constructed by the National Center for Health Statistics, which is a part of the Centers for Disease Control. To construct these charts, thousands of children of all ages were weighed and measured. Then the percentile curves were drawn based on the variations in growth that emerged in those thousands of children.

Charting Your Infant's Growth

When you take your child to the health clinic for regular check-ups, his height and weight are measured. These numbers are plotted on growth charts and become part of his records. Keeping track of the rate your child grows can be fun and interesting. But don't get compulsive and overreact to every little variation. Let the story unfold.

Children may be taller or shorter, heavier or lighter, but they usually grow in stature (or length) and weight in a predictable pattern. To understand how the growth curves work, let's try plotting some figures on them. Imagine we have a little boy— let's call him Kevin—whose weights in pounds and lengths in inches at his routine health visits are listed in figure 10.1:

FIGURE 10.1 KEVIN'S WEIGHTS AND LENGTHS

Age	Pounds	Inches	Age	Pounds	Inches
Birth	8.5	19.75	9 Months	21.75	28.75
1 Week	9	20	12 Months	24.5	30.25
1 Month	10.75	21.25	15 Months	26	31.5
2 Months	13	22.75	18 Months	27.6	33
4 Months	16	24.75	2 Years	30.25	34.75
6 Months	18.75	26.5			

Weight charts As we plot Kevin's weight against his age on the weight chart in figure 10.2, a pattern emerges. Notice that his data points follow pretty closely along the 75th percentile curve. That means if we took an average group of 100 boys his age, 25 of them would weigh as much or more than he does and 75 would weigh less. A child growing at a higher percentile curve is doing *no* better than one growing at a lower percentile curve—and no worse. Children vary enormously from one

FIGURE 10.2 KEVIN WEIGHT-FOR-AGE BIRTH TO 24 MONTHS

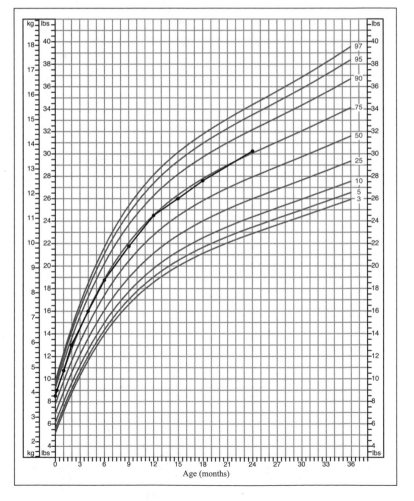

another in the way they grow—that's normal. The important comparison is with the child *himself.* Kevin is growing well, because his weights follow a consistent path. In his case, that path is along the 75th percentile curve.

Length charts Plotting Kevin's length measurements against his age in figure 10.3, we see that his length follows along right around the 50th percentile. His length measures about average. Since his weight plots out at a higher percentile curve than his

FIGURE 10.3 KEVIN LENGTH-FOR-AGE BIRTH TO 24 MONTHS

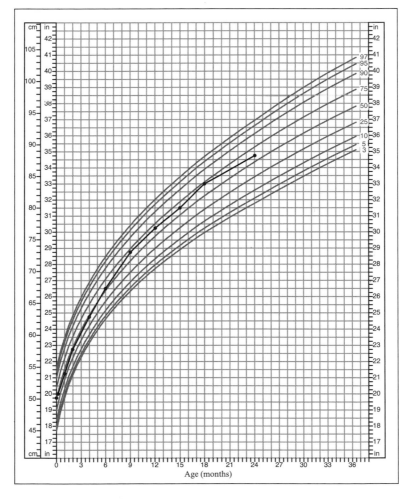

length does—75th on weight and 50th on length—he is a relatively heavy baby. He is totally normal. He is growing consistently
and predictably. He's just built more heavily—perhaps with
heavier bones and muscles or more fat—than another baby.

   Weight-for-length charts There's more. Another and better
way to know whether a child is relatively heavy or light is to
plot his weight against his length on a *weight-for-length* chart. In

FIGURE 10.4 KEVIN WEIGHT-FOR-LENGTH BIRTH TO 24 MONTHS

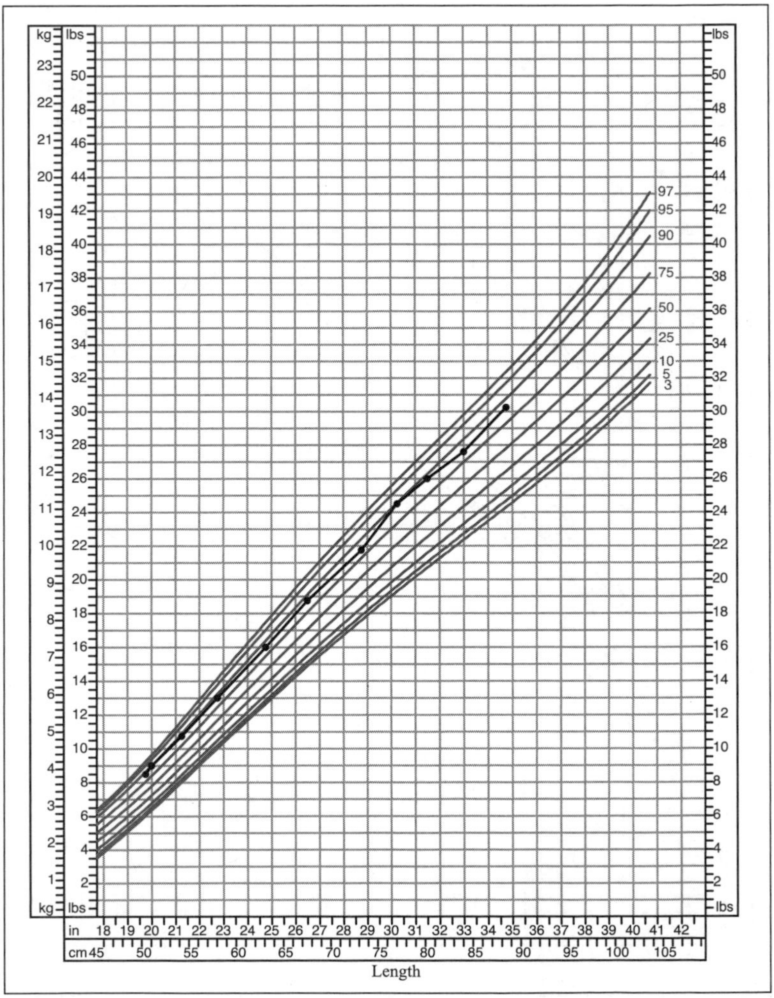

figure 10.4, we see that Kevin's weight-for-length measurements follow along just above the 85th percentile curve. He is relatively heavy for his length. Again, his consistent growth indicates he is growing normally. The data points confirm what we just said—he is built more heavily than other boys. The child who follows along at the 50th percentile weight-for-length curve has an average build. The one who follows along below the 15th

FIGURE 10.5 KEVIN WEIGHT-FOR-AGE 2 TO 18 YEARS

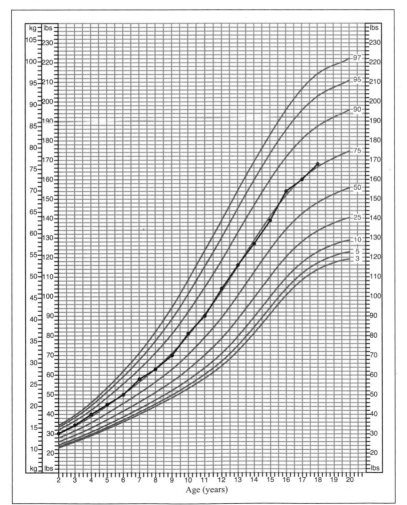

percentile curve has a relatively light build. All are normal. That is just the way they are.

Charting Your Older Child's Growth

The same charting principles apply to older children. Figures 10.5 through 10.8 show our same imaginary boy, Kevin, growing from age 2 to 18 years of age on the 2-to-20 years growth

FIGURE 10.6 KEVIN STATURE-FOR-AGE 2 TO 18 YEARS

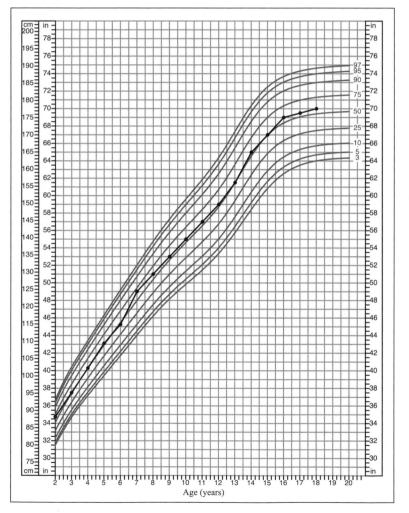

Age (years)

charts. Again, we can see he is growing consistently along his percentiles.

Standard health supervision guidelines for children and adolescents recommend a physical examination annually from age 2 years through age 18 years. We have plotted him accordingly. Kevin had more regular and frequent checkups than I generally see in clinical records. Imaginary parents, children,

FIGURE 10.7 KEVIN WEIGHT-FOR-STATURE 2 TO 7 YEARS

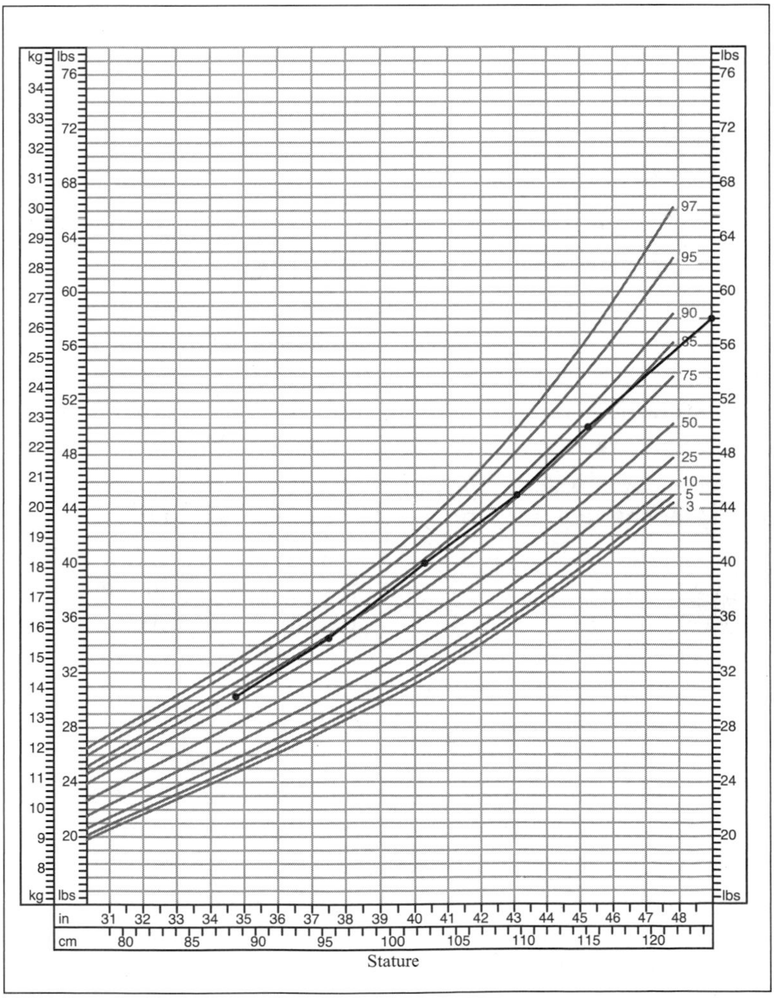

and health professionals are so much more predictable!

Weight-for-length charts plot a child's *length* while he is *lying down*. Weight-for-stature charts plot a child's *height* while he is *standing up*. We move from the *length* to the *stature* chart when we start measuring a child standing up, generally when he can stand still and stand up straight. Using the correct chart for the measurement is important because lying-down measurements are a bit greater than standing-up measurements. Gravity makes a child a bit shorter.

Kevin begins having his measurements plotted on the weight-for-stature chart at age 2. As when he was younger, his weight plots right along the 75th percentile (figure 10.5). Notice that his data points aren't always directly on the curve. Sometimes the points are a little above, sometimes a little below. That's normal growth.

Kevin's height also continues to plot just at or slightly above the 50th percentile (figure 10.6). Sometimes the data points are a little above, sometimes a little below the curve.

Kevin's weight-for-stature still plots right around the 85th percentile (figure 10.7). Like his weight and height, this measurement varies slightly over and under the curve. This weight-for-stature chart plots his growth from age 2 to 7 years.

BMI-for-Age Charts

For older children, BMI-for-age charts are added to the lineup. BMI, which stands for Body Mass Index, is calculated by dividing your child's weight in kilograms by his height in meters-squared. The resulting number—kilograms per meters squared—is similar in concept to a number that is more familiar to many readers—pounds per square inch.

Currently, the Centers for Disease Control recommends calculating and plotting BMI for all children over age 2 years. The BMI measurement is particularly promoted as a way of diagnosing overweight, as it is said to provide an approximation of body fat.[1] Many scientists object to this usage, saying BMI calculations don't match *actual* body fat percentages.[2] Those who object point out that many children are *dense*, not fat. Their relatively broad builds, heavy bones, and well-developed muscles make them weigh more and therefore plot relatively high on BMI curves. Children from some heritages tend to have shorter, denser bodies, like those of Mexican and Navaho descent.[3,4]

I prefer to finesse such arguments by looking at *practicality*. Whether the BMI charts measure *body density* or *body fat*, I still look for *consistency*. I find that the BMI charts provide a handy way of tracking weight-for-stature against age. The weight-for-

FIGURE 10.8 KEVIN BMI-FOR-AGE 2 TO 18 YEARS

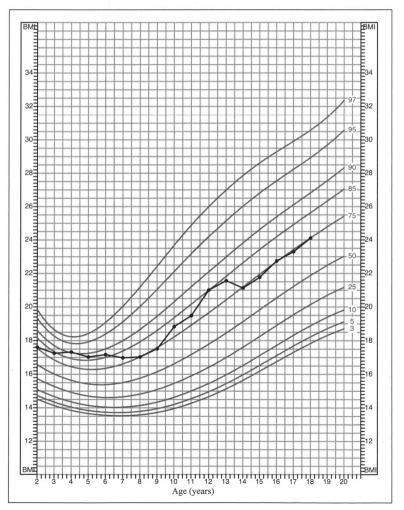

Age (years)

stature charts don't tell you age, and they make you do extra work to figure out the child's age at a given data point. I see BMI as measuring body *density,* not fatness, and I look for *tracking,* not absolute cutoff points.

I do, however, find my practical tolerance to be strained by the frequent exaggerations and distortions of BMI plots and curves, which make the results unnecessarily alarming. For example, Kevin's measurements plotted with only slight variations along his curves in figures 10.5, 10.6, and 10.7. In figure 10.7, his weight-for-stature values, which represented his measurements at 2 to 7 years of age, consistently plotted at the 85th percentile. In contrast, figure 10.8 shows that Kevin's BMI data points for the same ages vary considerably. Between 2 and 4 years of age, the data points in the BMI chart (figure 10.8) went up from the 75th to the 90th percentiles. Using currently recommended child-overweight diagnostic and treatment guidelines, that divergence would mean that Kevin is "at risk of overweight."*

Between 4 and 8 years of age, Kevin's BMI data points dropped back down from the 90th to the 75th percentile. Between age 9 and 12 years of age, his BMI again seemingly accelerated from the 75th to the 85th percentiles, once more putting him "at risk of overweight." In figures 10.5, 10.6, and 10.7, those divergences show up as slight variations around his usual percentiles. In all three sets of apparent divergences, nothing changed. The divergences were artifacts of the numbers. The BMI calculations exaggerated Kevin's slight variations in weight and height and made it look like his growth varied substantially.

To guard against errors in diagnoses based on such distortions, make sure your child's measurements are plotted on other charts, in addition to the BMI-for-age chart. Ask your health care provider to use a weight-for-stature chart as long as possible; then continue to keep a weight-for-age chart after that.

---

* In addition, some would diagnose a blip like this as "premature adiposity rebound," presumably a risk factor for later child obesity.

ACCURATE MEASUREMENTS ARE A MUST

Since so much information is conveyed by growth patterns, accurate measurements are essential. Properly weighing an infant requires a table-model balance or electronic scale checked periodically for accuracy and precision. Properly weighing your older child requires a balance beam or electronic scale, again checked periodically. Heights are trickier and are often taken improperly.

Accurately Measuring Length

Figure 10.9 shows how to measure an infant's length using a measuring frame, a specially constructed board with a fixed vertical head and movable vertical foot piece. Accurately measuring length requires two people: one to hold the baby's head straight against the head piece (you may be asked to do this), the other to straighten out his legs and hold his feet flat against the foot piece. Accurately measuring a wiggly, springy (and fully adorable) baby is tricky. Length measurements taken using the marks-on-the-paper and measuring-tape method are just not accurate.

FIGURE 10.9 MEASURING INFANT LENGTH

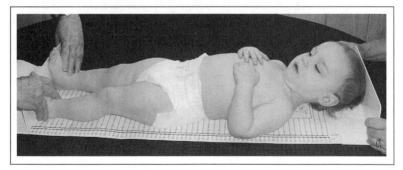

Figure 10.10 shows how to accurately measure the height of an older child. Use an accurate tape measure fastened to the wall or other flat vertical surface with no baseboard. Have the child stand up straight with his heels, backside, and head pressed against the wall. As he looks straight forward, place one edge of something square, like a book, flat against the top of his head and another edge flat against the wall. Make a mark

level with the top of his head, and read that on the tape.
Measurements taken using the rod that comes with stand-up
balance scales give only approximations.

FIGURE 10.10 MEASURING HEIGHT

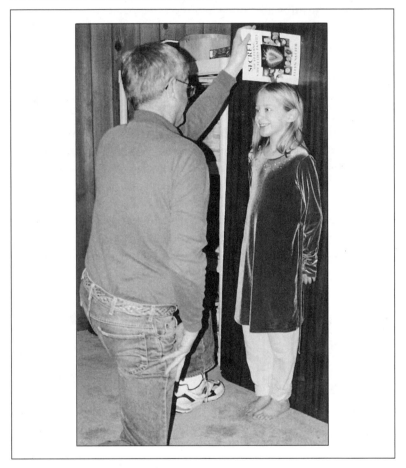

The Problem with Inaccurate Length or Height Measurements
Poorly taken length or height measurements don't let us draw
conclusions about long-term nutritional status, weight-for-
length, weight-for-stature, or BMI-for-age.

Plotting a child's weight against age tells us his short-term
nutritional status. While there are reasons for a child's growth

to shift naturally, in many cases acceleration from his usual weight-for-age curve could indicate that something is disrupting his energy regulation and making him gain too much weight. A deceleration in the child's growth from his usual weight-for-age curve could mean the opposite—interference is making him eat too little and grow too slowly.

Length and height measurements show a child's long-term nutritional status. Length or height acceleration or deceleration appears after several months of weight acceleration or deceleration. It seems that the body protects its linear self and surrenders linear growth only after weight divergence is well established. Head circumference is the very last measurement to show the consequences of nutritional problems. As far as I know, extreme energy excess does not increase head circumference, but *extreme* energy deficit decreases it.

Poorly taken length or height measurements make weight-for-length, weight-for-stature, and BMI-for-age data points worthless. A basic law in statistics states that your information is only as good as your *worst* data. Even if weight data are good, putting them together with poor length or height data spoils their accuracy and usefulness.

GETTING A FEELING FOR GROWTH CHARTS
By now you may be comatose rather than curious about growth charts. It will perk you up and help you get a grip on the information by doing a bit of plotting for your own child. You can get copies of the growth charts from your health professional. Alternatively, you can call the National Center for Health Statistics (NCHS) at (301) 458-4000 or write NCHS in Hyattsville, MD 20782.

You can go directly to the source of the charts by looking them up on the National Center for Health Statistics (Centers for Disease Control) Web site http://www.cdc.gov/growthcharts/. Click on either *Individual Growth Charts* (one chart per page) or *Clinical Growth Charts* (both weight-per-age and length-for-age or stature-for-age on the same page). Do a bit of selecting and scrolling to find the charts for your child's age and gender and you will find growth charts in all their variations: weight-for-

age, length- or stature-for-age, weight-for-length or -stature,
BMI-for-age. There are separate charts for boys and girls and for
boys or girls under age 3 years and from age 2 years on up. You
change from one chart to the other when your child begins
standing to have his height measured.

Print out the charts that are appropriate for your child and
plot whatever figures you have. Those figures may not be terribly accurate (depending on where they came from), but plotting
your child's data points will give you more of a feeling for what
the growth charts are all about and a general idea about your
child's growth.

Now take a little break. Our subject is about to get deeper.

THE BELL-SHAPED CURVE

Growth charts are based on the principle of the bell-shaped
curve, pictured in figure 10.11. Most biological measurements
are distributed in a population according to a symmetrical bell-

FIGURE 10.11 BELL-SHAPED CURVE

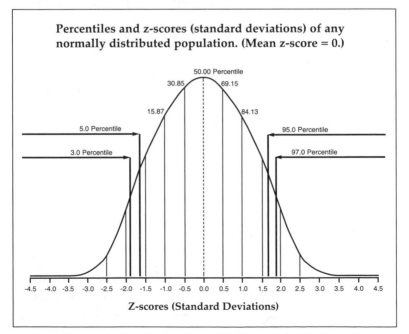

shaped curve. For instance, weights of children of a given gender and age distribute themselves on a bell-shaped curve. Most weigh an average amount. Only a few weigh considerably higher or lower than the average. The rest are somewhere in between. All are normal.

Go to http://acsweb.fmarion.edu/Pryor/bellcurve.htm for a bit of entertainment with your education. Then-graduate student Greg Pryor arranged men and women from one of his classes according to height, from shortest to tallest, on the steps of the football stadium. The two photographs show that the students arranged themselves in a bell curve—the men neatly, the women not as neatly. Other examples of biological measurements that make a bell curve are height, blood pressure, and heart rate.

Growth percentiles reflect the cumulative percentages of children's growth parameters on the bell-shaped curve. The weights of 15 percent of children plot at the 15th percentile or below, half at the 50th percentile or below, 85 percent plot at the 85th percentile or below, 95 percent plot at the 95th percentile or below, and so on. To belabor the point by working our way down from the top, weights of 5 percent of children plot at the 95th percentile or above, 15 percent at the 85th percentile and above, 50 percent at the 50th percentile above, and 85 percent at the 15th percentile or above.

If the percentiles were drawn that way, a child growing *way* out at the extremes could be growing at the 99.9th or the 0.1th percentile. Considering the figures in a slightly different way, one child in a thousand would plot at that extreme. That child would be highly *unusual*, but if he were growing consistently he would not be *abnormal*. He would still be under the bell curve. Children whose weight, height, weight-for-stature, or BMI plot near the average—the 50th percentile—are not necessarily growing any better than are children whose data points plot way out on the extremes. Nor is their growth any more likely to plot at a consistent percentile over time.

The alert reader will note a contradiction between this discussion and current statistics, which indicate that roughly 15 percent school-age and adolescent children plot at or above the 95th

BMI percentile.[5] The discrepancy arises out of the fact that the revised growth charts, which were published in 2000, were deliberately based on a previous, slimmer population of children.[6]

Arbitrary Cutoff Points

Despite the fundamental principles of biological variability, however, standard clinical diagnoses label as *overweight* or *at risk of overweight* children whose weight-for-length or BMI places them at the upper end of the bell curve. As you learned in chapter 6, "Optimize Feeding: Your School-Age Child," children whose BMI is at the 85th to 95th percentile are labeled by the Expert Committee as being at risk of overweight. Those whose BMI is at the 95th percentile or above are labeled overweight.[7] Parenthetically, children whose growth plots at the *lower* end of the curve are labeled as growing abnormally as well. Children whose weight-for-stature or BMI is *below* the 5th or 3rd percentile are labeled as suffering from failure to thrive or pediatric undernutrition.

The child growing at or above the 85th or 95th percentile or at or below the 3rd or 5th percentile is not necessarily growing abnormally—that child may simply be doing what nature told him to. Nor is the child growing at the 85th percentile necessarily at risk of overweight. The issue is growth *integrity,* and the child growing at the 85th or 95th percentile is no more or less likely to grow consistently than is the child whose growth plots closer to the mean.

In fact, labeling relatively large children as *overweight* or *at risk of overweight* is likely to undermine growth integrity by precipitating restrained feeding, reactive overeating, and weight gain. Even without being alarmed by a label, parents of exceptionally large children often unconsciously compensate and try to slim them down, especially if the child has a robust appetite and a great love of eating. The opposite holds true for parents of children growing at the lower percentiles. Labeling a child's growth as abnormal exacerbates parents' tendencies to be controlling with respect to feeding and is therefore disruptive of growth. However, if parents and professionals keep their nerve, feed children well, and trust them to grow in the way that nature intended, children at all percentiles grow well and predictably.

While arbitrary cutoffs are harmful for individual children, they are appropriate for statistical purposes. For *population-wide evaluation,* it is legitimate to use the 85th or 95th percentile cutoff point—or any percentile the epidemiologist chooses, for that matter. In conducting surveys and evaluating trends in *populations,* one can ask the question "What percentage of children currently plot at or above the 95th BMI percentile?" Statistical logic would lead us to expect 5 percent. Current data tell us that 10 to 20 percent of children plot at that level, depending on age and ethnic group. Thus, *as a population,* children are getting heavier. However, that observation tells us nothing at all about the individual child within that population.

As parents and clinicians, our concern is the *individual child,* not population-wide statistics.

EMPHASIZE GROWTH CONSISTENCY, NOT HIGH WEIGHT
If, when your child's weight is plotted for the first time, it is above the 95th or below the 5th percentile, your health care provider may raise concerns. The best course is to wait and see—to monitor his growth for a while to be sure it is consistent. For the individual child, you can't draw any conclusions from a single growth measurement or from plotting on the percentile charts and setting up arbitrary normal/abnormal cutoff points. To draw any conclusions, you need several data points over several months so you can see a pattern. Then you can determine whether that child's growth follows along a consistent percentile.[8]

To belabor the point, some children's weight data *consistently* plot at the 3rd percentile curve or even below. Those children demonstrate the ability to regulate food intake and grow predictably, and they are likely to be just fine. Some other children have data points that consistently plot at or above the 97th percentile curve or even above. They illustrate growth integrity and regulatory ability, and they are likely to be fine as well.

On the other hand, if a child rapidly *crosses* percentiles, making abrupt shifts up or down, it is important to unearth the

story behind the growth divergence. The abruptness and rapidity of the shifts make it *unlikely* to be a normal growth adjustment.
There may be a problem with feeding, parenting, or providing
the child with a positive environment. Finding out what causes
the growth acceleration gives an opportunity to solve problems
early.

The principle of identifying and intervening with growth
acceleration applies to children growing at any level on the
growth curve. A shift from the 50th percentile to the 95th may
be a concern. That concern is based on the child's growth *acceleration,* not on the current plotting at the 95th percentile per se.
The same principle holds for the child whose growth accelerates
from, say, the 5th to the 50th percentile or the 10th to the 75th.
The issue is rapidity and magnitude of change, not where the
growth ends up.

The same holds true for growth shifts in the opposite direction. In chapter 2, "Feed and Parent in the Best Way," you were
introduced to Mary and shown her growth charts (figures 2.1
and 2.2). Mary's mother had "successfully" forced her weight
down when she was an infant from above the 97th percentile to
the 50th percentile. If one were using the Expert Committee's
cutoff points for monitoring growth, even at her young age, her
original weight would have been concerning and her weight
drop-off a good thing. Mary got out of the "overweight" range
and into the "normal" range. Mary didn't actually *lose* weight.
Her weight just increased more slowly than it would have
otherwise so eventually it joined a lower percentile, just as the
guidelines encourage. However, that drop was the result of
dedicated and unrelenting underfeeding. In reality, Mary was
growing poorly. Review the rest of the story and you will see
that when Mary was 10 years old, her mother relaxed her vigilance and Mary gained all her weight back. Eventually, she
developed an eating disorder.

Why Distinguish Between Growth Tracking and Arbitrary Cutoffs?

Mary's story makes it all too apparent that you have to be able
to defend yourself from interference. You don't have to worry

about the theoretical arguments, professional posturing, and statistical squabbles. You have to worry about your *child*. If your child's weight plots high—on any of the curves, *even if he is an infant*—you may be told that he is overweight. If your child's weight plots out at the 85th percentile and you have a weight-zealous health professional, you are all too likely to be told that your child is at *risk* of overweight.

If you have an unusually enlightened health professional— I tend to call people who agree with me enlightened—you will leave his or her office without being alarmed by the statistics. In fact, you may even get the *enormous* help of being reassured about your child's consistent growth and encouraged to keep doing what you are doing. Such reassurance and support will help you resist pressure from neighbors, your extended family, the media, and strangers on the street. Everyone has an ax to grind about child overweight. The assertion that a large child is an overweight child and therefore a cause for grave concern is everywhere—on the radio, television, and Web, in newspapers and magazines.

Despite all the exposure, the messages are still *wrong*. In truth, a child growing at an upper percentile is highly likely to be just fine. What is critical is how *consistent* his growth has been over time. At all times, a child's growth *must* be interpreted in the context of *that child's own history*. It cannot be interpreted on the basis of an arbitrary cutoff. Making the distinction can save you from a great deal of unnecessary agony and keep you from making an intervention that can do more harm than good.

THE STORY OF THE SINGLE POINT

Because we are dealing with such a deeply ingrained misunderstanding, let's look at more growth charts. Figure 10.12 shows a plotting of a single weight-for-length point above the 97th percentile. It is for a child 37 inches in height, weighing 37 pounds. What can you tell about that child's growth? If one were diagnosing based on the child's plotting at the 95th percentile or above, the child would be diagnosed as overweight.

On the other hand, if we were considering longitudinal growth patterns rather than arbitrary cutoffs, we would have to reserve judgment until we got more growth data. Once we fill that in, that single point could tell quite a different story.

Curtis

Begin by looking at figure 10.13. Curtis's birth-to-36-month weight-for-length chart is smooth and consistent from one plotting to the next. Curtis appears to have been a large child since

FIGURE 10.12 WEIGHT-FOR-LENGTH SINGLE POINT

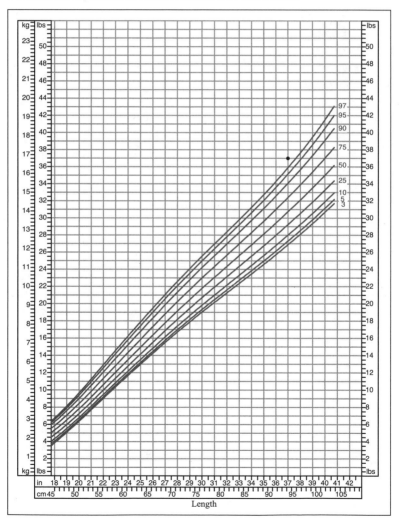

birth, and he remained large. The 37-pound, 37-inch single plotting in figure 10.12 was simply another point along his consistent growth curve.

Now look at the figure 10.14. As Curtis got older, his weight-
for-stature began diverging downward and eventually reached
the 50th percentile. Curtis's downward growth divergence
appeared to be normal because it was so smooth and slow. The

FIGURE 10.13 CURTIS WEIGHT-FOR-LENGTH BIRTH TO 36 MONTHS

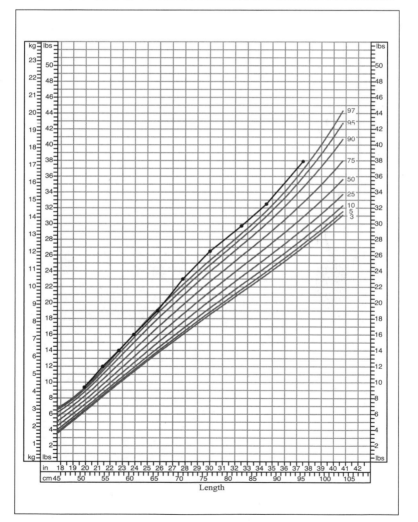

BMI plottings in figure 10.15 help us put ages on that divergence. It lasted about 9 years—from age 3 years to age 12 years.

Melissa

Now let's consider Melissa, another child whose 37-pound, 37-inch single measurements plotted in exactly the same place on figure 10.12. For Melissa, filling in the blanks around that single

FIGURE 10.14 CURTIS WEIGHT-FOR-STATURE 2 TO 6 YEARS

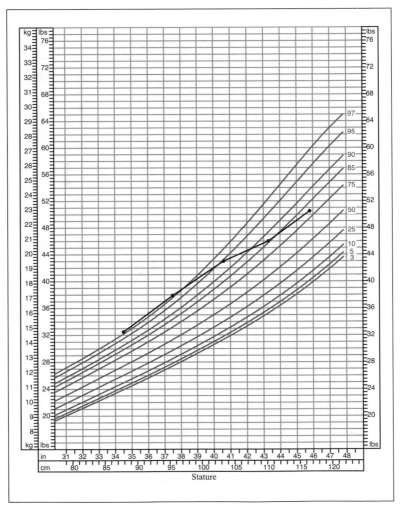

point gave quite a different picture. Figure 10.16, Melissa's birth-to-34-month weight-for-length chart, shows a pattern of unstable growth.

By the time she reached her 37-pound, 37-inch plotting at about age 34 months, Melissa showed what appeared to be a growth adjustment, a significant upward divergence, and two instances of leveling off. To put ages on the weight variations,

FIGURE 10.15 CURTIS BMI-FOR-AGE 2 TO 12 YEARS

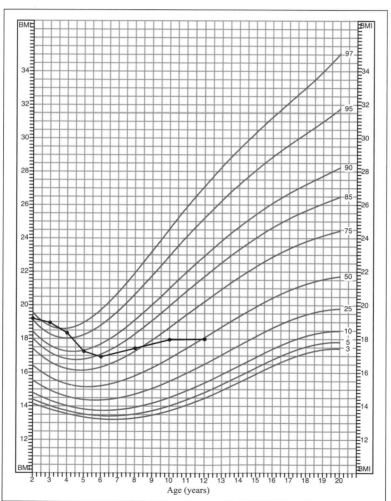

look at her weight-for-age pattern as shown in figure 10.17. The slow and smooth shift upward in weight from birth to age 10 months was likely a natural growth adjustment. Her weight leveled off between 10 and 18 months. Between 18 and 24 months it suddenly accelerated, then just as abruptly leveled off again, and stayed consistent for the next several months.

FIGURE 10.16 MELISSA WEIGHT-FOR-LENGTH BIRTH TO 34 MO.

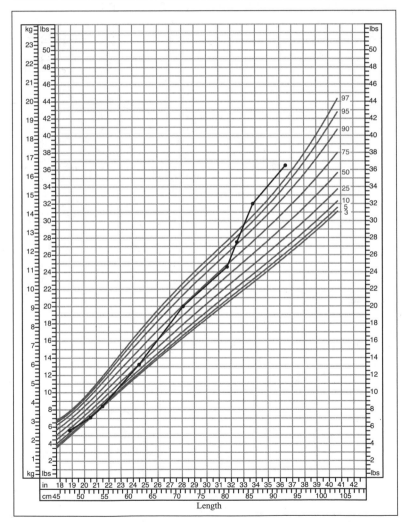

If I were seeing Melissa, I would use that growth pattern as a basis for asking questions—and for being cautious. I would wonder what caused her earlier weight instability. The early, gradual acceleration was likely normal—but I would check it out. I would also wonder what supported her weight *stability* between 10 and 18 months. The second weight shift starting at

---

FIGURE 10.17 MELISSA WEIGHT-FOR-AGE BIRTH TO 34 MONTHS

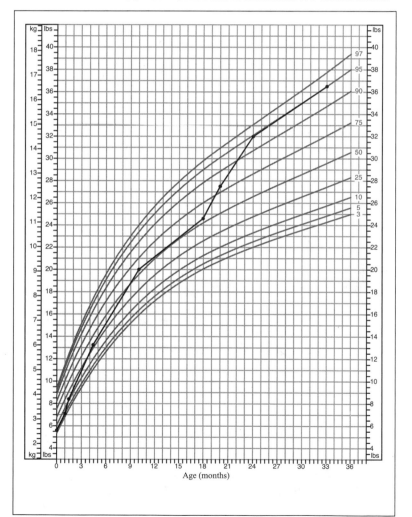

Age (months)

age 18 months may *not* have been normal because it was abrupt and contradicted earlier growth patterns. That rapid weight acceleration would warn me that that instability could be repeated unless the underlying causes were identified and corrected.

As we did for Curtis, let's look at what happened next for Melissa by examining her weight-for-stature, as shown in figure

FIGURE 10.18 MELISSA WEIGHT-FOR-STATURE 2 TO 6 YEARS

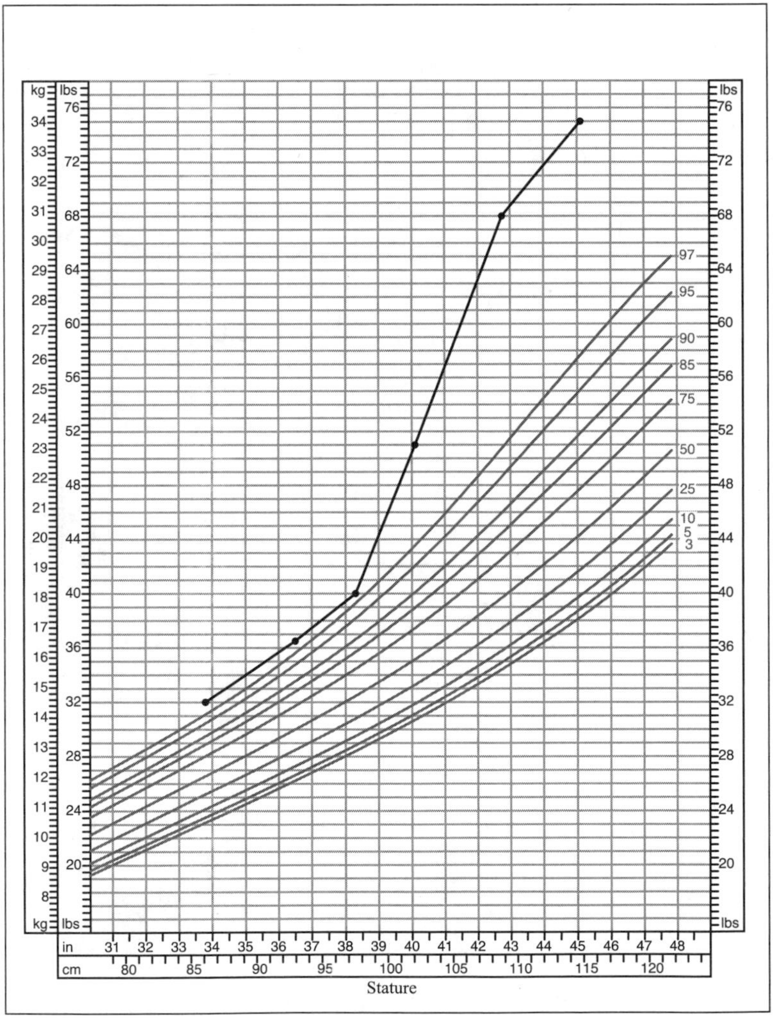

10.18. Soon after the 3-year-old single point we are using as a focus for our discussion, Melissa's weight-for-stature again accelerated markedly, continued to accelerate on a subsequent plotting, and then again leveled off.

To put ages on those divergences, let's take a look at Melissa's BMI chart in figure 10.19. Keeping in mind that while

FIGURE 10.19 MELISSA BMI-FOR-AGE 2 TO 6 YEARS

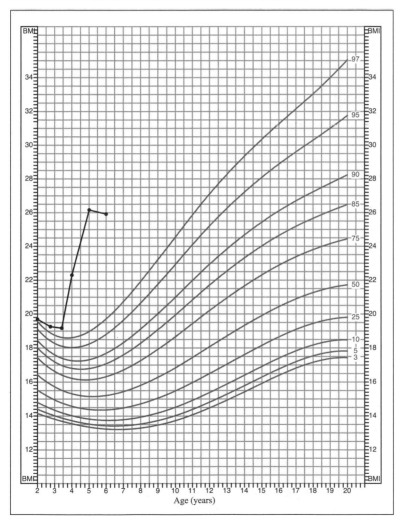

the BMI calculations introduce distortions in the *shape* of the curve, they do give us ages. Her rapid weight gain was between 4 and 5 years of age.

The Story Behind the Growth Charts
By now I hope you are absolutely *desperate* to find out the story behind these two children's growth charts.

FIGURE 10.20 CURTIS AGE 2 YEARS

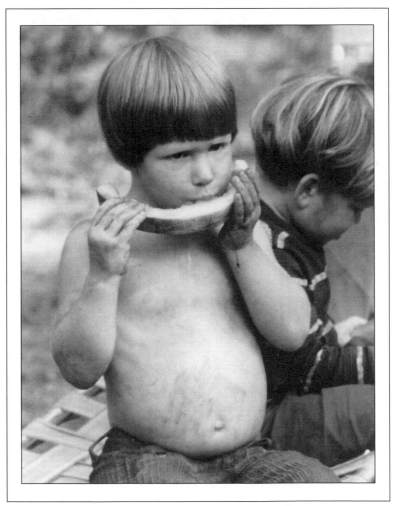

Curtis Curtis's story is instructive but unexciting. When things go well, everything looks easy and natural. Curtis's parents resisted interference with respect to his weight and maintained the division of responsibility in feeding throughout his growing-up years. On his own, Curtis maintained his weight consistently above the 97th percentile until he was 3 years old. By the time he was 4 years old, his weight had drifted down to

FIGURE 10.21 CURTIS AGE 15 YEARS

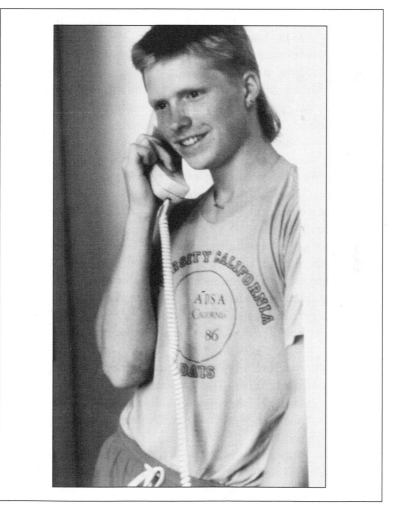

the 95th percentile. The annual drift continued, and by the time he was 12 years old, his weight-for-stature had reached the 50th percentile.

How do I know? Easy. He is my son! With his permission, I publish his pictures (figure 10.20 and 10.21) when he was about 2 years old and at age 15 years.

How did I feel about Curt's size and shape? I remember thinking, when Curtis was small, how cute I thought he was and how happy I was that I didn't feel I had to restrict him. He was a busy and robust child, and he *loved* to eat. From a very early age, he especially loved to feed himself mashed potatoes and gravy with his hands—oh the squishiness and absolute sensual pleasure of it all! Curtis's main eating problem was that he would get so busy playing it was hard to flag him down for snacks and meals. But if I neglected to feed him, he would run out of fuel, fall apart, yell and cry, and absolutely refuse to eat.

Thanks for asking.

Melissa Melissa's story, on the other hand, is far more interesting, but regrettable. Melissa was born somewhat prematurely. After a month of breastfeeding, Melissa's parents weaned her to the bottle. During her early months, her smooth and gradual increase in weight, followed by leveling off, indicated that feeding was going well.

Melissa's abrupt weight acceleration between 18 and 24 months (figure 10.17) raises questions about what was happening with her. What forces undermined Melissa's considerable ability to grow consistently? The reports from her parents were vague and circumstantial. The magnitude and rapidity of her weight gain, however, indicate that something serious was going on.

We *do* know from an understanding of child development that 18-month-old Melissa was navigating the tricky path of establishing herself as her own person. On top of that, Melissa's parents said they both were in alcohol treatment—first inpatient, then halfway-house—when Melissa was between 18 and 24 months old. During that time, Melissa was primarily cared for by her grandmother. From Melissa's perspective, she was abandoned by her parents. That abandonment took place at a critical time, a time when every toddler fears on some level that her parents will give up on her if she gets too bad.

According to Melissa's father, his mother, also an alcoholic, was a controlling and unreliable care provider. As a child, he wasn't sure if he would be fed, and when he *was* fed, his mother told him what and how much to eat. As he got older and his weight increased, she added food restriction and weight harangues to her feeding and parenting repertoire. In short, her parenting in general, and feeding in particular, was inconsistent, contradictory, and periodically downright cruel.

After that, the story goes from vague to frankly speculative. One scenario would have Melissa's grandmother overfeeding her. Rather than resisting the overfeeding, Melissa may have meekly eaten too much and gained too much weight. Why? Having been traumatized by one abandonment, Melissa would be unlikely to take chances with being abandoned a second time. Or she may have eaten too much in an attempt to provide for her own emotional needs.

Another scenario would have been that her grandmother was as inconsistent with feeding Melissa as she had been with her father. Like other children in similar situations, Melissa may have reacted to unreliable feeding by being preoccupied with food, putting pressure on her grandmother to feed her, eating as much as she could whenever she was fed, and gaining too much weight. She and her grandmother would have enacted the pattern of restraint and disinhibition that we have considered repeatedly in *Your Child's Weight.*

When Melissa was 2 years old and her parents took back their parenting jobs, Melissa's weight leveled off above the 97th percentile and paralleled that curve for the next year and a half. To me, that meant that things got better for Melissa—*lots* better. Melissa's parents said they were reliable about having family meals, and Melissa's consistent growth during that time substantiates that.

Now enter Melissa's doctor, who at her 3 ½-year office visit pronounced Melissa *obese* and instructed her parents to restrict her food intake. Her parents, having been disoriented already in the process of trying to improve themselves, asked no questions and attempted to do just that. Melissa's weight abruptly began to accelerate and continued its acceleration until Melissa was 5 years old. As you probably will have learned by now, whether a child's weight goes up or down with food restriction depends on who gets the upper hand. Clearly Melissa got the upper hand and was more effective at getting food out of her parents than they were at withholding it from her.

That was when I met the family and teased apart Melissa's story. Melissa's weight acceleration resulted from a combination of the same four causes we have discussed before, although in a different order. Her problems started with poor feeding practices at the time she went to live with her grandmother. Whatever the feeding distortion, Melissa lost eating capability and learned to use food for emotional reasons. After she got back with her parents, she was fed appropriately and recovered her ability to regulate food intake and grow consistently. However, the pediatrician misinterpreted her large size as overweight—he looked at her current weight level rather than her pattern of growth. Based on that narrowly focused assessment, he prescribed restrained feeding, and Melissa's weight again accelerated.

Melissa's growth pattern from birth gave me grounds for optimism. Twice before, Melissa had demonstrated her ability to regulate food intake and grow predictably. Given appropriate feeding, I was confident that she could do it again. Following my advice, Melissa's parents established a division of responsibility in feeding, and Melissa's rapid weight gain slowed down.

GROWTH DIVERGENCE CAN BE NORMAL OR ABNORMAL
Both Curtis and Melissa showed normal growth divergences— Curtis down from 3 to 12 years, Melissa up from birth to 10 months. Especially large or small, tall or short children often diverge toward the mean in growth, particularly if their parents are closer to the mean or at the opposite extreme from the child in weight or height. Generally, the growth adjustment is complete by the time the child is about 7 years old.[9]

Like Melissa, children may do catch-up growth right after they are born, particularly if they are small to begin with. My twin granddaughters, who each weighed about 6 pounds at birth, both did rapid catch-up growth during their first 18 months before their weight leveled off. Marin's weight accelerated to the 75th percentile, Adele's to the 95th percentile. I know from my own observations that they were fed appropriately and well, so I trust that those patterns were entirely their own and therefore normal.

Curtis's downward weight divergence was more typical than atypical. The weights of large children naturally diverge downward. Children who plot at the 95th percentile weight-for-length at birth have at least a 75 percent likelihood of dropping into a lower percentile as they get older.[10]

Distinguishing Normal from Abnormal Growth Adjustment
The trick is distinguishing whether a shift is a normal growth adjustment or an abnormal divergence. If it is abnormal, it may be caused by distortions in feeding dynamics or medical, nutritional, or psychosocial problems. Distortions in feeding dynamics are a frequent—and frequently overlooked—cause of abnormal growth divergence. Moreover, whether the original source of the problem is medical, nutritional, or psychosocial, feeding dynamics are likely to be distorted.

The *shape* of the growth curve gives another clue as to whether the divergence is normal or abnormal. Curtis's considerable downward weight shift appeared to be a normal adjustment because the shift was smooth and continuous and took several years. Melissa's birth-to-10-month weight acceleration appeared to be a normal adjustment for the same reasons: It was smooth and continuous and took several months. In contrast, her later weight-for-length and weight-for-stature shifts appeared *abnormal* because they were abrupt and crossed several growth percentiles in a relatively short time.

Asking Questions Is Best
I have found that the best way to test my speculation about whether a child's weight divergence is normal or abnormal is to ask parents questions about feeding and growth. How is feeding going? Is there anything about your child's eating that concerns you? How do you feel about your child's size and shape?

Growth? Simply examining the shape of growth curve doesn't allow drawing any conclusions.

It is also essential to teach parents about stage-appropriate feeding and to check whether they are feeding in a way that is developmentally and nutritionally appropriate.

Whether I think a growth shift is normal or abnormal, I ask questions. Even if everything is all right, the conversation gives an opportunity to support the parent.

Ask *Yourself* Some Questions

Asking questions to flesh out the data goes with the territory of being an advocate for children of *any* size and shape. If you are fortunate, you will have a tuned-in health professional who asks you the right questions. If you are not so fortunate, you will have to ask *yourself* some questions.

How can you distinguish abnormal from normal growth divergence? Think about feeding. How is feeding going? Are you observing the division of responsibility in feeding? Are you feeding in a stage-appropriate way?

How do you feel about your child's size and shape? About his weight? If you are uncomfortable about your child's size and shape, you may be unconsciously trying to compensate. Review what you have learned in this chapter and determine whether your child's growth is consistent. If it is consistent, you are doing just fine. If your child's growth is diverging for no apparent reason, get to the bottom of it. Either way, find a supportive health care provider to help you tease apart the causes and help you find direction.

How do you feel about your child's health and well-being? When children are ill or have had a rough start, unless parents get excellent anticipatory guidance, it is almost guaranteed that there will be feeding problems. Afraid and anxious parents get pushy with feeding, and pushiness backfires. The best way to help your ill child to eat well is to maintain the division of responsibility in feeding and to feed in a developmentally appropriate way. Taking over with respect to feeding, trying to get your child to eat more and grow faster, will make him eat less and grow more slowly.

Ill children frequently come out of their illness with eating problems. Then the task is restoring stage-appropriate feeding for whatever stage the child is in. Typically, newborns with medical problems are 2 or 3 years old by the time the medical problems stabilize. The first step is for health professionals to reassure parents that the child is no longer a fragile and ill child. Then parents can feed their child in a stage-appropriate fashion. Given patience, consistency, and a positive feeding environment, most children will bring themselves along with learning to eat.

Other Reasons for Growth Acceleration

While I have not ever seen it in actual practice, I suppose children's weight could conceivably accelerate because their diet is so extremely high in calories that it overwhelms their ability to compensate. More commonly, an extremely high-calorie diet is given in the context of poor feeding dynamics—the child is not provided with regular meals (or any meals at all), he is allowed to graze (or scavenges food as well as he can), and then he is harangued for eating so much.

Medical causes for child overweight are rare and generally are also associated with short stature.[11] Endocrine disorders include thyroid underactivity, Cushing's syndrome, and disorders of the pituitary gland or thalamus. The most common but still rare genetic condition that causes high body weight is Prader-Willi syndrome, a developmental disorder of moderate to severe cognitive impairment, reportedly voracious appetite, and metabolic efficiency that seemingly allows children to gain weight on very few calories. Down's syndrome is often said to cause excessive weight gain, but that tendency has not been objectively demonstrated. Weight acceleration with Down's syndrome is more likely to be the result of restrained feeding and disinhibited eating than because of to the condition itself.

BODY FAT IS NORMAL AND NECESSARY

In some clinical settings, a diagnosis of child overweight or obesity is reserved for children whose body fat is at or above a certain percentage. Body fat is measured using skin-fold calipers and any number of other methods that vary in sophistication and accuracy.

I have the same reservations about body fat percentage cutoffs as I do about arbitrary cutoffs on growth percentiles. No single measurement is valid in measuring the quality of a child's growth. That growth can be evaluated only by tracking a child's growth over time, evaluating it for consistency and predictability, and asking questions about feeding dynamics.

In addition to using statistical methods, you'll evaluate your child's growth the same way parents always have—by looking at him. During the first year, he gets longer and heavier; his body and arms and legs fill out. His stomach sticks out; his face gets rounder. That's fine. It's normal and desirable for your child to increase his body fat during the first year—from 11 percent at birth to 24 percent by age 1 year. This extra fat is important to his little body to support his internal organs and as a source of calories in case of illness.

During the second and third years, your child's body continues to change a lot as he moves through the chubbiness of the toddler stage to become a slimmer preschooler. Body fat drops to about 21 percent by age 2, and to 18 percent by age 3.

As he moves through the preschool and school-age years, your child's body fat percentage stabilizes. Then, just before the rapid growth spurt of puberty, like many preadolescents, he is likely to plump up. He will develop a padding of fat all over his body, he may develop a spare tire, his stomach will stick out, and his arms and legs will get fatter. This too is part of the normal growth process. Like a bird preparing to migrate, he is storing up energy for the nutritional challenges of the extremely rapid growth of puberty. Then he will slim down again.

Boys achieve most of their height by the time they are 18 to 20, and they continue to put on weight in the form of muscles for another couple of years. Girls get most of their height and their sexual development by age 16. After that, they continue to put on weight, primarily in the form of fat. That is likely the body's natural preparation for pregnancy and lactation. It is a perversion of our culture to consider the immature, slim-but-sexually-developed body of the adolescent girl to be the ideal shape for a woman.

DISCOVER THE STORY THAT GROWTH CHARTS TELL

The importance of understanding the stories behind the growth charts is born out in the stories of children you have met throughout *Your Child's Weight:* Mary (chapter 2, "Feed and Parent in the Best Way"), Haley (chapter 6, "Optimize Feeding: Your School-Age Child"), and Leane (whose story is serialized in chapters 2, 5, and 9).

Nineteen-year-old Mary's out-of-control eating and high body weight had its roots in food restriction when she was an infant. That restriction set her up for overeating and weight gain during a family crisis when she was 10. Her growth charts tell the story.

The seeds for 10-year-old Haley's accelerating weight were sown when her food was restricted when she was 10 months old. After that, Haley's nutritional fortunes—and her weight—went up and down depending on her life circumstances. When Haley was allowed to eat as much as she wanted, her weight gain was smooth and predictable. When her food intake was restricted, her weight accelerated. Her growth charts tell the story.

Leane's rapid weight gain and voracious appetite made her seem like a bottomless pit. Then it emerged that her food intake had been restricted and her weight held down almost from day one. Leane was afraid she wouldn't get enough to eat. After she got the upper hand with eating as a toddler, she kept eating as much as she could and kept gaining weight. Her growth charts tell the story.

All of these stories and the others in *Your Child's Weight* entail missed opportunities. What a lot of pain would have been avoided had an alert health professional been in the right place at the right time! That person could have responded to those early blips in growth by reassuring the parents about normal growth, teaching about appropriate feeding, and solving early feeding problems.

A CHILD OF EXTREME SIZE

I expect, like many in my audiences, you are still wondering about children of extreme size. Surely for them, weight-reduc-

tion dieting or even more drastic interventions are the only way
to go? I will answer that question by looking at one of those
children, 15-year-old Marcus, in detail. As is becoming more
frequent in our weight-obsessed society, it is a story of court-
ordered placement in foster care on the grounds of child obesity. Before I go any further, I want to tell you why I am spending
a fair amount of this chapter talking about this.

First, the story of Marcus illustrates an important theme of
Your Child's Weight: Rather than being a crisis of child overweight, our true crisis is one of providing for our children—
a crisis of parenting and of feeding dynamics. Child overweight
is just a symptom of that deeper crisis.

Second, Marcus vividly illustrates the point that the same
feeding principles apply even in extreme cases. In going far
beyond you and your situation, Marcus will demonstrate that
the division of responsibility in feeding is appropriate and
applies to *you* and *your child.* Extreme weight gain grows out of
extreme conditions; it does not call for extreme solutions.

Finally, the story of Marcus makes abundantly clear what I
have said throughout *Your Child's Weight:* Simplistic explanations and solutions do not suffice. The simplistic *explanation* is
that children get fat because they eat too much and exercise too
little. The simplistic *solution* is that the way to fix them is to get
them to eat less and exercise more. That explanation and solution are so unrealistic for Marcus that it boggles the mind.

The Valiant Marcus

Now, to the story of Marcus. Fifteen-year-old Marcus found his
way to me on the instigation of his foster mother, who was concerned about his food-preoccupation and overeating. We will
call his foster mother Fanny to differentiate her from his biological mother—Beatrice. (Get it? Fanny: Foster; Beatrice:
Biological. Soon you will be glad for the help keeping them
straight.) Child Protective Services had determined that Beatrice
was neglecting Marcus because she didn't restrict his food
intake and get him to lose weight. Marcus was placed in foster
care with Fanny in order to get his weight down.

In the 1$^1/_2$ years that Marcus had been living with her,

Fanny had managed to force his weight down by almost 150 pounds. However, in the several weeks before Fanny contacted me, Marcus had begun voraciously overeating. He snuck food, ate a great deal if he was alone in the house, stole food in grocery stores, even ate out of garbage cans. On one weekend visit with Beatrice, Marcus gained 12 pounds.

I knew at the outset that Marcus's current pressure on eating was coming from his weight loss. At 150 pounds below his previous weight, his biological pressure to eat and restore his usual weight had to be simply enormous. Maintaining that weight loss was extremely unlikely. I wasn't sure what could be done for Marcus, but I was willing to consider his case in detail to look for possibilities. I told Fanny—and the social services agency that coordinated his care—that I would be willing to do a careful evaluation and identify those possibilities. I describe that assessment in appendix E, "Assessment of Feeding/Growth Problems." Soon after we signed the agreement, a 5-inch-high box of medical, school, and social services records landed in my mailbox.

Marcus's Growth

Marcus's early records were sketchy. After careful and determined digging, I found data for his weight at birth and at one year (figure 10.22). Both of Marcus's early weights plotted in the same relative position-just below the 75th percentile, weight-for-age. With only two points, I couldn't draw a trend line, but it is reasonable to assume that his weight had tracked along the 75th percentile between those two points. For the first year, it appeared that Marcus regulated his food intake and grew consistently.

Figure 10.23 shows the plotting for Marcus from age 2 years until 6 1/2 years and illustrates his extremely rapid weight gain. Beyond giving us a visual representation of his growth, those data points are meaningless. There are no norms on the growth charts for children who plot outside the standard percentiles. Marcus was last plotted at age 6 1/2 years because his weight was too high at age 10 years old to fit on the graph. When he was 6 1/2 years old, he weighed 152 pounds. By age 10 years, he weighed 367 pounds.

Marcus's Weight Pattern

The growth chart in figure 10.23 makes it appear that Marcus's weight was accelerating rapidly and alarmingly. Was Marcus going to keep getting fatter and fatter, heavier and heavier until he weighed hundreds or even thousands of pounds? Achieving such enormous weight is extremely unusual, but it *does* happen. Since the growth charts weren't any help with determining

FIGURE 10.22 MARCUS WEIGHT-FOR-AGE BIRTH & 12 MONTHS

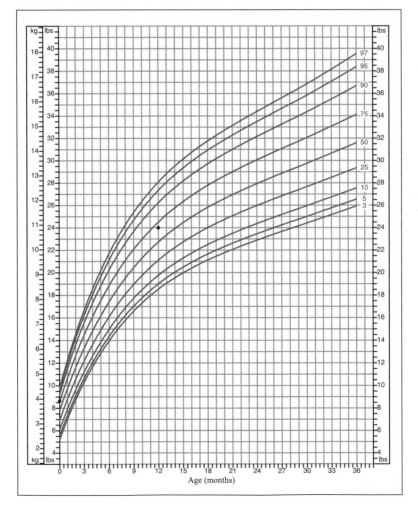

whether Marcus's weight was continuing to accelerate or leveling off, I resorted to another way of evaluating it: the Z-score.

The Z-score is a standard deviation. What's a standard deviation? Take another look at the bell curve in figure 10.11 on page 338. The horizontal line below the curve is marked off in points called *standard deviations*, or Z-scores. The mean is zero. The Z-scores are reported as numbers above or below the mean.

FIGURE 10.23 MARCUS WEIGHT-FOR-AGE 2 T0 6 ¹/₂ YEARS

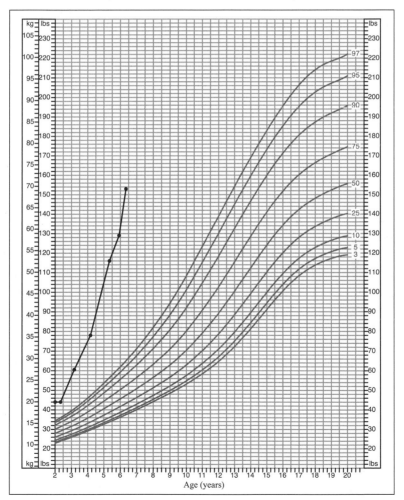

They are related to the percentiles that we have been looking at all along. One standard deviation above the mean, a Z-score of one, is the 84th percentile; one standard deviation below the mean, a Z-score of minus one, is the 16th percentile. The 95th percentile has a Z-score of about 1.6. It is 1.6 standard deviations above the mean. The 97th percentile has a Z-score of about 1.8.

So far, so good? Glad to hear it! Hang in there, because applying the Z-score clarifies things. Figure 10.24 lists Marcus's weight and Z-score from birth to age 15.* As we already know from his weight-for-age growth chart, Marcus's weight when he was born and at age 1 year were just above the mean. His Z-scores that first year, 0.8 and 0.5, were within one standard deviation above the mean.

FIGURE 10.24 MARCUS WEIGHTS AND Z-SCORES

Age	Weight	Z-score	Age	Weight	Z-score
0	8.6	0.8	8		
1	24	0.5	9		
2	44	4.0	10	367	4.0
3	61	4.6	11	366	4.1
4	78	4.5	12		
5	116	4.8	13	447	4.7
6	129	4.5	14	406	4.6
7			15	297	3.5

However, see what had happened by the time Marcus was 2 years old! His weight had precipitously increased until his Z-score was *four* standard deviations above the mean! It was *way* out under the right-hand tail of the bell curve.

Then the Z-score leveled off. That is, while he kept getting heavier, his weight followed a consistent trajectory. His subse-

---

* I have purchased a wonderful computer program that plots growth curves and calculates Z-scores. You can find that program at www.amshome.com. You can also do a Web search to find sites that calculate Z-scores, but they may be difficult to find. Since Web sites come and go, here is the search string we used: *weight Z-score calculator.*

quent assessments showed his Z-scores to consistently be around 4.5. If we had a curve that high, he would have been following it. Marcus was *not* getting fatter and fatter—his weight remained at a consistently high level. When he was 10 and 11 years old, his Z-score dropped a bit, but then it went back up to the usual level by age 13. Marcus's Z-score at age 15 years, 3.5, is where his weight was when I first met him. It had dropped by 150 pounds.

FIGURE 10.25 MARCUS Z-SCORE-FOR-AGE

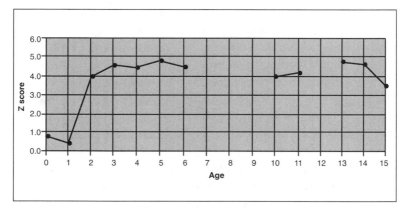

To get a picture of Marcus's Z-scores, let's do a simple graph. Figure 10.25 plots his age against his Z-scores. Clearly, the worst happened to Marcus between 1 and 2 years of age, the time for which his data were lost. What went on back then? His Z-score remained high from age 2 to age 6. What was his life like then? The data points are missing for ages 7, 8, and 9. Why was that? His Z-score *dropped* at age 10 and 11. What happened then? We don't know.

Family Interview
After I reviewed the clinical records and analyzed his growth, I met Marcus in a family interview. Included were both Beatrice and Fanny, as well as his grandmother—Beatrice's mother. I told Marcus where to sit so he didn't have to choose between Beatrice and Fanny.

Fanny appeared to love Marcus and gave every evidence of

looking out for him. Marcus appeared to love Fanny right back and depended on her to take care of him and help him figure things out. Being a new kid in a new community, Marcus had lots of social challenges, and Fanny supported and advised him and encouraged him to do the best he could. She saw to it that he was clean and well groomed when he went off to school, and she made sure he had his lunch money. After school, she sat down with him while he had his snack and kept up with what was going on with him.

Marcus clearly loved Beatrice as well and was glad to see her and her mother. Beatrice appeared glad to see Marcus as well and joked with him at the beginning of the session. Then Beatrice's discussion quickly centered around Marcus's eating and weight. According to Beatrice, Marcus had something the matter with his ability to stop eating. He had always been a voracious eater with out-of-control weight. He had weighed 18 pounds when he was 7 weeks old and 44 pounds by age 1 year.

Beatrice's report of Marcus's astonishing and early weight divergence was highly inaccurate, but nonetheless, that distorted story was reported over and over in his medical records. I can understand that—those records were so voluminous and confusing that it wasn't surprising that the data had been lost. However, it was a serious error, because it led medical people off on completely the wrong track—to the conclusion that Marcus's high body weight was biologically based. In fact, at the time I met him, Marcus had had repeated genetic testing to diagnose Prader-Willi syndrome. All the standard tests came up negative.

The steep pitch of Marcus's weight curve appeared to confirm his mother's report that Marcus was a voracious overeater on any food that was available. Beatrice said Marcus had "essentially no awareness of any satiety and will eat and eat and eat until whatever is there is gone—he does not have an off button in his system. He also has tended to hide and hoard food and has done it for a long time."

Other than his eating, Beatrice and her mother said Marcus was a good boy. They were matter-of-fact and proud in reporting that Marcus had taken on parental responsibilities from the time he was small. He "didn't give any trouble" and was "independent and good at occupying his time." Starting at about age 4, he had taken care of his infant brother.

When I spoke with Marcus privately, he remembered it being difficult and scary to have so much responsibility and so little support when he was small. He says he tried to take care of his little brother and see to it that they got fed, but there wasn't always food in the house. He remembered wanting to eat a lot so he could grow up fast.

Marcus's Early History

Seeing beyond surface impressions is what I do as a mental health professional. The child's *behavior* tells the real story. Marcus's behavior told me that things were not good in his home, and I looked for evidence of that. I could only guess what life was like for Marcus when he was a toddler. Based on Beatrice's self-absorption and the clues and chaos that peeked between the cracks in the family interview and in Marcus's reports, it must have been very hard for him. Beatrice was difficult to see through, because she was an attractive and well-groomed professional who lived in a middle-class suburb.

Beatrice had been a widow since Marcus was 4 years old, and her divorced mother often lived with her to help out. Beatrice's mother gave a clue to the chaos in the family when she described Beatrice as overwhelmed and needing help with providing for herself and her children. Beatrice's problems were attributed to her husband's death when Marcus was 4 years old. However, Marcus's growth acceleration between age 1 and 2 years of age indicated that life had been hard for Marcus when his father was still alive.

I knew from reading through the records that Marcus's family was chaotic. As is typical with chaotic families, Beatrice and her mother offered only the vaguest of information about Marcus's early months—or about any of his history. With her report that Marcus had been a "good boy" who "didn't give any trouble," who was "independent and good at occupying his time," Beatrice was likely to be telling quite a different story. Considered from Marcus's point of view, it was likely she didn't pay much attention to him and, in fact, neglected him. Secure children are troublesome and demanding or at least remembered by their parents as being energetic and curious. Frightened children who have given up on being provided for are consistently "good" and occupy their own time.

Beatrice proudly described Marcus at age 4 years as being "so responsible" and providing much of the care for his infant brother. Again, this is evidence of neglect. No 4-year-old child should have to be primarily responsible for *himself*, let alone responsible for an infant. Marcus had to have been a very frightened child who was doing whatever he could to get by.

The evidence indicated that Beatrice was a profoundly dependent and self-involved person who depended on Marcus to keep her going. Ironically, in failing Marcus, the system had also failed Beatrice. Had she been confronted when Marcus was small with the consequences to him of her actions, she may have been able to get better on his behalf. As it was, that opportunity was lost.

Eight to Thirteen Years

After moving several times, Marcus's family came to rest when he was 8 years old. Soon Marcus became the focus of an M-Team staffing at school. "M-Team" is the local language for a multidisciplinary planning meeting convened on behalf of a child who has particular needs. The report from that staffing showed Marcus to be in a world of trouble—frequently tardy for school and missing school, poorly groomed, tired and sleepy at school, explosive, impulsive, demanding too much attention. Soon after, the school social worker noted all of above plus poor hygiene—dirty, ripped clothing, fecal odor.

When Marcus was 11 years old, in a letter to child protective services, Marcus's principal echoed the social worker's observations. Marcus missed school a great deal and seemed exhausted when he was there. He often had no lunch money. When his mother was contacted—with difficulty—by the school, she urged school personnel to pay for his lunch. Child protective services visited the home and noted that Marcus and his younger brother were frequently left alone at night. Social services suspected that

Beatrice was abusing alcohol and noted that the house was filthy. Marcus's hygiene got so bad that his teacher and the principal arranged for him to shower at school. The plan failed because Beatrice didn't send along clean clothes from home.

A year later, a school social worker observed that Marcus's school absenteeism, exhaustion, and poor classroom performance had continued. At the time of her report, Beatrice had been jailed for failure to pay driving-while-intoxicated tickets, and Marcus and his brother had been placed in a residential treatment facility. The clinical records from the facility reported "no supervision at home."

I was tempted to summarize this litany but chose to go through it in detail to demonstrate to you that there was lots of evidence that Marcus was being neglected. From age 8 years old on, and probably before that, Marcus simply had not known that he would be provided for. He was trying to go to school and do what was expected of him with little or no support from home. At that point, Marcus's maintenance of high body weight was likely the result of three of the causes outlined in chapter 1: restrained feeding in the form of food insecurity, poor feeding practices, and stress.

Marcus himself told me that he missed school because he felt he needed to stay home from school to be sure Beatrice would be all right. He liked living with Fanny, and it felt good to him to have her taking care of him. However, he still worried about what would happen to Beatrice if he weren't there to look out for her.

All Blamed on Weight

The observations that were made of Marcus in the schools are the sort that teachers, school counselors, and principles use as indicators that a child is struggling. Schools have a protocol for reaching out to such a child and trying to help him. In the best of all worlds, they are able to see the child as just a child, no matter his weight, and apply the appropriate solution. In this case, the opposite happened. At every step along the way, Marcus's problems were blamed on his weight.

School absences, negative behavior: "High body weight."

Poor hygiene, dirty, ripped clothing? "Grave concern because of his extreme weight problems." According to the reports, smelling bad went with being fat.

Child protective service observations of neglect? Medical neglect based on his elevated body weight which was "non-environmental—not a result of omission on the mother's part."

School absenteeism, exhaustion, and poor classroom performance? "Our gravest concern is his weight."

No supervision at home? "Problematic on the grounds that it deprives him of outside control of his food consumption."

Finally, Marcus was placed in foster care on the grounds that "efforts to have his mother supervise his food intake in the home have not worked."

Tunnel Vision
Marcus's weight was the least of his problems. Rather than having his needs provided for, he had been given adult responsibilities from the time he was a toddler, or at least a preschooler. He was put in charge of providing for himself, his brother, and probably his mother as well. Rather than being helped by the people who were supposed to protect and support him, Marcus's teachers, principal, social workers, and health personnel profoundly failed him and exacerbated his difficulties by blaming him for his problems: He was too fat.

Rather than being willing or able to deal with the extreme neglect in his home situation, helping individuals and agencies overlooked Marcus's real dilemma and focused instead on his weight. Ironically, when Marcus was finally placed in a home where he could be provided for, it was for the purpose of weight loss.

What happened? Are schools and other agencies feeling so much pressure about child obesity that they are overlooking basic child welfare issues? Was Marcus's mother so formidable that no one wanted to take her on? Whatever the flaw in the process, Marcus paid the price.

My Impressions of Marcus
My conclusion was that Marcus *did* show an ability to regulate

his food intake and body weight. In fact, he had demonstrated that ability twice: first, from birth to age 12 months, when he appeared to grow consistently at the 75th percentile, and second, from age 2 to 13 years, when his weight remained stable at a Z-score of roughly 4.5. That evidence indicated that his high body weight was not the result of an intrinsic disability with food regulation but rather a response to the profound lack of support and extreme pressures in his home environment.

By age 3 years, the worst had happened to Marcus. His most marked weight gain was during a particularly vulnerable and dependent stage, between ages 1 and 3 years of age. The extreme magnitude of that early weight gain testified to the extreme degree of stress that he experienced.

After that exponential weight gain before he was 3 years old, Marcus's weight remained stable, if high. It wasn't his *weight,* but the salience and persistence of his *other symptoms* that manifested his distress. Those symptoms included school absenteeism, excessive fatigue, poor grooming, low frustration tolerance, explosiveness, impulsivity, and social immaturity.

Currently, Marcus was just plain *hungry.* As much as he wanted to please Fanny and stay on his diet, he couldn't help eating whatever he could get, whenever he could get it. He acknowledged that he often felt like he had two different people in him—the one who wanted to eat and the one who wanted *not* to eat.

How I Defined Marcus's Weight Issues

Getting a handle on a child's issues when weight is the presenting complaint is difficult because getting beneath the surface is contrary to the norms of assessment and treatment. Even without that barrier, it is a real mind-bender to explain the child's weight deregulation, examine underlying issues, and clarify how one relates to the other. Here is how I defined the issues for Marcus:

- Food insecurity from early childhood—inconsistent, unreliable feeding as well as food deprivation in the name of weight reduction.

- Disinhibition—a pattern of eating a great deal of food at any opportunity as a consequence of chronic food insecurity.
- In response to recent weight loss, current extreme biological pressure to eat large quantities of food and restore energy equilibrium.
- Based on long-term food insecurity and the pattern of disinhibition growing out of it, learned inability to regulate food intake based on internal cues of hunger, appetite, and satisfaction.
- Chaotic and unsupportive family environment.
- Poor self-esteem, high social anxiety growing out of a lifetime of being given tasks that were beyond his ability to achieve.
- Use, by Marcus and others, of food and weight issues to distract from or displace anxiety regarding other life issues.

My Recommendations for Marcus

Marcus needed to be taken care of and *fed*, he didn't need to be restricted. Food restriction simply mimicked the food insecurity and neglect from which he had suffered his whole life. As I said earlier, extreme weight gain grows out of extreme conditions. It does not call for extreme solutions. Marcus was a good boy who needed good parenting. For many years, Beatrice had demonstrated her inability to provide for Marcus. In my judgment, the placement in foster care was appropriate and long overdue. I do not agree, however, with the *grounds* for the referral. Beatrice was failing to *provide* for Marcus. The magnitude of his weight gain testified to the magnitude of that failure. It was *extreme* and provided reason for placement. Placing Marcus in foster care because of Beatrice's failure to *deprive* him and force weight loss was crazy.

Marcus would have been far better served if Fanny had been allowed and encouraged to follow the guidelines outlined in chapter 7, "Optimize Feeding: Your Adolescent." Providing Marcus with a positive and supportive eating environment would have positioned him to benefit from short-term treatment to help him learn to tune in to his internal regulators of hunger, appetite, and satisfaction. Had Marcus been reassured that he would get enough to eat, his eating would soon have settled down. For a while, he would have eaten great deal, but before long he would have come to trust that he would get enough to eat. He might even have lost some weight.

But the best didn't happen, and by the time I saw Marcus he had had a huge weight loss and his biological pressure to regain was intense. At that point, anything could happen. Even though Marcus was still fat, the fact that his body weight was so much lower than usual meant that he was in a starved state. Studies show that people recovering from starvation eat voraciously for a long time. Their hunger is powerful, and they have a strong and persistent need to eat far past the point of satisfaction.[12]

My treatment plan was the same as if I had seen Marcus before his weight loss:

- Optimize feeding and provide short-term treatment to recover internal regulators.
- Do a good job of parenting.
- Support Marcus's emotional and social growth and development.

Knowing that maintaining his current low weight was unlikely, I predicted that Marcus would regain a considerable amount before his weight leveled off. I hoped it would level off at a lower level, or even at the same level as it had been before he started losing weight, but I certainly wouldn't promise it. Many times, people regain to a higher level after weight loss. We had to wait and see what happened.

I never got to find out. Before I was able to complete the evaluation and make my recommendations, the courts knuckled under to Beatrice's pressure and sent Marcus back to live with her. It was unclear why this decision was made. The message to Marcus, however, was "Now your weight is down, we don't care what happens to you."

From what I know of other children, what would I predict for Marcus? That he would become depressed and grow up to be a marginal person—one of those who never gets a toehold on life. Chapter 7, "Optimize Feeding: Your Adolescent," explains about emotional competence. Having not developed that competence—having not had the life experiences he needed to learn to make his way—life will be overwhelming for Marcus, and he will get by as best he can. It is hard to know what will happen with his weight. Before, it appeared to stabilize at that high level, but that might not happen again. That enormous weight loss and his likely regain could make it go up higher than ever before.

As from the time he was very young, Marcus's weight will be the least of his problems.

Marcus's case is typical of the few children of extreme size whom I have evaluated. In every case, the child's Z-score had climbed to above 4.0 by age 4 years. In every case, the child had been profoundly neglected. My observations are very similar to those of Stanley Zlotkin, a respected physician and clinical nutritionist from Toronto. Using standardized testing of family functioning, Zlotkin found that family dynamics around massively obese 4- and 5-year-olds was substantially distorted. The preschoolers showed marked behavioral disturbances and were more likely than normal-weight preschoolers to have been reared in extremely disorganized or extremely rigid families.[13]

Clearly, the time to intervene with such children is with the first weight gain. That weight gain must be seen as a sign of profoundly disrupted parenting and failure to *provide*—failure to support the child's normal growth and development. Given the limitations in the current child-welfare system, that is unlikely to happen. However, another possibility would be to get a child like Marcus into Head Start or all-day child care. Certainly those agencies are not in a position to provide remedial care, but they could provide the care and support that appears, for whatever reason, to be beyond the parent. The same holds true for the schools. Marcus was clearly surrounded by caring school professionals who wanted to help him. Conceptualizing his problem as *weight* and the solution as *weight loss* handicapped them all in providing in the best way for him.

WHAT CAN WE LEARN FROM MARCUS?

Marcus's story is extreme, but the message with him is the same as the one presented throughout *Your Child's Weight.* Even in extreme cases, the cause of child overweight is the breakdown of the division of responsibility in feeding. Because of her personal limitations, Beatrice was unable to provide for Marcus in this fundamental and achievable way.

Base Treatment on Careful Assessment

With both extreme and not-so-extreme cases, teasing apart the stories behind the growth charts and assessing the history of a child's overweight brings us back to the same causes listed previously, all growing out of distortion in the division of responsibility in feeding: misinterpretation of normal growth, restrained feeding, poor feeding practices, and stress.

Much of the thinking that goes on around child overweight is muddled. In Marcus's case, the underlying cause was a breakdown in *parenting. Poor parenting* mandated the placement in foster care, not his weight. His weight was a *symptom* of the poor parenting. Without doing a careful assessment, the only legitimate intervention was to optimize feeding. The only legitimate *parenting* intervention was to optimize parenting. They are the same.

Drastic Interventions Without Assessment Are Unjustified

As explained in appendix E, "Assessment of Feeding/Growth Problems," any feeding advice that goes beyond basic good parenting, positive feeding, and supporting normal growth and development is *treatment.* Doing treatment absolutely mandates having a clear understanding of the underpinnings and antecedents of a child's eating problems and weight gain. Imposing a diet, placing a child in foster care for the purpose of weight loss, or doing weight-loss surgery to force weight loss are all drastic interventions. Those interventions can be justified only when a careful evaluation, including assessing feeding and family dynamics, shows that there is *absolutely* no other way of helping the child. In Marcus's case, there was enormous room for improvement before such drastic steps were necessary. I would wager a guess that in all but the rare minority of situations, that is the case.

Expense *Is* Justified

It is time-consuming and therefore expensive to do careful and complete assessments and set up focused treatment plans. However, compared with the cost of repeated weight-loss regimens, high-intensity interventions in obesity specialty clinics, long-term involvement in weight-loss programs and weight-loss surgeries, careful and complete assessment, followed by a focused treatment plan, is a real bargain.

At this time, insurance companies don't pay for doing these assessments. Social services paid part of my costs for Marcus's assessment, but that was unusual. Generally, parents pay for the assessment out-of-pocket and consider the money to be well spent.

In trying to solve their child's eating and weight problem, parents have most often been exposed to a piecemeal approach. Having all the pieces put together comes as a great relief to them. Understanding the stories behind the child's eating and growth puts a whole new perspective on parenting. But going into it, parents have to have great courage and commitment to invite such scrutiny. They do it because they love their children and want the best for them.

DEFINE THE PROBLEM IN A WAY IT CAN BE SOLVED
The story of Marcus highlights the message I have emphasized throughout *Your Child's Weight*. Defining the problem as overweight and the solution as weight loss presents a problem that can't be solved. Weight-reduction efforts are *not* successful, even the most energetic, highest-funded, most carefully constructed ones.[14] Nonetheless, parents, health professionals, teachers, child nutrition programs, mental health professionals, and social service agencies have been assigned the impossible task of slimming children down. On the other hand, the problem of child overweight *can* be solved if we remember that the overweight child is first and foremost a *child*. The primary tasks are *parenting* and *feeding* that child, not keeping or getting him thin.

Prevention of Child Overweight
Child overweight can be *prevented from birth* by feeding and par-

enting well to support the child's own normal growth and development. Both professionals and parents have a role to play.

- Parents can learn recommended feeding practice and *from birth* support their child in growing and developing well.
- Health professionals can teach recommended feeding practice to every parent, whether the child is large or small.
- Teachers can regard a child's size and shape as a given, just like intellect and learning style, and concentrate on what they do best—helping the child to make the most of what nature has provided.
- Child nutrition programs can focus on providing for the child, teaching recommended feeding practice, supporting nutritional status, and sustaining normal growth and development.
- Policy-makers can approach child overweight as a *wellness* issue, rather than one of *illness*. Policies can support normal growth and development rather than emphasizing the diagnosis and treatment of children arbitrarily defined as being overweight.
- Legislators can help parents provide for their children by working toward universal access to health care, funding child nutrition programs and Head Start, supporting minimum wage adequate to support a family, and providing subsidies for quality child care.

Treatment of Weight Acceleration

Rather than defining child overweight as high body weight per se, it can be defined as abnormal growth acceleration for the individual child. Given this redefinition, child overweight can be *treated* by identifying and correcting disruptive influences, restoring optimum feeding and parenting, and allowing the child to go back to growing normally.

For the child whose weight accelerates, a complete assessment can be done to determine the causes of that weight acceleration as outlined in appendix E.

Based on that assessment, a careful treatment plan with follow-up can be organized to help the family change the identified causes of the child's weight acceleration as outlined in appendix F.

Collaboration with other professionals can be arranged to address underlying or exacerbating circumstances. That professional might be a diabetes specialist to address the child's medical care, a family therapist to address patterns that are scapegoating, overprotecting, or neglecting the overweight child, or a social service agency to address issues of child welfare and child protection.

Wrestling with the technicalities of growth charts gives an anticlimactic, but necessary, ending for *Your Child's Weight: Helping Without Harming.* Marcus's story, along with the stories of the other children in this book, makes it abundantly clear: It is far better to prevent than to treat. Good parenting in general, and good parenting with respect to feeding in particular, are critically important in allowing children to grow and develop in ways that are right for them.

NOTES

1. Himes and Dietz, "Guidelines for Overweight."
2. Taylor et al., "Body Fat Percentages."
3. Ryan, Martinez, and Roche, "Socioeconomic Status and the Growth of American Children."
4. Eisenmann et al., "Growth and Overweight of Navajo Youth."
5. Ogden et al., "Prevalence and Trends in Overweight."
6. Ogden et al., "2000 Growth Charts for the United States."
7. Barlow and Dietz, "Obesity Evaluation and Treatment."
8. Hamill et al., "Physical Growth."
9. Tanner, Goldstein, and Whitehouse, "Standards for Children's Height."
10. Serdula et al., "Obese Children."
11. Legler and Rose, "Abnormal Growth Curves."
12. Keys et al., *Biology of Human Starvation..*
13. Zlotkin, S., and A. McGowan, "Family Dynamics Correlates with Massive Obesity in Preschoolers." Verbal communication, 1995.
14. Epstein et al., "Treatment of Pediatric Obesity."

APPENDIXES

SELECTED
REFERENCES

INDEX

APPENDIXES

APPENDIX
A

Position Statement

EATING MANAGEMENT
TO PREVENT AND TREAT
CHILD OVERWEIGHT

The position of the Ellyn Satter Institute is that the clinical definition of child overweight is not high weight per se, but *growth acceleration:* abnormal upward weight divergence for the *individual* child. Based on this clinical definition, each child is compared only to him- or herself, not to statistical cutoff points established for the purpose of population-wide evaluation. This definition avoids labeling as overweight the child whose weight, weight-for-height, or BMI is above a certain percentile but is growing consistently. It also allows identifying for early intervention the child whose measurements fall closer to the mean but who is nonetheless diverging from his or her previously established growth pattern.

Defining child overweight as growth acceleration reframes prevention. Rather than *avoiding overweight,* the emphasis becomes *supporting each child's normal growth.* Thus child overweight can be *prevented from birth* with appropriate feeding. Growth acceleration can be *treated* by examining the underpinnings and antecedents of the divergence, restoring positive feeding, and letting the child's own capability with respect to energy and growth regulation resolve the problem. Each child has a powerful and resilient ability to eat the right amount of food in order to grow in accordance with his or her genetic endowment. However, each child needs appropriate support from parents and other care providers in order to be able to eat and grow well—to manifest that genetic endowment.

Throughout the growing-up years, feeding demands the division of responsibility, with parents and other care providers providing appropriate food and children being allowed to eat as much or as little as they want of what their grown-ups provide. Depending on the child's stage of development, the division of responsibility plays out in different ways:

- The infant eats and grows best when he or she is fed on demand, with parents and other care providers guiding feeding based on information coming from the child with respect to timing, tempo, amount, and level of skill.
- The older baby eats and grows best when parents and other care providers observe the child's individual sequence of oral-motor development and provide appropriately modified food to support the child's gradual transition from semisolid food to soft table food.
- The toddler, preschooler, and older child eat and grow best when they have both structure and support. Parents and other care providers of older children are responsible for the *what, when,* and *where* of *feeding;* children remain responsible for the *how much* and *whether* of *eating.* This division of responsibility continues to be essential throughout the growing-up years.

Professionals who work with children are in a powerful position to teach and support parents in effective, stage-appropriate feeding. Moreover, professionals can help parents accept each child's consistent growth pattern, even when that pattern is outside statistical cutoff points. Finally, early-childhood professionals can do early intervention in response to feeding complaints or minor growth divergences. With early intervention, those minor issues can be kept from escalating into seriously distorted feeding and weight patterns.

For Further Information
Satter, E. M. "Internal Regulation and the Evolution of Normal Growth as the Basis for Prevention of Obesity in Childhood." *Journal of the American Dietetic Association* 96 (1996): 860-864.

Satter, E. M. "Your Child Knows How to Eat and Grow." In *Child of Mine: Feeding with Love and Good Sense,* pp. 31-83. Palo Alto, CA: Bull Publishing, 2000.

Satter, E. M. "Children and Food Regulation: The Research." In *Child of Mine: Feeding with Love and Good Sense,* pp. 478-81. Palo Alto, CA: Bull Publishing, 20000.

APPENDIX B

Principles and Practice

SATTER
FEEDING DYNAMICS APPROACH:
CHILD WEIGHT MANAGEMENT

- *Child overweight can be prevented from birth by optimizing feeding.*
- *Child overweight can be treated by correcting disruptive influences and restoring positive feeding.*

Principles for Practice
1. Emphasize prevention by supporting normal growth and development.
2. Maintain the division of responsibility in feeding.
3. Trust each child to regulate food intake.
4. Trust each child's natural growth tendencies.
5. Preserve each child's eating capability.

Philosophical Framework for Prevention (and Treatment) of Child Overweight
- It is normal for each child to eat the amount needed to grow pre-dictably in accordance with genetic endowment.
- To eat well and grow predictably, the child requires appropriate feeding—and parenting.

- *If that child does not eat and grow appropriately,* something is undermining and distorting the child's natural eating capability.
- *For one child at a time,* that something can be identified and remedied.

Implications for Child Overweight Prevention in Primary Practice
- Support the child's eating capability.
- Ask feeding questions—past and present.
- Teach and restore stage-appropriate feeding.
- Emphasize growth *tracking,* not arbitrary growth cutoffs.
- Support parents in accepting consistent growth, even extreme weight-for-height BMI.
- Make judgments based on *complete* growth history.

Implications for Child Overweight Treatment in Secondary or Tertiary Practice
- Determine the source and the level of the problem.
- Evaluate necessity for tertiary referral.
- Plan behavioral treatment and follow-up.
- Emphasize and restore the division of responsibility in feeding.

APPENDIX
C

CHILDREN
AND FOOD REGULATION:
THE RESEARCH

Children know how much they need to eat, and virtually from birth, they are resilient and resourceful regulators. University of Iowa physician Sam Fomon showed that when infants over age 6 weeks were fed either overconcentrated formula or overly dilute formula, they simply ate less of the concentrated or more of the dilute and grew consistently.[1] Until age 6 weeks, children compensated for variations in formula concentration, but not completely. From age 1 week to 9 months, Houston anthropologist Linda Adair followed the formula- and solid-food-intake of a little boy who was fed on demand. She found that although the infant ate three times as much some days as others, and even though his food intake was lower than 90 percent of other babies, his growth was consistent and his size and shape was average. When he started eating solid foods, he took less formula and continued to regulate well.[2]

From birth, to do well with food regulation, children depend on tuned-in and responsive feeding. In an Edinburgh, Scotland, study with normal, well-born infants, bottle-feeding parents of small babies were more active in feeding, and their babies grew less well than breastfeeding mothers of small babies; the breastfeeding mothers were not overactive in their feeding. Average-sized breast- and bottle-fed babies were fed similarly and grew equally well.[3] With children suffering from growth problems serious enough to be diagnosed as Nonorganic Failure to Thrive (NOFTT), in many if not most cases disruptions in the feeding relationship are at the root of the problem. Clinicians in a Buffalo, New York, hospital found that half of infants hospitalized with growth failure had feeding problems.[4] Feeding problems that can contribute to NOFTT range from too little support of feeding to too much control. Supporting the child in achieving developmental tasks is important in allowing normal eating and growth. In her work with infants and toddlers, Washington, D.C., Children's Hospital psychiatrist Irene Chatoor found that disorders of homeostasis, attachment, and separation/individuation can contribute to NOFTT.[5]

Children's considerable food regulation capability throughout their growing-up years depends on an appropriate division of responsibility in feeding. Both too much control of the child's prerogative in eating and too little support of the child's access to food can cause disruptions in food regulation and growth. Fima Lifshitz, a physician in a pediatric nutrition clinic on the upper east side in New York, has documented over 300 young patients who have eaten and grown poorly when their parents have restricted their food intake. Parents were doing what they thought was right based on scientific warnings about obesity or heart disease.[6] Letting children graze for food can *inadvertently* cause them not to get enough to eat as they fill up on small amounts and don't work up a good appetite for meals. Denver Children's Hospital psychologist Kay Toomey found in her clinical work with poorly eating toddlers that structured feedings allowed toddlers to voluntarily eat 50 percent more than when they were allowed to graze for food.[7] With grazing, the expectation is that children can be mobile and vocal enough to get food for themselves and see to it that they get fed. In an extreme cultural example of toddler grazing, Texas A&M anthropologist Katherine Dettwyler observed New Guinea toddlers roaming the village in groups and eating only if they happened to be present in a home when food was available. Adults did not, in any systematic way, see to it that toddlers got fed. Growth rates of children in New Guinea were very slow.[8]

Research in the University of Illinois preschool laboratories demonstrated that the amount children ate varied throughout the day. Furthermore, children were able to compensate for variations in the amounts they ate at mealtimes and snack times. Most children who got snacks before meals automatically ate less at mealtimes.[9] Colorado Public Health studies that followed children from year to year found that the amounts they ate varied considerably as well as the composition of their food intake. Some years, for instance, they ate far less fat, and other years they ate far more.[10] Even premature babies can regulate. A study conducted by newborn intensive care unit nurses showed that medically stable babies weighing as little as $3^{1}/_{3}$ pounds were able to give signs to their care providers indicating when they were hungry and when they were full. They grew well when they were fed on demand and, in fact, consumed fewer calories than schedule-fed babies and still grew well.[11]

You can't predict how much children will eat. Children of all ages who look alike and act alike may vary from one another in their calorie requirement by as much as 40 percent.[12] This is a result of the children's constitutional endowment, not because of poor patterns of food consumption or activity. Activity patterns, like food regulation and body size and shape, appear to be predominantly determined by genetics. Studies of young infants by Harvard nutritionist Jean Mayer showed that the fattest babies tended to eat the least and were the least active; the leanest babies ate the most and were the most active. The point? Being constitutionally determined, these tendencies can be changed only with extreme effort and at a high risk of destructive consequences.

Although children are good regulators, the way they are fed can undermine their ability to regulate and make them too fat. In my own clinical experience, children can *overeat* as well as undereat when they are allowed to graze for food and beverages. However, most of the research focuses on the negative consequences of *restricting* children's food intake. Most children given snacks before lunch compensated by eating less at lunchtime, but some did not. Those who didn't adjust their intake were children whose eating was controlled too much at home: parents and other adults controlled how much they ate by limiting quantities or by enforcing a clean plate policy.[9] Sometimes this overcontrol is documented indirectly. A 16-year longitudinal study conducted in the San Francisco Bay Area tried to identify differences between infants who became fat as teenagers and those who remained slim. There were no differences between the two groups with respect to family composition, calorie intake, early feeding patterns, and typical food selection, to name a few. However, children who became fat as teenagers were more likely to have had eating problems as preschoolers, and they were more likely to have had parents who were worried that their children would grow up fat.[13] From my clinical experience, I reason that these early eating problems came about when parents were overcontrolling and children were reacting to that control. Parents and children often have feeding struggles when parents try to restrict the amounts children eat. Eating struggles with parents can be so upsetting for children that they lose track of their internal regulators and have trouble eating the amount of food that is right for them.

The tactics parents use to control their own food intake rub off on children, for good or ill. Parents who overcontrol their own eating, with either amount or type of food, tend to throw away all controls from time to time and be fatter than they would be if they ate consistently. Studies at Pennsylvania State University show that children of parents who show this restraint and disinhibition pattern tend to overeat when they are given free access to "forbidden" food. Daughters of mothers who show this pattern are relatively fat.[14] Even without parental patterns of restraint and disinhibition, when children are not regularly allowed access to high-fat or high-sugar snack foods, they tend to overeat on those foods when they get the chance.[15] To head off this feast-and-famine pattern and still retain control of the family menu, serve high-fat foods like chips with the occasional meal or high-sugar foods like cookies for the occasional snack. Let children have as much as they want at those structured times.

Whether an underfed child eats too little, as in the Lifshitz studies,[6] or too much, as in the Pennsylvania State studies,[14,15] depends on who gets the upper hand. The submissive child of a controlling parent may get underfed. A more aggressive child who is able to beat down the parents' limits—at least at times—will likely be fed in a more erratic and inconsistent fashion and be at risk of gaining too much weight.

The point? Children know how much they need to eat, but they need help from adults if they are to act on and retain that capability. Children need to be able to tune in on what goes on inside of them and be aware of how hungry or how full they are. If adults give them insufficient support—don't offer food regularly or fail to offer appropriate emotional support at feeding times—children can have trouble knowing how hungry or how full they are and can eat too little or too much. If adults are too active and controlling in feeding, children experience so much static and interference from the outside that they can't tune in on their own sensations. Sometimes children go along with pressure from the outside and eat more or less than they really want. Sometimes they fight against that pressure and, again, eat more or less than they really want. Either way, they lose sight of how much they need and make errors in regulation. They eat too much or too little and get too fat or too thin.

NOTES

1. Fomon et al., "Influence of Formula Concentration."
2. Adair, "Infant's Ability to Self-Regulate."
3. Crow, Fawcett, and Wright, "Maternal Behavior During Breast- and Bottle-Feeding."
4. Sills, "Failure to Thrive."
5. Chatoor et al., "Non-Organic Failure to Thrive."
6. Lifshitz and Tarim, "Nutrition Dwarfing."
7. Toomey, "Caloric Intake of Toddlers."
8. Dettwyler, "Styles of Infant Feeding."
9. Birch and Fisher, "Appetite and Eating Behavior in Children."
10. Beal, "Dietary Intake of Individuals."
11. Saunders, Friedman, and Stramoski, "Feeding Preterm Infants."
12. National Research Council, *Recommended Dietary Allowances.*
13. Crawford and Shapiro, "How Obesity Develops."
14. Cutting et al., "Like Mother, Like Daughter."
15. Fisher and Birch, "Restricting Access to Food."

APPENDIX
D

This handout is posted at www.EllynSatter.com

  Cooking in
a Hurry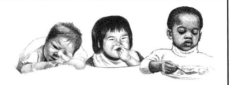

To feed your child–and yourself–well, you must have family meals. However, given the fact that time and energy are in short supply for most parents, remember that good cooking doesn't have to take a lot of time. In fact, it can't, or you simply won't do it. Make yourself into a thinking cook, where you use your head instead of your time and effort. But first of all, adjust your *attitude*. Good nutrition matters, but attitudes toward food are all important. If family mealtimes are regular and enjoyable, your child will enjoy eating, he'll get what he needs, and he'll eat well for a lifetime.

Planning ahead is the key
Do some advance planning for your family meals. That helps when the crunch is on and everybody's hungry and you're tired and you don't feel like cooking. Get things lined up for dinner the night before, while someone *else* does the dishes, so you don't have to tackle it when it's late and you're tired.

Your child can also get involved in preparing meals. If you think through your menus and teach him simple procedures, you'll find he can be a real help to you. You'll have fun together, and he'll be proud of himself.

Avoid common pitfalls in feeding children
Certain traps capture parents again and again and discourage them from making meals. *First*, catering–the feeling of having to please every eater with every food on the table. Instead, plan menus that combine liked and familiar foods with less popular foods, and make sure that there is at least one food on the table that each person *usually* eats. It's okay to be considerate. Plan menus that help you be successful with the meal. Don't, however, cater to whims or short-order cook for him. *Second*, don't try to get food into your child. You only have control over getting a meal on the table and over keeping mealtimes pleasant. You do not have control over whether or not your child eats. *Third*, be realistic about your child's mealtime behavior. He may be erratic and inconsistent with eating. But even if he doesn't eat much, he needs to come to the table, be pleasant to be around, say "yes, please," and "no, thank you," and act his age with eating. *Fourth*, remember

how important you are. The idea of meals is to *eat with* your child, not just *feed* him. Keep mealtimes pleasant–keep the conversation light and positive, don't badger him about eating. *Finally*, avoid over-and under-hunger. To eat well and to be willing to learn to like new food, children need to come to the table hungry but not starved–they need predictable mealtimes and planned snacks between meals.

Look for shortcuts
Today's supermarket is a great help to the busy parent trying to get a meal on the table. Elizabeth Jackson, a registered dietitian and savvy cook, advises, "Use *convenient foods* rather than *convenience meals*." There are many foods you can keep on hand to cut down on preparation time. Your home-cooked meals can be almost as quick–and probably more nutritious–than take-out fast food [see IS FAST FOOD GOOD FOOD?].

Here are some ideas to get you started. You probably won't earn a four-star rating, but the food will taste good and you'll be doing your part to get the family fed.

Grocery list: convenient foods
Meat, poultry, fish, dry beans, eggs, & nuts:
Chicken thighs, boned chicken breasts or stir-fry; frozen fish fillets, canned tuna, or salmon; lean ground beef; boneless pork chops, cutlets, or stir-fry; small ham roasts and slices; stew meat (needs to be cooked slowly); breakfast steaks; prepared meat patties. Canned baked beans, cans or jars of precooked navy beans, garbanzos, black beans, refried beans. Eggs. Peanut butter. Low-fat or regular-fat luncheon meats, sausages, hot dogs.

Milk, yogurt, & cheese:
Preshredded cheese, cheese slices, cheese spread in jars. Milk to drink. Instant and prepared puddings and custards. Plain and flavored yogurt. Canned or dried cream soups reconstituted with milk.

Vegetables:
Frozen potatoes, instant mashed potatoes, boxed scalloped potato mix, canned or frozen vegetables,

fresh cleaned and chopped vegetables from the produce section, preshredded coleslaw mix, peeled tiny carrots, cleaned salad fixings by the pound. Vegetable juices, like tomato juice, vegetable juice cocktail. Flavored canned tomatoes, like Italian, Mexican, Cajun.

Fruits:
Fresh, canned, or frozen fruits and fruit juices. Cleaned and portioned fruits from the produce section. Fruit nectars (apricot nectar is a good source of vitamin A). Dried fruits like raisins, prunes, apricots and peaches. Fig Newtons, raisin cookies.

Breads, cereal, rice, & pasta:
Enriched or whole grain bread. Noodles, macaroni, spaghetti. Rolls, frozen bread dough, corn bread mixes, muffin mix, Bisquick, pita bread and tortillas. Twist-can biscuits and roll dough. Instant plain or brown rice. Pizza bread. English muffins, bagels. Pancake mix.

Grocery list: convenient ingredients
Sauces and seasonings let you put together quick and tasty meals from ready-to-go foods. Ingredients you can keep on hand include spaghetti and other sauces in jars, cream soups, seasonings to sprinkle on (like lemon pepper), to mix in (like taco mix), or to serve on the side (like picante, tartar, or cocktail sauce).

Convenient meals from convenient ingredients and foods
• Spaghetti sauce in jars for spaghetti with meat sauce (you can throw in a few vegetables).
• Cream soups for mixing with cooked meat and rice or noodles.
• Dry taco mix to cook with ground beef for tacos or taco salad.
• Lemon pepper for cooking fish or chicken: use with a little butter or margarine, broil or cook in a frying pan.
• Omelets with microwaved frozen vegetables and grated cheese.
• Scrambled eggs with grated cheese topping.
• Baked potato with melted cheese spread.
• Brown chicken, add Cajun seasoning, simmer with Cajun tomatoes. Same goes for Italian.
• Add-your-own-meat soup mixes: beef vegetable with stew meat or chicken noodle with stir-fry chicken.
• Crock pot stew with stew meat and powdered stew mix or canned golden mushroom soup, and prepared vegetables.
• Homemade pizzas with ready-to-eat crust, canned

pizza sauce, preshredded cheese, prechopped vegetables, lean precooked sausage.
• Stir-fry chicken or pork with prepared vegetables. Season with bottled or dry oriental seasoning mix. Serve with instant rice.
• Scalloped potato mix and pieces of ham.
• Tuna salad with cheese slices on buns, wrapped and baked until the cheese melts.
• Ground beef cooked with mushroom soup and mixed vegetables. Top with Tater Tots and bake until the potatoes are done.
• Simmer chicken breasts ahead of time, cool them and cut them up for salads. Add pasta for a full-meal salad.
• Tuna noodle casserole made from canned tuna, cooked noodles and mushroom soup.
• Hot dogs and buns, baked beans, coleslaw made with preshredded cabbage and coleslaw salad dressing.

Have a variety to choose from
Some meals are complete in themselves; some require a salad, vegetable, or fruit to round them out. Always have bread, no matter what. Children never know what they are going to want to eat, so offer a modest variety. If the dinner is a casserole, offer bread and fruit with it. Your child might be more successful with eating, in fact, if you serve a casserole as a sauce-with-vegetables-and-meat-in-it and the noodles or rice on the side.

Always have something really good
If the meal isn't the greatest, have a wonderful bread. Toast some English muffins or bagels. Have some cream cheese to put on them. Make up a box of cornbread or muffins. If the meat isn't so popular, have corn for a vegetable. Offer a variety of snack crackers with the soup.

Don't make assumptions
Don't assume if a food is spicy, or challenging, or even gourmet, that your child won't like it. Mexican children prefer spicy foods. Brazilian children think black beans are everyday fare. Chinese children like sprouted seeds and beans. Russian children like borscht. Italian food is so much a part of our every-day cuisine that we expect children to learn to like it. If you serve something regularly, enjoy it yourself, and don't force your child to eat it, sooner or later he will learn to like it.

For more about planning and cooking enjoyable, fast and simple family meals, adapting meals for children *and* including your child in meal preparation, see Ellyn Satter's *Secrets of Feeding a Healthy Family*, Kelcy Press, 1999.

APPENDIX
E

ASSESSMENT OF
FEEDING/GROWTH
PROBLEMS

Any feeding advice that goes beyond basic good parenting, positive feeding, and supporting normal growth and development is *treatment*. Doing treatment absolutely mandates doing a careful and detailed assessment to provide a clear understanding of the underpinnings and antecedents of a child's eating problems and causes of weight divergence. I teach that assessment in detail in the "Feeding with Love and Good Sense VISIONS" workshop. Here, I will review that teaching briefly.

It is normal for children to eat well, grow predictably, and love and accept their bodies. When they do not, the organizing question is, "What is interfering with this child's normal ability?" Answering that question requires careful examination of the history and context of the child and the problem. For the younger child, the crosscutting task of the assessment is to explore factors that have contributed and continue to contribute to parents' inability to enact Ellyn Satter's Division of Responsibility in Feeding. For the older child and adolescent, it is to identify the child's capabilities with respect to eating and activity—or lack of them—and to explore the antecedents and underpinnings of those capabilities.

I took a preventive stance in writing *Your Child's Weight*—supporting parents in their task of responsibly and reasonably raising their children to get the body that is right for them. However, *Your Child's Weight* can be used as a *remedial* as well as a *preventive* book by evaluating a given child and situation in the light of optimum developmental and feeding recommendations and identifying and correcting gaps and errors in feeding or parenting. At times, parents can go through the remedial process on their own. Erica's parents, who were introduced in chapter 2, "Feed and Parent in the Best Way," took a clear look at themselves, identified their errors in feeding, and corrected them.

However, in many cases a problem is too established or too complicated for parents to understand and resolve it on their own, even aided by a self-help book such as this one. Typically, an established feeding problem has been dealt with in a piecemeal fashion. Parents have tried repeatedly to solve the problem, without success. They have been given much advice, often contradictory, generally poorly founded. Even in professional practice, feeding advice is often based on feeding lore rather than evidence-based feeding practice.

While all the clinical cases I discuss in *Your Child's Weight* are based on the careful assessment plan I outline here, in three stories the assessment process is particularly apparent. Review the stories of Haley in chapter 6, "Optimize Feeding: Your School-Age Child," and Melissa and Marcus in chapter 10, "Understand Your Child's Growth."

What Causes Established Feeding Problems?

Whatever the presenting complaint, I know at the outset that a major focus of the intervention will be restoring the stage-appropriate division of responsibility in feeding. However, before going ahead with a feeding intervention, it is important to identify the factors that have precipitated and may continue to exacerbate the distortion in feeding dynamics. Parents have reasons for feeding their child the way they do. To let go of their old ways, they need the security of knowing that the problem has been examined thoroughly; all the previous, partial, and counterproductive explanations reviewed and either ruled out or taken into account; and a treatment plan developed that incorporates all considerations. Doing a complete and systematic evaluation is essential to allow the parent to set aside unhelpful explanations and tactics and fully commit to the assessment and treatment plan.

Options for resolving puzzling and seemingly insoluble problems will emerge among the details generated by the assessment. Sally

Provence, a widely known pediatrician who worked in the Yale Child Study Center, encouraged physicians to "embrace complexity" rather than settle for simplistic answers. However, to gather the details, the health professional has to be able to tolerate the anxiety of *not knowing* until the interpretation and solution become apparent.

What could be behind an eating problem? The core of the problem may have been poor feeding practice, often based on unwise advice. The child's own characteristics may have contributed: Her normally large size may have been misinterpreted as overweight, restrained feeding instituted, and the consequently food-preoccupied child over-ate and gained too much weight. The child's continual hunger and food-preoccupation may have permeated her relationships with self and others. As a result, she has strongly learned to misuse food for emotional reasons.

The core of the problem might have been medical and physical. A child with an oral-motor limitation or medical problem was seen as being incapable with respect to eating or medically fragile. Her fright-ened parents responded naturally—and counterproductively—by pres-suring her to eat. The medical or oral-motor problem has since been resolved, but the distorted feeding interactions remain. The distortions have been exacerbated at each stage in development, as parents attempted to compensate for the faulty learning of the stage before.

The root cause of the problem might have been nutrition or food selection. The food might not have been appropriate for the child's oral-motor development at a given stage, or the food was so unappeal-ing, low in fat, or low in calories that the child wasn't interested in eat-ing or couldn't eat enough to grow well.

The problem may have grown out of the parents' agenda for their child's size and shape or their own relationship with food. Chronically dieting parents may have imposed their own food-restriction tactics on their child. Restraining and disinhibiting parents may have pulled their child along with their own cycles of going on and then falling off from diets.

What the Parents Must Provide

To ensure success with the assessment, it is essential to consider both *process* and *content*. Relative to *process*, parents must be clearly informed about the nature and process of the assessment, the reasons for the detailed examination, what they need to provide, and what it will cost. Then they must be supported in choosing to go ahead or not to go ahead at each stage of the assessment. However, parents must be

told that if they choose *not* to have the assessment, then they must settle for the general kind of advice about feeding and parenting that I
give in my books and teaching materials. It's neither possible nor ethi-
cal to give specific advice about particular problems without understanding those problems in detail.

Relative to *content,* issues that impinge on feeding are to be carefully examined: medical, developmental, nutritional, psychosocial, and
feeding dynamics. I explain each in detail below.

To do the assessment, I need complete medical records from birth,
including the narrative. This applies to adolescents as well as to infants
and to every age in between. I need a 7-day food-intake record with
enough detail to allow analysis; videotapes of three or four typical
family meals with all the principal people in place and visible on the
tapes; and information releases to the people who know the child well,
for instance, the physician, a preschool or home room teacher or school
counselor. If there are family meals, I ask for videotapes, no matter the
age of the child.

I analyze all the materials and then set up two or three interviews
with the parents and child. The first interview is with both parents and
child. The parents discuss their concerns with the child and give her an
opportunity to respond. Then I see the child alone, both to get the
child's view of the problem and to get a sense of the child's emotional
and social functioning. I spend a second interview with the parents
alone, getting more detail on the child's developmental history and the
nature of family functioning.

Content of the Assessment

Each part of the assessment has a role to play with respect to getting to
the bottom of the child's eating and growth problem.

- **Medical:** In addition to reviewing clinical records from birth, I
  depend on the child's physician to have done a recent and careful
  physical examination, with parents' concerns in mind, to assure
  us that any medical problems that may contribute to the difficulty
  have been identified. I also talk with the physician about the parents' concerns and get his or her perspective on the child and
  family.

  The narrative from birth in the clinical records often gives
  information about the child and family that parents have forgotten. It also notes medical interventions and advice that may have
  had an impact on feeding. Haley's parents did not remember

being told their 10-month-old daughter was obese and denied restricting her food intake from that time. However, from then on Haley's weight became unstable.

I replot growth data from the clinical record. Growth data may have been incorrectly plotted in the hurry of the clinical setting, and plotting it correctly will change the parents' perception of the child's ability to grow well.

Once the growth chart has been clearly delineated, the task is to tease apart the story the growth chart tells.

- **Developmental:** The growth chart often reflects the degree to which a child has achieved the tasks of each developmental stage. Using the growth chart as a basis for discussion, I ask the parent, "What happened here—and here?" A sudden shift up or down at a given stage generally signals disruption in developmental achievement of that stage. For instance, Haley's rapid weight gain as a toddler provided a clue that she had not fully achieved autonomy. When she got into school, rather than being able to join in comfortably with her peer group, she continued to struggle to keep herself the center of attention. Asking specific, stage-related questions helps bring forth detailed developmental information, although rigid or chaotic families have trouble providing details. The narrative from the medical record is helpful in filling in gaps.

  Because the developmental part of the assessment tends to deal with parenting in general, activity fits in this segment. Managing television use, encouraging and giving opportunities for developmentally appropriate active play, expecting the child to entertain himself, and being able to tolerate reasonable commotion are all parenting issues that can be assessed in a general discussion.

- **Nutrition and food selection:** Based on the interview with the parents and analysis and evaluation of a 7-day food intake record, the nutrition/food selection part of the assessment looks for past or present food- or nutrition-related clues to the child's eating/growth problem. This part of the assessment determines the source of the child's nutritional support (for instance, eating or grazing voluntarily, naso-gastric tube, force-feeding), assesses the child's energy intake and nutritional status, determines whether the food is developmentally appropriate, and looks for evidence of restrained feeding (unusually narrow day-to-day calorie variation or food servings in round numbers) or restraint and disinhibition (unusually wide day-to-day calorie variation).

  Previous, counterproductive nutrition or food selection advice and tactics can contribute to a child's eating and growth problem. Frequently parents have limited the finicky child's menu to food she readily accepts or limited the "overweight" child's menu to drab, unexciting, very low-fat food. While this part of the assessment gives clues for ways parents can improve menu planning, its primary benefit is in ruling out food selection as the basis for the problem and the intervention. Despite the struggles around feeding and the child's erratic eating, most children do well nutritionally. The finicky child's nutrient intake is generally at or near adequate levels; the large child's energy intake is generally well within or even at the low end of normal ranges.

- **Psychosocial:** The psychosocial assessment has to do with the *context* of feeding: the child's overall social and emotional environment as provided by the parent. Since I most often teach this model to health professionals, the goal is to identify dysfunction that is pronounced enough to interfere with eating management and require a referral to social services or to a mental health provider. I encourage my trainees to look for "red flags," such as evidence of abuse or neglect, overly involved or controlling parents, or those who are not involved enough and even laissez-faire. Parents may have rigid agendas, lack empathy for their child, or have little sensitivity for how their own behavior contributes to the problem. Both parents' and children's emotional responses may be out of proportion to the situation at hand. The whole family may overreact to moderate issues or underreact to serious ones.

  Some family dysfunction may be temporary, precipitated by crisis. For instance, when a child has first been diagnosed with a severe illness, otherwise functional parents may become enmeshed and overprotective at the one extreme or may distance themselves emotionally from the child at the other. They may become more rigid and controlling than usual or go to the other extreme and become chaotic.

- **Feeding/eating dynamics:** Whatever the precipitating or exacerbating causes of the eating and growth problem, the feeding relationship will be affected. Parents and children will be crossing the lines of the division of responsibility in feeding. For the younger child, accurate assessment requires *observation* of the feeding interaction; parent report is not accurate or sufficient. Such observation is also helpful for the older child, but in the absence of family meals, it is necessary to make do with extrapolating from in-office interactions. Parents who are controlling or disengaged in office interactions are likely to be the same with respect to feeding and parenting overall.

Since parents' eating attitudes and behaviors impinge directly on the child's feeding problem, I assess parents' eating competence as well, using my own questionnaire, "About Your Eating." The questionnaire assesses eating attitudes, food regulation, and food-acceptance behaviors and the ability to manage food context: feeding themselves (and their family) regularly. I use the same questionnaire with teenagers, although I assume scores on food context will be low.

Detecting and explaining feeding distortions draws on information gleaned from the rest of the evaluation. Child temperamental characteristics such as negativity, irritability, or exaggerated caution may call out overactive or intrusive feeding behaviors. Medical issues, particularly life-threatening ones, are virtually guaranteed to distort feeding dynamics as frightened parents try to ensure their child's nutritional well-being or even survival. Parents' own learning about nutrition, food selection, or eating may be faulty. An exceptionally large or small child may challenge parents' ability to be trusting with respect to feeding.

Once the assessment and the treatment plan is in place, parents can be told in detail what caused the problems with their child's eating and growth. Growing out of that detailed problem identification, they can be provided with a detailed treatment plan. That treatment plan and its enactment will be reviewed in appendix F, "Treatment of Feeding/Growth Problems."

APPENDIX
F

TREATMENT OF
FEEDING / GROWTH
PROBLEMS

For parents of children with long-standing eating problems, making fundamental changes requires a leap of faith and steady nerves. The child will most likely eat a considerable amount before he rediscovers his internal regulators of hunger, appetite, and satiety. During the transition, parents have to resist the urge to compensate for their child's eating extremes and instead must continue to maintain Ellyn Satter's Division of Responsibility in Feeding. Holding steady with respect to feeding in the presence of the child's eating extremes assures the child that his parents truly will feed him as much as he wants to eat. Then he will regain his sensitivity to his internal regulators of hunger, appetite, and satiety, and his eating will moderate.

To initiate and persist with such fundamental change, parents have to be fully satisfied that all issues have been considered and that they are doing the right thing. Giving them—and yourself—that reassurance requires the thorough assessment described in appendix E, "Assessment of Feeding/Growth Problems."

Ten follow-up sessions are generally enough to help parents and children through the transition. Parents need weekly follow-up for 6 or 7 weeks until they establish positive feeding. Within that time their child will have had time to show clear evidence of food regulation. After that, the task is consolidating change. Then biweekly sessions, and toward the end, even monthly sessions are adequate. Parents must give careful attention to the detail of the treatment plan for at least 3 months before the child accepts that the change is there to stay and truly develops new patterns. However, parents can't revert to the old ways of feeding or the child will revert to the old eating problems.

The Treatment Plan
The details of the treatment plan, of course, vary depending on the details of the assessment. However, figure F.1 lists the fundamental features of every treatment plan.

Doing Follow-up
In follow-up, I support parents in sorting out and maintaining the division of responsibility in feeding, help them detect and eliminate their patterns of food restriction, help them find ways to reassure to their child that he will be fed, and help them detect evidence of their child's internal regulation.

Sort Out the Division of Responsibility in Feeding Here are some typical questions that arise in follow-up.

- **Isn't it controlling to be so rigid about meal and snack times?** No, it is taking responsibility for what is yours. Your child needs the structure and still has lots of room for choices.
- **Isn't it restrained feeding to not let a child eat between times?** No, he isn't being deprived. He has plenty of opportunity to get as much as he wants at regular eating times.
- **How much bread should we put on the table?** A *lot*.
- **Is it all right if our child eats that much bread?** Yes. He will tire of it and eventually eat something else.
- **Shouldn't the child be eating his vegetables?** He will eat vegetables when he is ready. In the meantime, keep including them in meals and enjoying them yourself.
- **Is it restrained feeding if we don't have enough strawberries to let everyone eat their fill?** No, as long as there is something else to fill up on.
- **Is it really all right to let him fill up on cookies at snack time?** Yes. At first he will eat a lot, but after the newness wears off he will be satisfied with fewer cookies.

FIGURE F.1 TREATMENT PLAN: THE PARENTS' TASKS AND THE CHILD'S

The Parents' Tasks
- Restore the stage-appropriate division of responsibility in feeding.
- Provide regular and predictable meals and sit-down snacks.
- Make mealtime and snack time pleasant by eating and being companionable with the child.
- Plan menus with a variety of appealing food; don't exclude high-calorie food.
- Let the child eat much or little or nothing at all from what parents provide.
- At every regular eating time, give the child strong permission to eat what and how much he wants from what parents provide.
- Provide rewarding and filling food for snacks, including "forbidden" food.
- Don't allow grazing for food or beverages (except water) between times.
- With the child older than about age 10, provide treatment to help him to recover his sensitivity to his internal regulators of hunger, appetite, and satiety.
- Limit television watching to one or two hours daily.
- Help the child find ways to enjoy moving his body, experiencing himself as physically capable.
- Let his weight do what it will based on positive parenting and feeding.

The Child's Tasks
Starting at age 8 to 10 years, the child has jobs as well. Here is a typical list of those jobs:

- Do your eating at mealtime and snack time.
- Pick and choose from the foods your parents offer you for meals and snacks.
- Go to the table hungry and eat until you are satisfied.
- Pay attention while you eat.
- Be good company at the table.
- Ask your parents to include the "forbidden" food you like.
- Sneak up on new food and learn to like it.
- Point out to your parents—politely—when they are taking over your jobs with eating.

Detect Tendencies to Restrict Food Intake Parents' tendencies to restrict food intake are so deeply ingrained, automatic, and culturally reinforced that it can be surprising and even discouraging for parents to detect and get rid of those tendencies. If the child continues to be food-preoccupied or periodically disinhibits, parents are restricting in some way, perhaps without realizing it. Identifying and discontinuing that restriction is absolutely essential or treatment will fail.

- **Is it all right to run out of our child's favorite food so he will eat something else?** No. Deliberately running out of his favorite food is manipulative, and your child will catch on and not trust you.
- **Is it all right to use low-calorie salad dressing and margarine?** No. Your child depends on your including high-fat food with meals in order to eat the calories he needs and get pleasure and satisfaction from his meals. Using low-fat foods to get your child to eat fewer calories is restrained feeding.
- **He forgot his snack. Shall I just let it go?** You have to be the one to remember the snack. Remind him: "It is time for snack. If you don't have it now, you will have to wait for dinner."
- **He eats so *fast*. He guards his plate and just wolfs his food down. Shouldn't I make him slow down?** Once he learns to trust you to give him as much as he wants and not to be critical, he will slow down and stop guarding his plate.
- **Is it all right to just give him fruit for snack? Otherwise, he won't eat his dinner.** He needs something more substantial than fruit. Move snack time earlier so he has time to get hungry for dinner.
- **What about a bedtime snack? It seems like he shouldn't have that if he doesn't eat his dinner!** Using snacks to put leverage on meals makes your child overeat. He isn't trying to get around you—he does the best he can with his dinner. Young children especially find grown-up dinnertime food challenging. They are tired, and they have been eating all day. Have your dessert at dinner; then have the bedtime snack be good but unexciting— cereal and milk, cheese, crackers, and juice. Then trust your child to do well with his eating.

Reassure the Child He Will Be Fed Finding ways to reassure the child that he will be fed—*and really meaning it*—speeds the child's process of learning to trust and therefore being able to detect his internal regulators. In order to stop eating when he is comfortably full but not stuffed, he has to be sure that another meal or snack is coming soon and he can again have as much as he wants to eat. How can parents provide that reassurance?

- Put the food on the table in serving bowls so the child can help himself.
- Make sure there is *plenty* of food. Leftovers provide reassurance that everyone has had enough to eat.
- Offer more food, but don't urge or insist.
- Be prompt and matter-of-fact about giving second and third helpings, even if he seems to eat *a lot.*
- Don't worry at first about wasting food. After your child is fully reassured that he will get enough to eat, he can learn ways to cut down on waste. Remember, however, that food waste is an inevitable part of feeding children.
- When in doubt, ask yourself, "What would I do if I weren't worried about his weight?" If you would do it in parenting a "normal" child, it is likely to be okay.

Detect the Child's Internal Regulation Finally, parents depend on follow-up to help them detect evidence of their child's internal regulation. An early sign of internal regulation might be that a child leaves a little food on his plate or forgets about snack time. Rather than celebrating leftover food and skipping the snack, the parent can reassure the child by saying "Are you sure you have had enough? That's it until snack time," or "It's time for your snack." In a backward sort of way, being firm about structured eating times reassures the child that his hunger is not the fearsome thing it once was. He can tolerate his hunger because he can count on being filled up at the next meal or snack. A child might show evidence of internal regulation by not finishing his food and then reassure himself that he will be fed by asking to save something for a snack.

Together or Apart?
The age of the child determines the structure of treatment sessions-whether you treat parents alone, parents and children together, or parents and children separately.

Children Up to Age 10 Years For children up to about 10 years of age, treatment goes best with parents alone. With younger children, parents have enough control of the child's eating environment that they can turn the situation around on behalf of the child. Once positive feeding is restored, children evolve sensitivity to their internal regulators on their own.

Children Age 10 to 12 Years For the child from roughly 10 to 12 years old, it works best to have sessions with both parents and children together. These older children have more autonomy and are learning to manage some food selection and schedule keeping on their own. They benefit from the discussions in the sessions.

In addition, parents and children can be helpful to each other in sorting out the boundaries of the division of responsibility and arriving at reasonable rules and expectations. Of course, parents must remember that while school-age children can be good collaborators in working out rules, it is up to parents to enforce them. Children still try to get around even their own rules. Parents must also remember their own authority—they don't have to stand over their child to enforce the rules. The school-age child is on his own for lunch and after-school snack. It is legitimate for parents to expect him to use the lunch money they provide for the regular school lunch menu, not the a la carte menu, and to have a get-your-snack-by-this-time rule.

Adolescents Since adolescents are working on autonomy, and since parents are working on playing a supportive role, parents and adolescents benefit from having separate sessions, with the occasional session together. The focus of parents' sessions is essentially what I detailed earlier: Sort out the division of responsibility in feeding, detect tendencies to restrict food intake, find ways to reassure the child he will be fed, and learn to detect evidence of the child's internal regulation. If parents lack eating competence, they also benefit from recovering their internal regulators.

The focus of the child's sessions is recovering eating competence, initially around internal regulation of food intake. While the child's food acceptance may also be severely impaired, focusing on that too soon turns the intervention into a diet rather than an initiative toward eating competence. Individual sessions help the adolescent tune in on hunger, appetite, and satisfaction. To support their internal regulators, adolescents can learn to take responsibility for timing and food selection to provide themselves with structured and rewarding eating times throughout the day. They can also learn to depend on parents to provide them with a reliable evening meal.

Negotiating the timing, content and process of afternoon snacks and the evening meal demands joint sessions. Children and parents differ on when and what to eat, emotional climate, and who gets to say what shall and shall not happen. All of those issues can and must be sorted out in order to preserve the family meal.

APPENDIX
G

FEEDING AND PARENTING IN
THE SCHOOL SETTING

This is a *yay-boo* story. Concern about child weight issues has focused energy and interest on the school nutrition program. *Yay!* This concern often translates into restrained feeding. *Boo!* Restricting children's food intake makes them food-preoccupied and prone to overeat when they get the chance. Chapter 2, "Feed and Parent in the Best Way," and chapter 4, "Help Without Harming: Food Selection," cover many of the forms restrained feeding can take: restricting dietary fat, trying to get children to fill up on vegetables and fruit, emphasizing "proper" portion sizes, urging children to eat healthy foods.

Making slimming children down the priority of school nutrition programs distorts their true mission. Our first responsibility with respect to feeding children is nurturing them: reassuring them that we will take care of them and providing them with the nutrients and energy they need to be healthy and grow well physically, emotionally, socially, and mentally. For children to learn well, they must be fed.

Restriction Doesn't Work
Instituting restrained feeding in a school setting to slim children down

has been tried, and it doesn't work. In an intervention with third- to fifth-grade children in the public schools of Kearney, Nebraska, school lunch fat percentage in intervention schools was cut to 25 percent and school physical activity and school nutrition education increased. At the end of 2 years, study children were no slimmer and, based on 24-hour observations, ate no less fat and were no more active than children in control schools. In those control schools, fat percentage was 35 percent and school physical activity was the same as usual. Children compensated at home for the interventions at school. In fact, they even compensated at school. Children who were offered 25 percent fat lunches actually ate 31 percent of their calories as fat. Children offered 35 percent ate 33 percent.[1] Children are excellent regulators and compensate intuitively and nimbly for variations in their nutritional environment.

Using essentially the same interventions as the Kearney study, the highly funded 3-year Pathways study targeted almost 1,800 third-through fifth-grade native American children in 41 schools in four western states. The intervention resulted in no significant changes in energy intake, physical activity, or percentage body fat, although the percentage of fat *served* to the children in school meals was reduced. The children *did* have an increase in food- and health-related *knowledge.*[2] In other words, they knew what they were *supposed* to be doing, even if they weren't doing it. While this seems to be a desirable outcome, the reality is that the children had been taught that what they usually ate—or what their parents fed them—was undesirable and nutritionally inferior. They learned to be ashamed of their food.

Still another study was the highly funded Child and Adolescent Trial for Cardiovascular Health (CATCH) study, sponsored by the National Institutes of Health. In 56 schools, 5,106 third-grade children were targeted with school food service modifications, enhanced physical education, and classroom health curricula teaching children to avoid dietary fat and become more active. The goal was to improve children's blood pressure, blood cholesterol, and body weight. The outcomes of the CATCH intervention were virtually identical to the those of the two studies just cited. Over the 3 years of the trial, the percentage of energy from fat in school lunches decreased (from 38.7 percent to 31.9 percent) compared to lunches in control schools (fat percentage fell from 38.9 percent to 36.2 percent). The intensity of physical activity in CATCH-targeted physical education classes increased compared with the control schools. Unlike the Kearney study, there were no 24-hour assessments of food intake or activity, assessment of at-home changes, or 24-hour changes. The CATCH curriculum taught third- through fifth-graders to avoid dietary fat. Then the children were asked how much fat they ate. They said they ate less. The target children were taught to pursue vigorous physical activity; then they were asked how much time they spent being vigorously active. They said they spent more. Blood pressure, body size, and cholesterol measures did not differ significantly between treatment schools and the control schools.[3] Because they want to achieve and to please their grown-ups, asking third- to fifth-graders about their changes in food selection and physical activity is not an adequate outcome measure. Only observation is accurate, but those data were not collected.

Coercion Doesn't Work Either

If we try to encourage, pressure, reward, or educate children to eat certain foods, they get turned off to those foods and are less likely to eat them.[4] If we try to deprive children of certain foods, they become more interested in those foods and are inclined to overdo on them when they get the chance, even when they aren't hungry. Compared with children who are not deprived, treat-deprived children are heavier.[5] If we manage children's portion sizes, they lose track of their internal eating capability—they learn to eat the amount that is on the *plate*, rather than the amount they are *hungry for*.[6]

Standard approaches to nutrition education teach children to go by the rules of food selection and regulation rather than continue to depend on their internal regulators of hunger, appetite, and satisfaction. Children are taught the Food Guide Pyramid, portion size, the dos and don'ts of food selection, and the nutritional desirability of eating right. After an enormous review of nutrition education programs for children, university specialists found that such coercive, restrictive programs didn't work. The few programs that were successful in bringing about even minor changes in the way children ate were programs that were not coercive. Those programs took significant time to let children eat or work with food and involved families, schools, and communities.[7] After a thorough review of environmental influences on children's eating, other nutrition educators reminded readers that basic respect for the family unit was the essential means of ensuring children's health and well-being.[8]

Basic respect for the family unit means honoring what the family eats and is able to provide. Nutrition lessons can introduce children to new and different food. Children can go home and talk about that food with their parents, and some parents may choose to include new foods on the family menu. If nutrition messages are kept neutral, the family is involved without being criticized. But nutrition lessons that say "ice cream is bad" or "fat is bad" (or "broccoli is bad," for that matter) undermine the family and the child as well.

If Deprivation and Coercion Don't Work, What Does?

What is the likelihood that the average school district will be able to slim children down when ambitious, multimillion-dollar programs have not? Slim to none. In fact, none. On the other hand, what is the likelihood that the average school district can optimize feeding and opportunities to be active and support children's natural growth processes? Lots better, but these tasks aren't easy either. As you learned in chapter 1, "Help Without Harming," here is what that optimizing would look like:

- Feed and parent in the best way, including providing filling, well-timed meals and safe places for children's natural activity.
- Maintain Ellyn Satter's Division of Responsibility in Feeding. Adults do the *what*, *when*, and *where* of feeding; children do the *how much* and *whether* of eating.
- Let each child grow up to get the body that is right for him or her.
- Maintain Ellyn Satter's Division of Responsibility for Physical Activity. Adults are responsible for *structure, safety,* and *opportunities;* children are responsible for *how much* and *whether* they are active.
- Love children just the way they are—fat, thin, or in between—and raise them to be capable.
- Do what schools do best: Teach children to make the most of what they have.

Set Clear and Collaborative Policies About Food Selection

People rarely come right out and say this, but the two major philosophies about school menu planning are give-them-what-they-will-eat at the one extreme and school-nutrition-as-education at the other. Give-them-what-they-will-eat school nutrition programs make pizza, chicken nuggets, and tacos menu mainstays. The school-nutrition-as-education programs make an effort to introduce children to a variety of food and help them to increase their mastery with food acceptance. They might even experiment with salad bars or taco buffets.

While I will make no bones about preferring the second, children get regular and reliable meals either way. The bottom line is that children must be fed. Children with disorganized families and those of limited economic circumstances depend on school nutrition programs to provide for them.

School-nutrition-as-education programs are more empowering for children. Schools can help children and parents by exposing children to foods they don't get at home and by teaching them food acceptance skills. Throughout life, people do best nutritionally when they have these skills—when they can be relaxed in the presence of new foods, gradually learn to like those foods, and throughout life increase their repertoire of preferred foods.

However, committing to school-nutrition-as-education is a collaborative process in which everyone has to be on board. School nutrition personnel play the key parental role with respect to feeding by maintaining the division of responsibility and providing a positive mealtime environment. However, they can play this role only if they are backed up by parents, school board members, teachers and aids, administrators, support and office personnel, and the janitor. I am not kidding about the janitor. He or she is a high-status person in most schools and is in a position to support or undermine the learning that goes on there.

Anybody who has worked toward collaboration and consensus on any issue knows that such work is a time-consuming, delicate, and potentially acrimonious process. For that matter, making the give-them-what-they-will-eat choice requires commitment and cooperation from all the major players as well. However, since the give-them-what-they-will-eat approach most closely resembles current feeding norms, instituting it does not require as much learning and cooperation on everyone's part. But keep in mind that even if schools take this approach, every school nutrition program is mandated by law to provide one-third of a child's daily nutritional requirement at lunch, one-quarter at breakfast. And they do it, on budgets so tight they squeak.

Adults Agree and Support the Program

To optimize feeding in school nutrition programs, each of the major players listed earlier must be willing to put aside his or her personal food preferences, dietary hobbyhorses, and cherished school-nutrition criticisms and support the program on behalf of the children. We have a long tradition of picking on school nutrition programs—"too much starch," "too much grease," "not enough vegetables"—everyone has an ax to grind. We all have our food traditions and feel strongly about them, but when we criticize or disdain the food they depend on, children feel ashamed of eating it and liking it.

I realize that asking for everyone's support is asking a lot. It means that nobody gets catered to—not the meat-and-potato eaters or the tortilla eaters or the chapati eaters or the low-carbohydrate dieters or the vegetarians. Parents are certainly entitled to follow their convictions and preferences at home, and children learn to eat and prefer the foods their parents provide. However, schools can't do their job of feeding children and still cater to each child all the time.

Establish the Primary Goal of Helping Children Grow Up with Respect to Eating

School nutrition programs can expose children to nutritious foods they don't get offered at home. Children benefit from learning to manage unfamiliar food and to respect foodways that are different from their own. Challenges with food acceptance are the same as every other challenging life circumstance. Children can cope. In the Head Start program, where teaching children mealtime skills is an important part of the curriculum, children who have never sat at a table learn mealtime skills. They learn to be polite about turning down food they don't want to eat, to eat food that is not catered specifically to their individual likes and dislikes, to respect what their friends like, and to like those foods as well. Children in school settings can do the same.

However, in order for children to learn, their grown-ups must be clear about expectations. Since we can't take children any further than we have gone ourselves, either we must have mastered those capabilities or we must take ourselves out of the running as role models. In the best of all possible worlds, school personnel would eat in the lunchroom. That is undoubtedly the impossible dream, but being positive about the nutrition program and withholding criticism is not.

Children can grow up with respect to food regulation as well. If all has gone well at home, children come to school with a well-established intuitive ability to eat the right amount of food to grow well. Grown-ups put a meal on the table. The child eats until she is satisfied; then she stops, knowing another meal or another snack is coming and she can do it again—and again—and again. Rather than teaching children food restriction and portion size, the school can teach children about internal regulation-to consciously identify and preserve their internal regulators of hunger, appetite, and satisfaction. See chapter 10, "Raising a Healthy Eater in Your Community," of *Secrets of Feeding a Healthy Family* for more on teaching food acceptance and food regulation.

Evaluate the Program in the Context of Children's Eating Behavior
As children learn to cope, all the major players must know what to
expect from their eating behavior. Otherwise, they will assume children are doing poorly with respect to eating and lose courage about
supporting the program.

Children eat erratically. Some days they eat a lot; other days they eat
only a little. Some days they eat some of everything that is put in front
of them; other days they eat only one or two foods. Some days they *love*
a particular food; other days they ignore that food completely. They eat
what *tastes* good to them on a given day at a given meal. They don't eat
a food because they have been taught that it is good for them. They eat
only what tastes good, and that varies from one day to the next.

Some children come to school with limitations in their mealtime
and food acceptance skills and need extra help in order to be successful. Consider Kenny, who was freaked out by the tacos at school lunch.
Consider Kenny's mother, a good home cook who was offended by the
strange food at school and incensed that the lunch ladies wouldn't just
give her son meat and potatoes like she did.

Why was Kenny so freaked out about the tacos? Why didn't he
just not eat them? Because the rule in his family was that you had to
eat what was on your plate. He could clean his plate at home because
everything was familiar. At school, it was a different matter. Kenny and
his mother both settled down when they understood that every meal
would have something that Kenny could fill up on and that he didn't
have to eat anything he didn't want to.

Plan Menus to Support Children's Eating Capabilities
The National School Lunch Program mandates that participating
schools must serve lunches with 30 percent or less of calories from fat.[9]
In my view, that percentage is too low*. Relative to health issues, I
have supported my arguments elsewhere.[10,11] Relative to supporting
children in learning food acceptance, higher-fat food tastes better.
Relative to practicality, it is far easier and less expensive for food service personnel to provide appealing and varied menus if they have
more fat to work with.

Rather than trying to control children's overall fat intake, I would

---

* Fat intake would still be moderate if programs aimed for 35 percent fat overall, 12 to 15 percent saturated fat. Even better, limiting saturated fat could be
accomplished by using a variety of fat sources, including those that provide
monounsaturated and saturated fat.

recommend offering a range of mealtime food—high-fat, moderate-fat, low-fat—and letting children pick and choose from what we have made available. This recommendation is in line with the Centers for Disease Control *School Health Index,* which encourages the *inclusion* of low-fat items.[12] Research shows that when children's energy needs are high, they automatically eat higher-calorie foods. When their energy needs are low, they eat lower-calorie foods.[13] The children in the Kearney, Nebraska, study mentioned earlier in this appendix[1] demonstrated this principle.

The practice of selling a la carte foods interferes with planning menus that support children's eating capabilities. Against their better judgment and wishes, nutrition programs sell a la carte foods item-by-item on the lunch line to make money to support their programs. They are forced into taking advantage of children in order to keep their programs going. Because a la carte foods tend to be high-sugar, high-fat, familiar and therefore easy for children to like, they compete unfairly with the standard menu. It is like having a dessert buffet at every family meal. How interested will your child be in learning to eat vegetables if he can fill up on unlimited amounts of dessert?

Consider Competitive Foods in the Context of Child Development

Competitive foods—foods in vending machines, snack bars, school fund drives, and parties—undermine children's ability to do well nutritionally. Like a la carte foods, competitive foods exploit children as a way of funding programs. However, unlike the a la carte foods, these competitive foods are sold to support any number of school programs totally unrelated to child nutrition.

The main problem with competitive foods is that they interfere with structure. Children who are allowed to eat all the time don't get hungry enough to do a good job at mealtime of eating the amount they need and learning to like new food. Instead of going to the table hungry and eating until they are satisfied, they just top themselves up. Children who are allowed to graze and spoil their appetites for meals have no reason to sneak up on new food and learn to like it.

Children who are allowed to eat off and on all day often have trouble eating the right amount to grow appropriately. Some eat too much and get fat. Some eat too little and get thin. Some have so much capability with food regulation that they eat what they need and grow the same. Since we don't know which child is which, we have no choice but to provide all children with structured mealtimes.

Nutritious foods spoil children's appetites for lunch at school and dinner at home just as much as nonnutritious ones do. Juices are as filling as soda, and they are equally likely to rot teeth. Fruit is not as calorically dense as candy, but children who fill up on fruit are still not interested in lunch. Vending machines, snack bars, and parties tend to offer the same foods over and over again. If familiar, easy-to-like, filling food is readily available, children take the path of least resistance. They don't experiment with the food in the school nutrition program and at the family dinner table.

Feed in Developmentally Appropriate Ways

Policies on competitive and a la carte foods must differ depending on children's developmental stage. Grade-school and middle-school-age children are still forming their food habits. Developmentally, they depend on their grown-ups to give them guidance in what they need to learn. Keeping control of the menu and holding down on competitive and a la carte foods supports their learning to like a variety of foods.

High school-age children, on the other hand, have developed their food habits, for good or ill. For them, the next step is defining identity with respect to eating. In order to take those developmental steps, children of this age experiment and even do risky things with respect to their eating, just as they do in every other part of their lives.

For adolescents, it is wise to liberalize guidelines on competitive and a la carte foods and structure. Using commercial franchises in the school cafeteria is not so bad at this age. Why? Because if children don't get it at school, they leave school to get it. High school-age children need a greater scope for experimentation; children in grade school and middle school need grown-ups to provide for them.

High school-age children have such a strong drive for autonomy and identity that they defy restriction. Schools that try to tightly control the high school food environment will precipitate students' breaking the rules and support a black market in forbidden food.

How Is This Approach Different?

Readers familiar with the standard School Nutrition Program policies and tools are likely to be comparing and contrasting my recommendations with existing guidelines. These instruments come from the United States Department of Agriculture, the Centers for Disease Control, the American School Food Service Association, and the National Association of State Boards of Education.[9,14-16] Those organizations emphasize food selection as their primary intervention, control portion size and fat content of meals, and teach and persuade children to eat certain foods and not to eat others.

I emphasize feeding behavior and positive parenting with respect to food (including choosing menus and maintaining structure). Then I trust children to bring themselves along with food acceptance and to do a good job with food regulation. It is a subtle but enormous difference. The standard approach sees children as being defective—as needing to be restrained so they don't get too fat. My approach sees children as being competent. Based on experience and the research, my absolute conviction is that if we put children in a positive food environment, we can trust them to eat and grow in a way that is right for them.

NOTES

1. Donnelly et al., "Nutrition and Physical Activity Program."
2. Caballero et al, "Pathways."
3. Luepker et al., "Field Trial to Improve Children's Dietary Patterns."
4. Birch, Johnson, and Fisher, "Children's Eating."
5. Fisher and Birch, "Eating in the Absence of Hunger."
6. Johnson and Birch, "Parents' and Children's Adiposity."
7. Lytle and Achterberg, "Changing the Diet of America's Children."
8. Crockett and Sims, "Environmental Influences on Children's Eating."
9. Food and Nutrition Service, "Team Nutrition, National School Lunch Program." Web page [accessed 16 January 2004]. Available at http://www.fns.usda.gov/cnd/lunch/.
10. Satter, "Children, Dietary Fat, and Heart Disease."
11. Satter, "Moderate View on Fat Restriction."
12. Centers for Disease Control and Prevention, *School Health Index for Physical Activity, Healthy Eating, and a Tobacco-Free Lifestyle: A Self-Assessment and Planning Guide. Elementary School Version, Module 4: Nutrition Services.*
13. Kern et al., "The Postingestive Consequences of Fat."
14. Centers for Disease Control and Prevention, *School Health Index for Physical Activity, Healthy Eating, and a Tobacco-Free Lifestyle: A Self-Assessment and Planning Guide. Middle School and High School Version.*
15. American School Food Service Association, "Keys to Excellence." Web page [accessed 16 January 2004]. Available at http://www.asfsa.org/.
16. National Association of State Boards of Education, "Healthy Schools."

APPENDIX
H

DEVELOPMENT OF
PHYSICAL SELF-ESTEEM:
BIRTH THROUGH
ADOLESCENCE

As in other areas of their lives, children develop physical self-esteem step-by-step. What they discover and come to feel about themselves when they are little provides the foundation for their learning and attitudes at each stage of development. If all goes well, as children grow and mature, their attitudes and capabilities with respect to physical self-esteem become more and more empowered—and empowering.

Toddlers and Preschoolers
Toddlers and preschoolers want to know what their bodies *are*. They don't make value judgments. Young children accept their bodies as a given; they are curious about them and find out about them by *moving* them. If they contrast and compare their own body with another person's, it is to learn more about themselves. They learn words for their body parts; they examine their belly buttons, toes, and genitals. As they get older, they learn about the broader aspects of shape and size. Kindergartners love to draw around their hands or have their friends draw their outlines on big pieces of paper. They don't make judgments. For young children, being critical of their own or others' size

and shape is a perversion introduced by adults—by parents, teachers, or coaches.

Parents and other adults can help by liking and accepting the child's body just the way it is—skinny or fat, short or tall, big or little, and protecting the child from judgments. They can help by being realistic and tolerant of young children's levels of activity. They can give structure, safe and interesting places for children to move, and limits so children don't overwhelm themselves and other children with their energy and aggression.

Throughout the growing-up years, parents also help children with physical self-esteem by liking and accepting their *own* bodies. Children are very tuned in to their elders and constantly try to figure things out. It is not lost on children when parents make derogatory remarks about their own bodies, go on weight-reduction diets, or decry their inability to lose and maintain weight. Those actions and attitudes introduce children to the idea that, rather than accepting and getting to know their body, they should be assessing and criticizing it and trying to change.

School-Age Children

School-age children want to know what their body can *do*. In contrast to younger children, who learn by doing, they *think* about that capability and deliberately *work* on it. They try out their strength, speed, and coordination. They experiment with various activities to find out what appeals to them. Once they choose, they practice an activity over and over again to get it right.

If all goes well, school-age children are unselfconscious about size and shape. They eat the food that is put in front of them, accept their size and shape as givens, use their body in ways that feel good, master activities that they value, and live in the body they have. On the other hand, school-age children's drive to *do* makes them vulnerable to the idea that their body must be *changed* in order for them to achieve. A gymnastics teacher or soccer coach might introduce that notion by suggesting that they could do better—or look better doing—if they were thinner.

The saving grace as well as the pitfall for the school-age child is that he respects his grown-ups and uses them as models in working toward being grown up. Parents are helpful in protecting children's physical self-esteem when they do consciousness-raising with coaches and teachers and even pull children out of activities in which that self-esteem is being undermined. Parents *can* make a difference, because they continue to be of primary importance. Children pick up their parents' attitudes and convictions and learn whether their interests, capabilities, and characteristics are satisfactory. Parents are *not* helpful when they criticize their own bodies and diet to change them.

Young Adolescents

Early in adolescence, children become concerned with whether their body is *acceptable to peers*. The major theme is *autonomy*, as a child learns to make it in a teenage world. Early adolescence challenges physical self-regard as children strike out on their own from parents and focus on peers. They get more concerned about size, shape, and physical attractiveness as they evaluate themselves and others, often in the midst of rapid bodily changes.

The young adolescent wants to know what her body *looks like*. Toward the end of the school-age years-around ages 11 to 13 or now even as early as age 9—children begin to look in the mirror a lot and wonder what nature will do for—or to—them. During these early adolescent years, interest in size, shape, and sexual development begin to merge with social consciousness and revolve around self-esteem overall. Children continue to try things out and find out what is a good fit, from playing sports to learning to use the computer to playing a musical instrument to "going together." As you may know, going together at this age involves saying they like each other and might go so far as to include standing together on the playground. Children this age want to have boy-girl parties; then they spend the whole time in sex-segregated groups, showing off and making occasional sorties across the room.

For children and their parents, holding steady through this period of fluctuating capabilities, interests, size, and shape is complicated by the fact that almost all children gain fat as they approach puberty. Getting chubby is common and a normal part of the growth process. First the child stores energy; then he uses it up during the big push in height. Getting taller requires depositing considerable amounts of organ, muscle, and bony tissue and requires a lot of energy. Moreover, between 11 and 13 or 14, adolescents don't feel as good about themselves as they did before. They become more self-conscious, their positive and negative feelings about themselves come and go, and their overall self-esteem goes down significantly. Little wonder that preadolescents often seize on issues of size and shape as a ready-made explanation for their distress.

The market adds additional pressure at this stage. Because they have money—lots of it—Madison Avenue calls late school-age children and young adolescents *Tweens* and targets a *lot* of advertising at them. Beverage, food, clothing, and music companies are out to convince children in the 9-to-13-year-old age group that they have to eat, dress, and listen right in order to be popular.

Parents are still centrally important at this stage, and they do not have to be overruled by advertising and peer pressure. They can provide firm leadership without being arbitrary, maintain realistic standards, and be accepting and encouraging. Parents do best when they gradually dole out independence as a child demonstrates she is capable of handling it. So she wants to go out on her own to buy her clothes? First she has to demonstrate that she is able to resist extreme, too-tight, overly exposed, and sexualized fashion and capable of staying within a budget. So she wants to study ballet? First she has to demonstrate that she is capable of standing up to the pressures to thinness that lead to distorted eating attitudes and behaviors. The same holds true for a boy who wants to wrestle—or study ballet.

Children become aware of themselves sexually at this stage, and parents are the first mirrors for a child's sexual attractiveness. If a mother finds a son attractive, that child will find himself to be attractive. If a father finds a daughter attractive, that child will find herself to be attractive. Finding a child attractive and letting her know that is not perversion—it is good parenting. It only becomes perversion when those feelings are acted upon. Telling a child "You look great!" is a wonderful gift—but only if you mean it. If you *can't* say it and mean it, get help for yourself.

Adolescents

The theme for later adolescence is *identity*, as children come up against the reality of what adult role their body will allow, equip, or coerce them to do. Will she be a ballerina or a firefighter? Will he be a football player or a jockey? Coming to terms with what one is or is not and can or can't do is essential for living a contented and productive life.

Adolescence is a tough time, as peers are unpitying in their assessments and arbitrary in the judgments and pressures they put on each other. In the high school world, it is prized to be slim, good-looking, athletically gifted, successful with the opposite sex, socially facile, and perhaps even ruthless in achieving social prominence. It is not prized to be sturdy or fat, ordinary-looking, intellectually gifted, socially awkward, considerate and inclusive of others. In short, most ordinary values get turned upside down.

Adolescents put others down as a shortcut to feeling better about themselves. Appearance is a battering ram that is ready to hand. Adolescents have always been preoccupied with appearance, and in today's world they are preoccupied to the point of obsession. Putting others down based on appearance is a short-term self-esteem fix that is most readily available to the gifted. Take heart. In a perverse sort of way, less physically gifted children have the greater opportunity to develop true self-esteem—of finding more enduring ways to feel good about themselves and their relationships with others at no one else's expense.

Adolescence is a risky time and one that is hard on parents as well as children. Will the adolescent be loyal to his own feelings and perceptions, persist in finding in ways that are right for him, cultivate friends who appreciate and support him, and develop rewarding ways of being with other people? To do that, he will have to hang in there with himself, tolerate his upsets, make realistic judgments of the social group he belongs to—or aspires to belong to. Little wonder that given the difficulty of the task, many adolescents stumble, turning to scholastic failure (or rigidly defined success), delinquency, promiscuity, social isolation, or a fixation on size and shape as an unconscious distraction from their malaise. As we say in the family therapy world, it's a matter of symptom selection. Anxious children seize on the issue that is prominent in their lives in order to act out their distress. If parents pass along the societal preoccupation with size and shape in their attitudes toward themselves and their children, is it any wonder that during adolescence some children become body builders, others anorexics, still others gain a lot of weight? What is common to all is that they see size and shape as being at the root of their problems.

Adolescents with high BMI often want to diet and lose weight. Putting your child on a diet or his putting himself on a diet will make him fail and preserve his conviction that his true self is thinner. Remember, for the adolescent a major task is coming to terms with identity. Maintaining the myth of some other, thinner identity simply postpones achieving that task. In our culture, many people diet their whole lives and go to their graves without ever coming to terms with their size and shape. You don't have to collude with that.

Physical Self-Esteem and Sexual Maturation Sexual maturation puts enormous pressure on all adolescents. It particularly puts pressure on those who are unusual in any way. Hormone levels shoot up, and along with that come insistent sexual feelings. As her body changes, the adolescent has to cope with a new size and shape and distressing side effects, like physical awkwardness and pimples.

Today's children are being pushed along sexually. Beginning with preadolescents, the media and manufacturers exploit children by making them feel they have to market their wares—before they even know what those wares *are* or *mean*. Children are sexualized while they are still trying to achieve the school-age tasks of trying themselves out and finding out what they are good at. Both boys and girls have their particular challenges. Boys who mature late and girls who mature early are likely to be especially distressed by their physical development, or lack of it. Late-maturing boys may feel less capable than friends, self-conscious, and out of the social mainstream. Early-maturing girls might be perceived as being boy-crazy and snobbish by their classmates as their sexual maturation and interests carry them beyond the level of the other girls. They may be seen as being older and more mature than they are and be overwhelmed by attention they get from older boys and men. That is particularly the case for girls who are very pretty or have considerable breast development.

Parents must be careful to set limits to protect their children from situations that overwhelm them, taking stands about what is sexually okay and not okay. They must be careful not to push—or let anyone else push—children any further or faster than they want to go. Today's children, who learn their sexual lessons from the media and take direction from their peers, pressure and overwhelm themselves. What kind of message does it give to children to allow—or even encourage—them to wear sexually provocative clothing? Date before they are ready? Let them jump into sexually dangerous situations? Take a too-enthusiastic interest in their sexual experimentation? Once again, good parenting can make all the difference.

On the other hand, be careful not to be overprotective or to see your child as being socially fragile. Children whose size and shape do not conform to the standards may blame their body for their sexual anxiety. As a consequence, rather than pushing themselves along to learn and grow, they turn to dieting. It's a handy excuse for avoiding an issue that every child has to learn to deal with sooner or later. As one of my patients said ruefully, "I guess I am not fat enough to ward off that kind of attention." She needed to learn to consider what she wanted and stand up for it, rather than just going along with others' pressures.

APPENDIX
I

HEALTH RISKS OF CHILD OVERWEIGHT

The model I present in this book, the Satter Feeding Dynamics Approach to Child Weight Regulation, is a *wellness* model. It teaches optimum feeding to support normal growth and development. Normal growth is, by definition, the child's genetically determined growth potential. The approach advocates the acceptance of a child's consistent levels of body weight, even if that weight is above the current diagnostic cutoffs for child overweight. Like any wellness model, this one advocates identifying problems early and correcting those problems promptly. The feeding dynamics approach targets weight *acceleration*, not high weight per se, and encourages early identification of abnormal growth acceleration. Then, rather than advocating weight-reduction efforts, the model emphasizes identifying and *correcting distortions* and *restoring optimum* feeding—and parenting.

Throughout *Your Child's Weight: Helping Without Harming*, I have encouraged parents to resist outside interference that would lead them to impose weight-reduction efforts on their child. One of the most potent sources of interference—for both parents and professionals—is the relentlessly repeated message that children defined as "overweight" or "at risk of overweight" have serious health problems, both as children and as adults. The admonition, of course, that follows from such health warnings is that children must lose weight. The conviction with which that advice is given appears to be unfazed by the reality that weight-reduction efforts have only with extreme rarity produced lasting weight loss.[1]

To take this wellness approach, I have had to satisfy myself that my recommendations are legitimate and responsible and that they do no harm. My careful examination of the research studies indicates that, while overweight is modestly correlated with health issues, the health picture for child overweight is not as bad as we have been led to believe. The exception to this statement is that children whose weight is profoundly elevated—far beyond the 95th percentile cutoffs in most studies—*do* have significantly elevated disease.

Moreover, there is evidence that if weight *is* a culprit with respect to disease, it is *accelerating* weight, not *high weight per se,* that is most likely to cause problems. That evidence is sparse. Only a few of the researchers who study children with high weight or BMI distinguish between children whose weight is high and stable and those whose weight is accelerating. They tend to lump all children of a given size into the same category.

My conclusion, that there are only modest correlations between child overweight and disease, is quite different from what you generally hear. Why is that? This review considers research studies that are not generally included in literature reviews. It also looks in detail at the data in commonly cited studies and arrives at somewhat different conclusions than those indicated by the summaries and caveats of the study authors. In many cases, it is a matter of spin—interpretations given for the data. My spin is that health issues related to overweight are notable but not cataclysmic. The spin of the prevailing thought is that health risks are very high and extremely serious. I will illustrate how that spin works in my review of the studies.

Spin, of course, has to do with politics, and politics enters into the scientific process. In any field of endeavor, favored theories and practices become the politically correct ones. Right now, it is politically correct to assume that high body weight is equivalent to disease. That conviction, as with any other theory that represents prevailing thought, is so strong that it tends to squelch outcomes that find otherwise. Studies questioning favored theories and practices are severely criticized or, worse, ignored altogether. For the most part, I am not saying this is a deliberate obfuscation of the truth. Rather, it is just the way the scientific process *works*. Once a given theory is in place, it takes a *lot* of evidence to topple it.

Now to the studies. This summary of the research addresses the most common issues that are embedded in the topic of health risks of child overweight:

- Do overweight children become overweight adults?
- Conversely, do slim children remain slim adults?
- Do children of size have higher disease predictors?
- Are overweight children less healthy as adults?
- What is the consequence of weight acceleration?

Do Overweight Children Become Overweight Adults?

1. *The tendency is to slimming.* This study was a meta-analysis—an analysis of other studies. The authors reviewed 17 studies, each of which had followed children for decades. The consensus of the studies was that, up to preadolescence, the fat child has no greater risk of growing up fat than the thin one. In fact, until about age 9 to 12 years, the likelihood of slimming down was greater than the likelihood of growing up fat. The percentage of "overweight" infants and toddlers (those whose weight was at the 95th percentile and above) who were obese as adults was less than 25 percent. The percentage of "overweight" preschoolers who were obese as adults was 26 to 41 percent. The percentage of "overweight" school-age children who were obese as adults was 42 to 63 percent. The percentage of "overweight" adolescents who were obese as adults was 60 to 70 percent. The researchers also reviewed studies that considered the weight histories of obese adults to determine whether they had been obese as children. Only 5 to 20 percent of obese adults had been obese as children.[2]

   Whether you consider these research results reassuring or alarming is a matter of the spin you choose to put on them. The authors' remarks emphasized that "overweight" children are "at higher risk for obesity as adults." I interpret this article to mean that the tendency is to slimming: 75 percent of infants and toddlers slim down by the time they are adults, as do roughly 60 percent to 75 percent of preschoolers and 50 percent to 60 percent of school-age children. It is hard for me to wrap my mind around the authors' logic, but it appears to be this: Large children have a certain likelihood of remaining large in later life. Since current policy makes largeness synonymous with *overweight*, *likelihood* of remaining large is synonymous with *risk*. Ergo, children's large size at birth means they are at "risk" of overweight later in life. Forgive me if this logic doesn't hold up. It's not my interpretation.

On the other hand, consider these findings in the light of the principles of growth conservation. Children's growth tends to track—to follow a consistent percentile curve. Based on that principle, it is reasonable to expect that an infant or toddler whose weight or BMI stabilizes at the 25th percentile (or the 95th, or any other percentile) is likely to remain in that percentile throughout life. As a consequence, it would be valid to expect the correlation between "overweight" (or any weight category) in the child and in the adult to be *100 percent*. This article found that not to be the case. Children tended to *disobey* the laws of growth conservation. They slimmed down as they got older.

If you remember only one study in the maze of discussion and data you are about to enter, remember this one. Properly interpreted, it says, *do not interfere*. Hysteria about child overweight and the pressure to intervene is getting directed toward younger and younger children, even toward infants. In pointing out clearly that *the tendency is to slimming*, this study illustrates that such overconcern at young ages is misplaced.

2. *Build persisted from childhood to adulthood, but percentage of body fat did not.* In 412 Newcastle, England, adults followed from 1947, body mass index at age 9 years was significantly correlated with body mass index at age 50. However, there were *no* correlations between *body fat percentages* between ages 9 and 50 years. After age 13 years, body fatness began to be correlated with adult fatness. Most fat adults were not fat as children.[3]

What does this mean? BMI is generally used as a proxy for body fat, although there is considerable disagreement about whether there is enough association between BMI calculations and actual body fat measurements to warrant that use.[4] *Build* refers to body density and is determined by the broadness of the body and the thickness and heaviness of bones, muscles, and organ tissue. The authors in the Newcastle study used BMI, not as a measure of body *fat*, but as a measure of *build*. Instead of using BMI as a proxy for body fat, they measured body fat directly using an accepted method, *bioelectrical impedence*. As I said earlier, build tracked, but body fat didn't. Ergo, this study indicated that fat children had no greater likelihood of growing up fat than the thin ones did. However, blocky, solidly built children were likely to grow up blocky and solidly built.

Relative to our earlier discussion about the politics of scientific inquiry, readers of this article fretted about whether the results contradicted prevailing thought. Wrote one, "We are concerned that the media and editorial coverage of Wright's article may have left the erroneous impression that obesity in childhood does not predict obesity in later life, and is not a cause for concern." There was nothing erroneous about that impression. It was exactly what the research showed. Other writers on child obesity tend not to cite this article, which calls the current thinking into question. At this writing, the 2001 Newcastle study was cited by other authors only 19 times.

The author's reply to her detractors was instructive: "We have found no evidence that being a thin child is of long-term health benefit. We thus argue that efforts to turn the tide of adult obesity will be misdirected if they are directed primarily at turning plump children into thin ones."

3. *Most obese adults were not obese as children.* Only 21 percent of 3,000 obese British adults first surveyed in 1946 had been obese at age 11 years, and 79 percent of obese 36-year-olds first became obese in early adult life. Subjects showed a pattern of increasing incidence of obesity throughout life. The older the subjects were when they became obese, the greater their likelihood of remaining obese. On the other hand, individuals who became obese between ages 11 and 36 years were often not the most overweight in early childhood.[5]

4. *Roughly half (or perhaps 60 to 70 percent) of adolescents with high BMI tended to have a high BMI in later life.* As indicated by the Newcastle study (no. 2), build tends to remain the same from childhood through adulthood. This is a normal, not an abnormal process. In spite of that, only 54 percent of 485 Norwegians followed from age 15 to 33 years remained in the same BMI categories when they were older as they had been when younger.[6] The meta-analysis I discussed previously (no. 1) indicated that 60 to 70 percent of adolescents whose BMI were above the 95th BMI percentile remained in that percentile as adults.[2] Was it *build* or body *fat* that tracked? That study did not distinguish one from the other.

Do Normal-Weight or Slim Children Remain Slim as Adults?

5. *Getting out of childhood slim offered no protection against adult obesity.* In a 36-year longitudinal study in Britain, 79 percent of obese 36-year-olds became obese in adult life. Thirty-nine percent of men

and 46 percent of women who were obese at age 36 were normal weight or below at age 11 years.[5]

6. *Extreme levels of thinness are associated with increased risk of adult disease.* The Newcastle study (no. 2) showed that the thinnest children tended to have the highest adult health risk at every level of adult BMI. Underweight children were less healthy as adults.[3]

Do Children of Size Have Higher Disease Predictors?
Depending principally on genetics, people of all sizes are more or less prone to degenerative diseases like diabetes, heart disease, and stroke. The question is whether that risk is elevated for children of size.

7. *Abdominal fatness correlated with degenerative disease, but it doesn't follow that fatness causes disease.* A study of 2,996 children, ages 5 to 17 years, in Bogalusa, Louisiana, found increasing abdominal fatness to be correlated with higher blood lipid and insulin concentrations. Circulating insulin doubled between the 50th and the 90th BMI percentiles of abdominal fat measures. LDL cholesterol and triglycerides increased by 35 to 50 percent.[7]

What do these tests mean? Generally, studies of this type are interpreted to mean that overweight *causes* diabetes and a tendency to heart disease. In reality, the studies do *not* illustrate cause and effect, but only *covariance:* As one goes up, the others go up. Since all three characteristics are genetic conditions, it is just as likely that a common metabolic underpinning causes them all. For instance, consider the calcium and vitamin D research presented in appendix J, "Dairy Products, Bone Health, and Weight Management."

8. *High BMI correlated with degenerative disease, but it doesn't follow that fatness causes disease.* A study of 9,167 children, ages 5 to 17 years, also enrolled in the Bogalusa study, examined BMI instead of abdominal fatness to detect a relationship with disease predictors. The percentage of overweight children who showed elevated lipid and insulin concentrations was higher for those in the 95th to 97th BMI percentiles compared with those whose BMI was closer to the average. The comparisons were as follows: triglycerides—17 percent versus 10 percent; low-density lipoproteins—15 percent versus 9 percent; circulating insulin—10 percent versus 3 percent. In reporting their data, the authors *compared overweight children with children who have no risk factors* and stated that triglycerides of overweight children were 7.1 times higher, low-density lipoproteins were 3.4 times higher, and circulating insulin was 12.6 times higher.[8]

Again, the interpretation is a matter of spin. When the results are reported as percentages, they are concerning but not alarming. The data showed, for instance, that the percentage of children whose circulating insulin was elevated was 10 percent, versus 3 percent of children whose weight was closer to the mean. However, in their summary of the data, the authors said the circulating insulin of overweight children was *12.6* times *higher*. To get that figure, they compared the large children with still another group of children, those who showed *unusually low* disease predictors. Presented that way, the data are horrifying. Same data, different spin.

9. *For* extremely *large children, there was a marked correlation between high BMI and degenerative disease.* In the Bogalusa BMI study just cited, (no. 8), children characterized as being of *extreme* size (at and above the 97th percentile) more often had elevated lipid and insulin concentrations. Twenty-five percent had high triglycerides, 23 percent had elevated low-density lipoproteins, and 27 percent had high circulating insulin. Compare these figures with those for children whose BMI is closer to the median: 10 percent, 9 percent, and 3 percent, and figures given in no. 8 for children whose BMI was above the 95th percentile, *including those of extreme size* were 17 percent, 15 percent, and 10 percent. While health risks were not calculated for children whose BMI was at the 95th percentile range, it is clear that their health data were exaggerated by combining them with the data from children of extreme size.[8]

There is little doubt that extremely high body weight—4 or 5 or more standard deviations above the mean—carries health consequences. "Morbidly obese" children achieve extremely high body weight through extreme circumstances that are rare. Basing health policy on child overweight on the needs of such unusual children is like basing population-wide nutrition policy on the needs of people with congestive heart failure.

10. *Obese children with asthma had no more or no more severe symptoms.* A 9-month study of 3,222 inner-city children from seven cities found no significant differences between obese and nonobese children. The obese group had a higher mean number of days of wheezing per 2-week period (4.0 versus 3.4), and a greater proportion of obese children had unscheduled emergency room visits (39 percent versus 31 percent). There were no differences between the groups in terms of frequency of hospitalization or in waking up at night (presumably because of breathing problems).[9]

As so often happens when results do not confirm the prevailing thought, these authors concluded with a caveat: "It is puzzling that the obese children did not experience more nocturnal awakening, limitation of play, or more hospitalization than the nonobese."

11. *Obese children were more likely to be* diagnosed *with asthma.* A study based on the National Health and Nutrition Examination Survey found that children diagnosed with asthma were almost twice as likely to be at or above the 95th BMI percentile.[10]

As indicated with an earlier study, this study finds covariance—as one goes up, so does the other. However, one does not necessarily *cause* the other. Unlike in the previous study, there is no distinction of whether the asthma *caused* the obesity, or vice versa, or whether they covaried.

12. *Overweight children had no more or more severe asthma, nor did they have more trouble breathing.* No differences in asthma incidence and severity were found between 80 overweight children compared with 80 average-weight children. When the data were analyzed in the opposite direction, it appeared that more children with asthma had a BMI at or above the 95th percentile. In other words, obesity did not appear to increase the likelihood that children would get asthma. However, asthma may have increased the likelihood that children would become obese.[11]

Any study of asthma and obesity is subject to the bias of the diagnostician. Does the child have asthma, or is he or she short of breath because of poor conditioning? The common *assumption* that obese children have a higher incidence of asthma can weight the diagnosis in favor of asthma.

Are Overweight Children Less Healthy as Adults?

13. *Being overweight in childhood did not increase adult obesity and risk of disease.* The Newcastle study (no. 2) showed that when child fatness persisted into adulthood, overweight adults showed no more disease indicators than average-weight adults. They had no greater incidence of high blood pressure and no higher concentrations of low-density lipoprotein, triglyceride, and fasting insulin. The exception was adult women. For them, persistence of body fat between childhood and adulthood was correlated with *lower* triglycerides and total cholesterol.[3] That is not a mistake—the word is *lower.*

These results indicated that women who were fat all their lives had lower levels of disease indicators than those who became fat in later life. This study considers the difference in health outcome between people whose weight is high but consistent and those whose weight accelerates. Subjects were healthier when their weight was high and consistent.

14. *Adult levels of disease indicators did* not *vary with child weight status.* A study that followed 2,617 Bogalusa study participants from age 2 to 17 years to age 18 to 37 years showed that although many obese adults had higher than average levels of lipids, insulin, and blood pressure, levels did not vary with childhood weight status or with the age of obesity onset.[12]

These authors appeared to have trouble with their results, which did not confirm the prevailing thought. Their caveat was "Additional data are needed to assess the independent relationship of childhood weight status to coronary heart disease morbidity."

15. *Adult males who showed exceptionally high or low BMIs at age 18 had increased mortality at age 50.* The 3 percent of 78,612 Dutch men who had the highest BMI at age 18 years had twice the risk of premature death of men in other categories . The 5 percent of men having the lowest BMI had $1^{1}/_{2}$ times the risk.[13]

What does this mean? A twofold risk in mortality sounds alarming, but it is actually a modest increase. To put the numbers in perspective, consider that smokers compared with people who have never smoked have 12 times the risk of premature death.

16. *Risk of mortality was modestly elevated for men whose weight had been high as children.* Premature death of 13,146 Maryland subjects after 22 years was 1.5 times higher for 2- to 18-year-olds who started out in the highest weight group compared with median-BMI groups.[14]

This large study and the previous one, also large, found very similar levels of risk.

17. *Mortality and morbidity in adults was higher when men where obese as adolescents.* This was a 22-year follow-up study of 508 Harvard Growth Study participants who were enrolled at ages 13 to 18 years. Among overweight compared with lean enrollees, mortality was 1.8 times higher for all causes, 2.3 times higher for heart disease, 13.2 times higher for atherosclerosis, and 9.1 times higher for colon cancer.[15]

This study, with its alarming statistics for atherosclerosis and colon cancer, was small, and the statistical analysis was eccentric. In contrast to the standard 95th percentile cutoff for overweight, or even the 85th percentile cutoff for *risk of overweight,* the researchers established the cutoff at the 75th percentile. That cutoff gave a greater number of overweight subjects and therefore higher mortality and disease figures.

Despite the small numbers of subjects and limitations in study design and statistical analysis, this study is often quoted and used as definitive proof of the serious health risk presented by high BMI in childhood. As of January 27, 2004, the Harvard study had been cited 479 times in other articles, compared with 97 times for the Maryland study (no. 16) published the same year and 87 times for the Dutch study (no. 15) published four years previously.

In this instance, we are seeing scientific politics at work. It is a natural human tendency to pay more attention to information that confirms our own biases. It appears that scientists writing journal articles fall prey to this tendency.

What Is the Consequence of Weight Acceleration?

The following studies demonstrate that weight acceleration is a risk factor in adult disease. However, the studies must be treated as *preliminary* studies and regarded as being helpful in raising questions for further testing. Why? Because the studies test *covariance*, not *cause-and-effect*. They are also *morbidity* studies. They assess disease incidence and are therefore subject to diagnostic and reporting bias. Mortality studies are more reliable because there is no bias. Either subjects die or they don't.

18. *Overweight adults who were underweight as children had higher health risks.* When adults became overweight in later life compared with adults who were overweight since childhood, they had a greater incidence of bone demineralization, diabetes, insulin resistance, and elevated blood lipids and hypertension.[16-19]

19. *Children who were underweight at birth and showed rapid weight gain prior to their teens had higher health risks.* Adults who had been underweight at birth and rapidly gained weight in early life showed a higher risk of type 2 diabetes, coronary heart disease, and hypertension.[20-23]

In summary, the data on the health consequences of childhood overweight give us cause for concern but not reason to panic. Health concerns do not support taking drastic, health-threatening, and potentially weight-destabilizing approaches to lose weight.

The solution must not be worse than the disease. Child overweight presents a modest level of risk. Weight-loss efforts are almost without exception unsuccessful and are highly likely to do harm. Social and emotional harm aside, the health risks of weight-loss efforts include negating natural tendencies to slimming, destabilizing body weight, and increasing disease risk associated with weight acceleration.

NOTES

1. Epstein et al., "Treatment of Pediatric Obesity."
2. Serdula et al., "Obese Children."
3. Wright et al., "Implications of Childhood Obesity."
4. Taylor et al., "Body Fat Percentages."
5. Braddon et al., "Onset of Obesity."
6. Kvaavik, Tell, and Klepp, "Predictors and Tracking of Body Mass Index."
7. Freedman et al., "Relation of Circumferences and Skinfold Thicknesses."
8. Freedman et al., "Relation of Overweight to Cardiovascular Risk."
9. Belamarich et al., "Obese Inner-City Children with Asthma."
10. von Mutius et al., "Relation of Body Mass Index to Asthma and Atopy."
11. Gennuso et al., "Relationship Between Asthma and Obesity."
12. Freedman et al., "Relationship of Childhood Obesity to Coronary Heart Disease Risk Factors."
13. Hoffmans, Kromhout, and De Lezenne Coulander, "Impact of Body Mass Index."
14. Nieto, Szklo, and Comstock, "Childhood Weight and Growth Rate."
15. Must et al., "Long-Term Morbidity and Mortality of Overweight Adolescents."
16. Abraham, Collins, and Nordsieck, "Relationships of Childhood Weight Status."
17. Holbrook, and Barrett-Conner, "Association of Lifetime Weight and Weight Control Patterns."
18. Sinaiko et al., "Relation of Weight and Rate of Increase in Weight During Childhood."
19. Lauer and Clarke, "Childhood Risk Factors for High Adult Blood Pressure."
20. Bhargava et al., "Relation of Serial Changes in Childhood Body-Mass Index."
21. Forsen et al., "Fetal and Childhood Growth."
22. Eriksson et al., "Early Growth and Coronary Heart Disease in Later Life."
23. Eriksson et al., "Fetal and Childhood Growth."

APPENDIX
J

DAIRY PRODUCTS, BONE HEALTH AND WEIGHT MANAGEMENT

Accumulating research indicates that consuming milk and other dairy products may help both adults and children to be moderately slimmer. I do not like writing this. My long career as a dietitian has made me reluctant to credit any one food with offering a cure for anything, but there it is.

Don't get me wrong. While my scientific scruples make me hesitate to acknowledge the connection, my concerns about children's nutrition and bone health make me willing to embrace any means, fair or foul, to encourage milk consumption. Milk consumption has decreased seriously in recent years, and children's bone health is suffering.

From the research, it appears that with respect to milk consumption and your child's weight, milk drinking can't hurt, and it may even help. With respect to your child's bone health, milk consumption is absolutely essential. However, milk is losing its place as a primary beverage for children. In the last 20 to 30 years, soda and other sweetened beverages have replaced milk in our children's diets.[1] Whether or not the research on milk consumption and weight holds up, the idea is that

milk is important. Toddlers, preschoolers, and school-age children
need 2 to 3 cups a day. Adolescents need 3 to 4 cups.

Milk Consumption and Bone Health

Children are suffering the nutritional consequences of low levels of milk
consumption. Compared with children who regularly consumed milk,
New Zealand children who didn't drink milk had considerably lower
calcium intakes, were shorter, and had smaller bones with a lower density of bone mineral. Furthermore, children who didn't drink milk sustained a higher number of bone fractures.[2,3] The incidence of forearm
fracture has increased in the last 30 years.[4] Teenage girls who drink more
carbonated beverages and therefore less milk have more bone fractures.[5]
Women with low milk intake during childhood and adolescence have
less bone mass in adulthood and greater risk of fracture.[6]

This research reinforces what we already know: Children need
milk, and so do the rest of us. Milk is our most reliable food source of
calcium in the United States. It is also a primary source of vitamin D
along with protein and a wide variety of other vitamins and minerals
also necessary for building strong bones. At this writing there are
many products fortified with calcium and even an orange juice fortified with calcium and vitamin D. Unless it is milk, however, it doesn't
give milk's high-quality protein, vitamins, and minerals, all of which
are important for bone health.

The rumors (and even press conferences by seeming authorities)
that go around every so often saying that milk is bad for people in general and for children in particular are simply wrong. Such ideas about
drinking milk are based on flimsy evidence by people on crusades.
Their evidence does not hold up to careful scrutiny.

Milk Consumption and Weight

Now let's turn to the research connecting milk consumption with
weight. Tennessee children whose dietary intake and weight were followed from ages 2 months to 8 years old were leaner when milk was a
regular part of their diet. Children who drank more milk also consumed more fruits and vegetables and fewer sweetened beverages.[7] A
nationwide survey of children in the United States showed that children who more often ate ready-to-eat cereal (with milk) were leaner
and had better nutrient profiles than those who did not.[8] Since ready-
to-eat cereal is typically a breakfast food, presumably those children
also ate breakfast more frequently than did children who did not consume cereal. Girls ages 9 to 14 who consumed diets rich in calcium

weighed less and had less abdominal fat than did girls who consumed less calcium. For every 300 milligrams of calcium consumed, girls were on the average 1.9 pounds lighter.[9] Eight ounces of milk gives 300 milligrams of calcium.

Girls ages 5 to 9 years drank more milk if their mothers did. Naturally, girls who consumed adequate amounts of calcium had better bone mineral status than those who did not. Furthermore, the girls who consumed adequate amounts of calcium ate more total calories but were no heavier than the girls who did not.[10]

Children who drank more sweetened drinks consumed less milk, took in more calories overall, and were heavier than children who consumed milk. Naturally, the milk-drinking children had better diets as well. They took in more protein, calcium, magnesium, phosphorus, and vitamin A than the children who drank soda and Kool-Aid.[11]

Is Milk a Marker for Meals?

It is quite possible that the key connection between milk and slimming is structured feeding, not milk consumption per se. Remember that early in chapter 3, "Make Family Meals a Priority," you learned that nutritionists use consumption of breakfast, milk, fruits, and vegetables as markers of nutritional quality. In turn, those consumption patterns act as measures of participation in family meals. Milk drinking may have offered an indirect way of measuring the degree to which children participated in family meals. None of the researchers asked about structured meals and snacks versus grazing.

Or Maybe It Slims on Its Own

On the other hand, milk may have some attribute that conveys a positive regulatory effect. Dairy consumption in overweight young adults appears to be protective against insulin resistance, considered to be a warning sign of adult-onset diabetes.[12] Women who consumed more calcium, mostly from dairy products, weighed less than women who consumed less.[13]

Arguing metabolically in favor of a direct slimming role for milk, studies with mice and with human fat cells—in petri dishes—have identified a biochemical role for calcium in decreasing body fat deposition.[14] Parathyroid hormone and 1,25 dihydroxy vitamin D (an intermediate metabolite in the body's conversion of ingested vitamin D to biologically active vitamin D) both increase in response to low calcium intakes (low serum calcium). Increase of those two metabolites leads to increased calcium in the fat cell, increases in fat storage, and decreases in fat breakdown. Increasing the amount of calcium in the diet suppresses both metabolic agents and decreases calcium and therefore fat storage in the fat cells.

The moral of the story? In the cells, anyway, calcium exerts an antiobesity effect. However, this is all preliminary and a long way from telling us about ourselves. Studies in mice and isolated human cells do not necessarily apply to whole people. If you must jump to conclusions, drink your milk. To keep an eye on the research as it accumulates, go to the American Dairy Council Web site: http://www.nationaldairycouncil.org/healthyweight/index.asp

The Bottom Line
Does drinking milk help with weight maintenance? It can't hurt. It might help. Certainly with respect to the bone health of all family members, it can help a great deal.

NOTES
1. Nicklas, "Calcium Intake Trends."
2. Goulding et al., "Children Who Avoid Drinking Cow's Milk."
3. Black et al., "Children Who Avoid Drinking Cow Milk."
4. Khosla et al., "Incidence of Childhood Distal Forearm Fractures."
5. Wyshak, "Teenaged Girls, Carbonated Beverage Consumption."
6. Kalkwarf, Khoury, and Lanphear, "Milk Intake During Childhood and Adolescence."
7. Skinner et al., "Longitudinal Calcium Intake."
8. Albertson et al., "Ready-to-Eat Cereal Consumption"
9. Novotny, "Higher Dairy Intake."
10. Fisher et al., "Meeting Calcium Recommendations During Middle Childhood."
11. Mrdjenovic, and Levitsky, "Nutritional and Energetic Consequences of Sweetened Drink Consumption."
12. Pereira et al., "Dairy Consumption, Obesity, and the Insulin Resistance Syndrome."
13. Davies et al, "Calcium Intake and Body Weight."
14. Zemel, "Mechanisms of Dairy Modulation of Adiposity."

APPENDIX
K

BOOKS AND RESOURCES
BY ELLYN SATTER

Books by Ellyn Satter

Available in book stores, on the web at www.EllynSatter.com, and by direct order from Ellyn Satter Associates at 800-808-7976.

Child of Mine: Feeding with Love and Good Sense Bull Publishing Co., Palo Alto, CA, 2000. A warm, supportive, and entertaining book that tells how to parent with respect to food and feeding in a wise, loving, and tuned-in way. In her usual engaging and conversational style, Satter empowers parents to make their own judgments about nutrition and feeding from infancy through preschool. The first edition of this book has become bedside-table reading for parents as well as a classic in the nutrition world. It has firmly built the bridge between nutrition and feeding and made the feeding relationship a primary focus of nutrition intervention.

How to Get Your Kid to Eat... But Not Too Much Bull Publishing Co., Palo Alto, CA, 1987. Both parents and professionals rely on this book to solve feeding problems such as "Why won't my child eat?" "Why does my child like food one day but not the other?" "How can I stop having these battles around food?" and "How can I get my child to eat vegetables?" As a basis for solving feeding problems, *How to Get Your Kid to Eat* discusses normal feeding, child development, family dynamics, psychology, and parent-child relationships.

Secrets of Feeding a Healthy Family Kelcy Press, Madison, WI, 1999. Helps adults choose food joyfully, appealingly, and wisely; manage eating; and establish a positive feeding relationship with children. Recipe, planning, and shopping chapters offer the reader a kitchen primer: food preparation for the "thinking cook," fast tips, night-before suggestions, in-depth background information, ways to involve kids in the kitchen, and guidelines for adapting menus for young children. Satter's comment that "you are a family when you begin taking care of yourself" makes this a book for all.

Teaching materials by Ellyn Satter

FEEDING IN PRIMARY CARE PREGNANCY THROUGH PRESCHOOL: Easy-to-Read Reproducible Masters Ellyn Satter Associates, Madison, WI, 53711, 2004. Obesity and other childhood eating problems can be prevented from birth by optimizing feeding. These remarkably crafted, easy-to-read (fourth-grade) handouts identify key information for each developmental stage. Distilled without being diluted, handouts empower health professionals to establish relationships with parents on behalf of children and embody Ellyn Satter's conviction that observing the child trumps all other advice given to parents. Copying the masters on office machines gives a cost-effective price of $.02 per copy! Highly recommended for purchase by agencies that serve clients with limited reading ability, including WIC, Head Start and Early Head Start, CACFP, medical and nutrition clinics.

NUTRITION AND FEEDING FOR INFANTS AND CHILDREN: Handout Masters Ellyn Satter Associates, Madison, WI, 53711. These reproducible handout masters skillfully weave together the elements of child development, nutrition, and emotionally healthful parenting to highlight the key issues in feeding, food selection, and growth. Well suited for handing out to parents who can comfortably read newspapers, these handouts also act as a concise reference and resource for health professionals doing counseling with parents of all reading levels. Copying the masters on office machines gives a cost-effective price of $.02 per copy! Quantity discount prices allow placing a copy in each agency office! Recommended as a resource for WIC, Head Start and Early Head Start, CACFP, Extension, EFNEP, feeding teams, early childhood programs, medical clinics, nutrition clinics.

ELLYN SATTER'S FEEDING WITH LOVE AND GOOD SENSE: Video and Teacher's Guide Ellyn Satter Associates, Madison, WI, 1995. The classic feeding dynamics video, these ever-popular vignettes are of real parents and children at feeding time. Videos demonstrate positive and negative feeding, inspire parents and health workers to take feeding seriously and show them how to be successful. Ready-to-use lesson plans and easy-to-read copy-ready masters (fourth-grade reading level) help the busy teacher combine nutrition, feeding dynamics, child development, and parenting. Recommended for parents' classes in pediatrics and obstetrics, WIC, Head Start, CACFP, EFNEP, Extension.

Training materials for professionals

Ellyn Satter's Montana FEEDING RELATIONSHIP Training Package Ellyn Satter Associates, Madison, WI, 53711, 1997. Highly popular one-day primary intervention feeding dynamics workshop on videotape. The economical way to train nutrition staff in understanding feeding dynamics, child development as it relates to feeding and developmentally appropriate feeding practices. This outstanding package makes it simple to put a presentation together because the handouts and lectures are ready to go. Best taught by a graduate of the *Feeding with Love and Good Sense VISION Workshop.*

One-day training for professionals in feeding dynamics and child overweight prevention

Children, the Feeding Relationship, and Weight This highly successful workshop demonstrates the concepts presented in Ellyn Satter's *Your Child's Weight: Helping Without Harming,* Kelcy Press, 2005. Using detailed case studies, the workshop illustrates how appropriate feeding dynamics supports appropriate growth and how distorted feeding dynamics produces distorted growth. The workshop equips participants to approach child overweight as a behavioral and parenting issue rather than a problem of food selection and activity management.

The Feeding Relationship: An Introduction to the Possibilities This highly sought-after workshop introduces the concept of feeding dynamics, then coaches audience members in identifying behavioral issues in feeding problems. The first step in feeding dynamics training is thinking in behavioral terms. This workshop is an essential first step for agencies working toward a collaborative approach to feeding dynamics education as a routine part of health education. Agencies that have sponsored this workshop found it extremely effective with multidisciplinary groups to get people started thinking in terms of feeding dynamics and moving themselves along.

Feeding Dynamics Education and Intervention in Primary Care This training workshop is the perfect next step for agencies that have introduced their staff to feeding dynamics, made policy, and acquired educational materials. This workshop briefly reviews feeding dynamics, then moves on to tools for intervention. In the problem-solving segment, participants are taught developmental and feeding principles, then apply them to specific case studies. Then participants go one step further and think through approaching parents with impressions and recommendations. Again, to do well with this workshop, students must be well-grounded in basic feeding principles.

Helping Children to Eat and Grow Well in Child Care and Head Start This popular workshop is ideal for audiences who work directly with children. Professionals such as child care providers and Head Start teachers are already tuned in to behavioral issues and ready to consider them in a workshop. They want to know what to do to get children to eat well. Their challenge is replacing feeding lore with recommended feeding practice. This workshop is short on the theoretical and long on the practical and applied. Much of the content is woven into the examples for problem solving. In addition, since part of the issue in solving problems is working with the parents, each of the case studies goes on to talk about approaching parents with recommendations.

Three-day training in eating and feeding

TREATING THE DIETING CASUALTY: Intensive Workshop The missing piece for treating those with disordered eating, this powerful, step-by-step approach resolves inner conflicts about eating and teaches positive, competent eating based on internal regulators. There is far more to normal eating than not dieting! This workshop teaches an in-depth, theoretically sound understanding of eating attitudes and behaviors and approaches to treatment. For health, education, and mental health professionals.

FEEDING WITH LOVE AND GOOD SENSE: Intensive Workshop
Using Ellyn Satter's approach, established feeding problems can be treated effectively in general practice on an outpatient basis. Training for professionals in assessing and solving childhood feeding problems integrates the principles of nutrition, feeding, child development, and parenting. Specific problems covered in the workshop are the child who eats poorly, the finicky child, and the obese child. For health, education, child care, and mental health professionals.

SELECTED REFERENCES

Abraham, S., G. Collins, and M. Nordsieck. "Relationships of Childhood Weight Status to Morbidity in Adults." *HSMHA* Health Reports 86 (1971): 273-84.

Adair, L. S. "The Infant's Ability to Self-Regulate Caloric Intake: A Case Study." *Journal of the American Dietetic Association* 84, no. 5 (1984): 543-46.

Adelson, J. "Friendship and the Peer Group in Adolescence." In *Handbook of Adolescent Psychology*, ed. J. C. Coleman. New York: Wiley, 1980.

Albertson, A., G. Anderson, S. Crockett, and M. Goebel. "Ready-to-Eat Cereal Consumption: Its Relationship with BMI and Nutrient Intake of Children Aged 4 to 12 Years." *Journal of the American Dietetic Association* 103, no. 12 (2003): 1613-19.

American Dietetic Association (ADA). *Nutrition and You: Trends 2000.* Chicago: American Dietetic Association, 2000.

American School Food Service Association. "Keys to Excellence." Web page [accessed 16 January 2004]. Available at http://www.asfsa.org/.

Anderson, R. E., C. J. Crespo, S. J. Bartlett, L. J. Cheskin, and M. Pratt. "Relationship of Physical Activity and Television Watching with Body Weight and Level of Fatness Among Children: Results from the Third National Health and Nutrition Examination Survey." *Journal of the American Medical Association* 279 (1998): 938-42.

Anderson, S. E., L. G. Bandini, W. H. Dietz, and A. Must. "Relationship Between Temperament, Nonresting Energy Expenditure, Body Composition, and Physical Activity in Girls." *International Journal of Obesity and Related Metabolic Disorders* (2003): 300-306.

Anliker, J. A., M. J. Laus, K. W. Samonds, and V. A. Beal. "Mothers' Reports of Their Three-Year-Old Children's Control Over Foods and Involvement in Food-Related Activities." *Journal of Nutrition Education* 24, no. 6 (1992): 285-91.

Barlow, S. E., and W. H. Dietz. "Obesity Evaluation and Treatment: Expert Committee Recommendations." *Pediatrics* 102, no. 3 (1998): e29.

Barlow, S. E., F. L. Trowbridge, W. J. Klish, and W. H. Dietz. "Treatment of Child and Adolescent Obesity: Reports from Pediatricians, Pediatric Nurse Practitioners, and Registered Dietitians." *Pediatrics* 110, no. 1 (2002): 229-35.

Baumrind, D. "Current Patterns of Parental Authority." *Developmental Psychology Monograph* 4, no. 1, pt. 2 (1971): 1-103.

Beal, V. A. "Dietary Intake of Individuals Followed Through Infancy and Childhood." *American Journal of Public Health* 51, no. 8 (1961): 1107-17.

Belamarich, P. F., E. Luder, M. Kattan, H. Mitchell, S. Islam, H. Lynn, and E. F. Crain. "Do Obese Inner-City Children with Asthma Have More Symptoms Than Nonobese Children with Asthma?" *Pediatrics* 106, no. 6 (2000): 1436-41.

Bell, E. A., and B. J. Rolls. "Energy Density of Foods Affects Energy Intake Across Multiple Levels of Fat Content in Lean and Obese Women." *American Journal of Clinical Nutrition* 73 (2001): 1010-1018.

Bhargava, S. K., H. S. Sachdev, C. H. D. Fall, C. Osmond, R. Lakshmy, D. J. P. Barker, S. K. D. Biswas, S. Ramji, D. Prabhakaran, and K. S. Reddy. "Relation of Serial Changes in Childhood Body-Mass Index to Impaired Glucose Tolerance in Young Adulthood." *New England Journal of Medicine* 350, no. 9 (2004): 865-75.

Birch, L. L., and J. O. Fisher. "Appetite and Eating Behavior in Children." *Pediatric Clinics of North America* 42, no. 4 (1995): 931-53.

Birch, L. L., and J. O. Fisher. "Mothers' Child-Feeding Practices Influence Daughters' Eating and Weight." *American Journal of Clinical Nutrition* 71 (2000): 1054-61.

Birch, L. L, J. O. Fisher, and K. K. Davison. "Learning to Overeat: Maternal Use of Restrictive Feeding Practices Promotes Girls'

Eating in the Absence of Hunger." *American Journal of Clinical Nutrition* 78, no. 2 (2003): 215-20.

Birch, L. L, S. L. Johnson, and J. O Fisher. "Children's Eating: The Development of Food-Acceptance Patterns." *Young Children* 50, no. 2 (1995): 71-78.

Birch, L. L., L. S. McPhee, J. L. Bryant, and S. L. Johnson. "Children's Lunch Intake: Effects of Midmorning Snacks Varying in Energy Density and Fat Content." *Appetite* 20 (1993): 83-94.

Black, R. E., S. M. Williams, I. E. Jones, and A. Goulding. "Children Who Avoid Drinking Cow Milk Have Low Dietary Calcium Intakes and Poor Bone Health." *American Journal of Clinical Nutrition* 76, no. 3 (2002): 675-80.

Borra, S., L. Shirreffs, M. Kelly, K. Neville, and C. Geiger. "Developing Health Messages: Qualitative Studies with Children, Parents, and Teachers Help Identify Communications Opportunities for Healthful Lifestyles and the Prevention of Obesity." *Journal of the American Dietetic Association* 103, no. 6 (2003): 721-28.

Braddon, F. E. M., B. Rodgers, M. E. J. Wadsworth, and J. M. C. Davies. "Onset of Obesity in a 36 Year Birth Cohort Study. " *British Medical Journal* 293 (1986): 299-303.

Braet, C., I. Mervielde, and W. Vandereycken. "Psychological Aspects of Childhood Obesity: A Controlled Study in a Clinical and Nonclinical Sample." *Journal of Pediatric Psychology* 22, no. 1 (1997): 59-71.

Buhrmester, D., and W. Furman. "The Development of Companionship and Intimacy." *Child Development* 58 (1987): 1101-13.

Caballero, B., T. Clay, S. M. Davis, B. Ethelbah, B. H. Rock, T. Lohman, J. Norman, M. Story, E. J. Stone, L. Stephenson, and J. Stevens. "Pathways: A School-Based, Randomized Controlled Trial for the Prevention of Obesity in American Indian Schoolchildren." *American Journal of Clinical Nutrition* 78, no. 5 (2003): 1030-1038.

Centers for Disease Control and Prevention. *School Health Index for Physical Activity, Healthy Eating, and a Tobacco-Free Lifestyle: A Self-Assessment and Planning Guide. Middle School and High School Version.* Atlanta, GA: 2002.

Centers for Disease Control and Prevention. *School Health Index for Physical Activity, Healthy Eating, and a Tobacco-Free Lifestyle: A Self-Assessment and Planning Guide. Elementary School Version Module 4: Nutrition Services.* Atlanta, GA: 2002.

Chatoor, I. "Feeding Disorders in Infants and Toddlers: Diagnosis and Treatment." *Child and Adolescent Psychiatric Clinics of North America*

11, no. 2 (2002): 163-83.

Chatoor, I., S. Schaefer, L. Dickson, and J. Egan. "Non-Organic Failure to Thrive: A Developmental Perspective." *Pediatric Annals* 13, no. 11 (1984): 829-43.

Committee on Public Education. "Children, Adolescents, and Television." *Pediatrics* 107, no. 2 (2001): 423-26.

Committee on School Health. "Soft Drinks in Schools." *Pediatrics* 113, no. 1 (2004): 152-54.

Coon, K. A., J. Goldberg, B. L. Rogers, and K. L. Tucker. "Relationships Between Use of Television During Meals and Children's Food Consumption Patterns." *Pediatrics* 107, no. 1 (2001): e7.

Council of Economic Advisers to the President. *Teens and Their Parents in the 21st Century: An Examination of Trends in Teen Behavior and the Role of Parental Involvement*. 2000.

Crawford, P. B., and L. R. Shapiro. "How Obesity Develops: A New Look at Nature and Nurture." *Obesity & Health* F. M. Berg, 40-41. Hettinger, ND: Healthy Living Institute, 1991.

Crockett, S. J., and L. S. Sims. "Environmental Influences on Children's Eating." *Journal of Nutrition Education* 27 (1995): 235-49.

Crow, R. A., J. N. Fawcett, and P. Wright. "Maternal Behavior During Breast- and Bottle-Feeding." *Journal of Behavioral Medicine* 3, no. 3 (1980): 259-77.

Cutting, T. M., J. O. Fisher, K. Grimm-Thomas, and L. L. Birch. "Like Mother, Like Daughter: Familial Patterns of Overweight Are Mediated by Mothers' Dietary Disinhibition." *American Journal of Clinical Nutrition* 69 (1999): 608-13.

Davies, K. M., R. P. Heaney, R. R. Recker, J. M. Lappe, M. J. Barger-Lux, K. Rafferty, and S. Hinders. "Calcium Intake and Body Weight." *Journal of Clinical Endocrinology and Metabolism* 85, no. 12 (2000): 4635-38.

Davison, K. K., and L. L. Birch. "Weight Status, Parent Reaction, and Self-Concept in Five-Year-Old Girls." *Pediatrics* 107 (2001): 46-53.

Demo, D. H., and A. C. Acock. "Family Structure, Family Process, and Adolescent Well-Being." *Journal of Research on Adolescence* 6 (1996): 457-88.

Dettwyler, K. A. "Styles of Infant Feeding: Parental/Caretaker Control of Food Consumption in Young Children." *American Anthropologist* 91 (1989): 696-703.

Donnelly, J. E., D. J. Jacobsen, J. E. Whatley, J. O. Hill, L. L. Swift, A. C. Cherrington, B. Polk, Z. V. Tran, and G. Reed. "Nutrition and Physical Activity Program to Attenuate Obesity and Promote

Physical and Metabolic Fitness in Elementary School Children." *Obesity Research* 4 (1996): 229-43.

Eisenberg, M. E., R. E. Olson, D. Neumark-Sztainer, M. Story, and L. H. Bearinger. "Correlations Between Family Meals and Psychosocial Well-Being Among Adolescents." *Archives of Pediatric and Adolescent Medicine* 158, no. 8 (2004): 792-6.

Eisenmann, J. C., P. T. Katzmarzyk, D. A. Arnall, V. Kanuho, C. Interpreter, and R. M. Malina. "Growth and Overweight of Navajo Youth: Secular Changes from 1955 to 1997." *International Journal of Obesity* 24 (2000): 211-18.

Elder, G. H. "Structural Variations in the Childrearing Relationship." *Sociometry* 25 (1962): 241-62.

Epstein L. H., M. D. Myers, H. A. Raynor, and B. E. Saelens. "Treatment of Pediatric Obesity." *Pediatrics* 101 (1998): 554-70.

Epstein, L. H., B. E. Saelens, M. D. Myers, and D. Vito. "The Effects of Decreasing Sedentary Behaviors on Activity Choice in Obese Children." *Health Psychology* 16 (1997): 107-13.

Erikson, E. H. "Eight Ages of Man." In *Childhood and Society*, 2nd ed., 242-74. New York : W. W. Norton.

Eriksson, J., T. Forsen, J. Tuomilehto, C. Osmond, and D. Barker. "Fetal and Childhood Growth and Hypertension in Adult Life." *Hypertension* 36, no. 5 (2000): 790-94.

Eriksson, J. G., T. Forsen, J. Tuomilehto, C. Osmond, and D. J. Barker. "Early Growth and Coronary Heart Disease in Later Life: Longitudinal Study." *British Medical Journal* 322, no. 7292 (2001): 949-53.

Faith, M. S., M. A. Leone, T. S. Ayers, M. Heo, and A. Pietrobelli. "Weight Criticism During Physical Activity, Coping Skills, and Reported Physical Activity in Children." *Pediatrics* 110, no. 2, pt. 1 (2002): e23.

Fisher, J. O., and L. L. Birch. "Eating in the Absence of Hunger and Overweight in Girls from 5 to 7 y of Age." *American Journal of Clinical Nutrition* 76, no. 1 (2002): 226-31.

Fisher, J. O., and L. L. Birch. "Parents' Restrictive Feeding Practices Are Associated with Young Girls' Negative Self-Evaluation of Eating." *Journal of the American Dietetic Association* 100 (2000): 1341-46.

Fisher, J. O., and L. L. Birch. "Restricting Access to Food and Children's Eating." *Appetite* 32 (1999): 405-19.

Fisher, J. O., D. C. Mitchell, H. Smiciklas-Wright, M. L. Mannino, and L. L. Birch. "Meeting Calcium Recommendations During Middle Childhood Reflects Mother-Daughter Beverage Choices and

Predicts Bone Mineral Status." *American Journal of Clinical Nutrition* 79, no. 4 (2004): 698-706.

FMI Research Department. "Nature of Concern About Nutritional Content, 1989-1998." *Trends in the United States: Consumer Attitudes & the Supermarket*, 72. Washington, DC: Food Marketing Institute, 2003.

Fomon, S. J., L. J. Filer Jr., L. N. Thomas, T. A. Anderson, and S. E. Nelson. "Influence of Formula Concentration on Caloric Intake and Growth of Normal Infants." *Acta Paediatrica Scandanavica* 64 (1975): 172-81.

Food and Nutrition Service. "Team Nutrition, National School Lunch Program." Web page [accessed 16 January 2004]. Available at http://www.fns.usda.gov/cnd/lunch/.

Forsen, T., J. Eriksson, J. Tuomilehto, A. Reunanen, C. Osmond, and D. Barker. "The Fetal and Childhood Growth of Persons Who Develop Type 2 Diabetes." *Annals of Internal Medicine* 133, no. 3 (2000): 176-82.

Fredricks, J. A., and J. S. Eccles. "Children's Competence and Value Beliefs from Childhood Through Adolescence: Growth Trajectories in Two Male-Sex-Typed Domains. " *Developmental Psychology* 38 (2002): 519-33.

Freedman, D. S., W. H. Dietz, S. R. Srinivasan, and G. S. Berenson. "The Relation of Overweight to Cardiovascular Risk Factors Among Children and Adolescents: The Bogalusa Heart Study." *Pediatrics* 103, no. 6, pt. 1 (1999): 1175-82.

Freedman, D. S., L. K. Khan, W. H. Dietz, S. R. Srinivasan, and G. S. Berenson. "Relationship of Childhood Obesity to Coronary Heart Disease Risk Factors in Adulthood: The Bogalusa Heart Study." *Pediatrics* 108, no. 3 (2001): 712-18.

Freedman, D. S., M. K. Serdula, S. R. Srinivasan , and G. S. Berenson. "Relation of Circumferences and Skinfold Thicknesses to Lipid and Insulin Concentrations in Children and Adolescents: The Bogalusa Heart Study." *American Journal of Clinical Nutrition* 69, no. 2 (1999): 308-17.

Gennuso, J., L. H. Epstein, R. A. Paluch, and F. Cerny. "The Relationship Between Asthma and Obesity in Urban Minority Children and Adolescents." *Archives of Pediatrics and Adolescent Medicine* 152, no. 12 (1998): 1197-200.

Gillman, M. W., S. L. Rifas-Shiman, A. L. Frazier, H. R. Rockett, C. A. Camargo, A. E. Field, C. S. Berkey, and G. A. Colditz. "Family Dinner and Diet Quality Among Older Children and Adolescents."

Archives of Family Medicine 9 (2000): 235-40.

Glanz, K., M. Basil, E. Maibach, J. Goldberg, and D. Snyder. "Why Americans Eat What They Do: Taste, Nutrition, Cost, Convenience, and Weight Control Concerns as Influences on Food Consumption." *Journal of the American Dietetic Association* 98 (1998): 1118-26.

Goulding, A., J. Rockell, R. Black, A. Grant, I. Jones, and S. Williams. "Children Who Avoid Drinking Cow's Milk Are at Increased Risk for Prepubertal Bone Fractures." *Journal of the American Dietetic Association* 104, no. 2 (2004): 250-253.

Hamill, P. V. V., T. A. Drizd, C. L. Johnson, R. B. Reed, A. F. Roche, and W. M. Moore. "Physical Growth: National Center for Health Statistics Percentiles." *American Journal of Clinical Nutrition* 32 (1979): 607-29.

Himes, J. H., and W. H. Dietz. "Guidelines for Overweight in Adolescent Preventive Services: Recommendations from an Expert Committee. The Expert Committee on Clinical Guidelines for Overweight in Adolescent Preventive Services." *American Journal of Clinical Nutrition* 59, no. 2 (1994): 307-16.

Hofferth, S. L. "How American Children Spend Their Time." *Journal of Marriage and the Family* 63, no. 295-308 (2001).

Hoffmans, M. D., D. Kromhout, and C. De Lezenne Coulander. "The Impact of Body Mass Index of 78,612 18-Year-Old Dutch Men on 32-Year Mortality from All Causes." *Journal of Clinical Epidemiology* 41 (1988): 749-56.

Holbrook, T. L., and E. Barrett-Conner. "The Association of Lifetime Weight and Weight Control Patterns with Bone Mineral Density in an Adult Community." *Bone and Mineral* 20 (1993): 141-49.

Hood, M. Y., L. L. Moore, A. Sundarajan-Ramamurti, M. Singer, L. A. Cupples, and R. C. Ellison. "Parental Eating Attitudes and the Development of Obesity in Children. The Framingham Children's Study ." *International Journal of Obesity* 24 (2000): 1319-25.

Ikeda, J. P., P. Lyons, F. Schwartzman, and R. A. Mitchell. "Self-Reported Dieting Experiences of Women with Body Mass Indexes of 30 or More." *Journal of the American Dietetic Association* 104, no. 6 (2004): 972-74.

Jahns, L., A. M. Siega-Riz, and B. M. Popkin. "The Increasing Prevalence of Snacking Among US Children from 1977 to 1996." *Journal of Pediatrics* 138 (2001): 493-98.

Johnson, C. M. "Helping Infants to Sleep." *Pediatric Basics* 65 (1993): 10-16.

Johnson, S. L., and L. L. Birch. "Parents' and Children's Adiposity and Eating Style." *Pediatrics* 94 (1994): 653-61.

Johnston, L. D., P. M. O'Malley, and J. G. Bachman. *Monitoring the Future: National Survey Results on Drug Use.* Bethesda, MD: National Institute of Drug Abuse, 2002.

Jones, S. J., L. Jahns, B. A. Laraia, and B. Haughton. "Lower Risk of Overweight in School-Aged Food Insecure Girls Who Participate in Food Assistance: Results from the Panel Study of Income Dynamics Child Development Supplement." *Archives of Pediatrics and Adolescent Medicine* 157, no. 8 (2003): 780-784.

Kalkwarf, H. J., J. C. Khoury, and B. P. Lanphear. "Milk Intake During Childhood and Adolescence, Adult Bone Density, and Osteoporotic Fractures in US Women." *American Journal of Clinical Nutrition* 77, no. 1 (2003): 257-65.

Kaur, H., W. Choi, M. Mayo, and K. Jo Harris. "Duration of Television Watching Is Associated with Increased Body Mass Index." *Journal of Pediatrics* 143, no. 4 (2003): 506-11.

Kern, D. L., L. McPhee, J. Fisher, S. Johnson, and L. L. Birch. "The Postingestive Consequences of Fat Condition Preferences for Flavors Associated with High Dietary Fat." *Physiology and Behavior* 54 (1993): 71-76.

Keys, A., J. Brozek, A. Henschel, O. Mickelsen, and H. Taylor. *The Biology of Human Starvation.* Minneapolis: University of Minnesota Press, 1950.

Khosla, S., L. J. Melton 3rd, M. B. Dekutoski, S. J. Achenbach, A. L. Oberg, and B. L. Riggs. "Incidence of Childhood Distal Forearm Fractures Over 30 Years: A Population-Based Study." *Journal of the American Medical Association* 290, no. 11 (2003): 1479-85.

Klesges, R. C., M. L. Shelton, and L. M. Klesges. "Effects of Television on Metabolic Rate: Potential Implications for Childhood Obesity." *Pediatrics* 91, no. 2 (1993): 281-86.

Knol, L., B. Haughton, and E. Fitzhugh. "Food Insufficiency Is Not Related to the Overall Variety of Foods Consumed by Young Children in Low-Income Families." *Journal of the American Dietetic Association* 104, no. 4 (2004): 640-644.

Kvaavik, E., G. S. Tell, and K. I. Klepp. "Predictors and Tracking of Body Mass Index from Adolescence into Adulthood: Follow-Up of 18 to 20 Years in the Oslo Youth Study." *Archives of Pediatrics and Adolescent Medicine* 157, no. 12 (2003): 1212-18.

Lauer, R. M. , and W. R. Clarke. "Childhood Risk Factors for High Adult Blood Pressure: The Muscatine Study." *Pediatrics* 84, no. 4

(1989): 633-41.

Lean, M. E., T. S. Han, and J. C. Seidell. "Impairment of Health and Quality of Life Using New US Federal Guidelines for the Identification of Obesity." *Archives of Internal Medicine* 159 (1999): 837-43.

Legler, J. D., and L. C. Rose. "Assessment of Abnormal Growth Curves." *American Family Physician* 58 (1998): 158-68.

Leopold, A. K. "'Functional Fitness' Means Training for Your Real Life." *New York Times,* 6 June 2004, sec. 15, col. 1, p. 2.

Lifshitz, F., and O. Tarim. "Nutrition Dwarfing." *Current Problems in Pediatrics* 23 (1993): 322-36.

Lissau, I., and T. I. Sorensen. "Parental Neglect During Childhood and Increased Risk of Obesity in Young Adulthood." *Lancet* 343 (1994): 324-27.

Luepker, R. V., C. L. Perry, S. M. McKinlay, P. R. Nader, G. S. Parcel, E. J. Stone, L. S. Webber, J. P. Elder, H. A. Feldman, C. C. Johnson, et al. "Outcomes of a Field Trial to Improve Children's Dietary Patterns and Physical Activity. The Child and Adolescent Trial for Cardiovascular Health. CATCH Collaborative Group." *Journal of the American Medical Association* 275, no. 10 (1996): 768-76.

Lytle, L., and C. Achterberg. "Changing the Diet of America's Children: What Works and Why?" *Journal of Nutrition Education* 27 (1995): 250-260.

Lytle, L. A., A. L. Eldridge, K. Kotz, J. Piper, S. Williams, and B. Kalina. "Children's Interpretation of Nutrition Messages." *Journal of Nutrition Education* 29 (1997): 128-36.

Maccoby, E. E. *Social Development: Psychological Growth and the Parent-Child Relationship.* New York: Harcourt Brace Jovanovich, 1980.

Mackin, M. L., S. V. Medendorp, and M. C. Maier. "Infant Sleep and Bedtime Cereal." *American Journal of Diseases in Childhood* 143 (1989): 1066-68.

Mayer, J., P. Roy, and K. P. Mitra. "Relation Between Caloric Intake, Body Weight, and Physical Work." *American Journal of Clinical Nutrition* 4, no. 2 (1956): 169-75.

Moore, L. L., D. Gao, M. L. Bradlee, L. A. Cupples, A. Sundarajan-Ramamurti, M. H. Proctor , M. Y. Hood, M. R. Singer, and R. C. Ellison. "Does Early Physical Activity Predict Body Fat Change Throughout Childhood?" *Preventive Medicine* 37, no. 1 (2003): 10-7.

Mrdjenovic, G., and D. A. Levitsky. "Nutritional and Energetic Consequences of Sweetened Drink Consumption in 6- to 13-Year-Old Children." *Journal of Pediatrics* 142, no. 6 (2003): 604-10.

Must, A., P. F. Jacques, G. E. Dallal, C. J. Bajema, and W. H. Dietz. "Long-Term Morbidity and Mortality of Overweight Adolescents. A Follow-Up of the Harvard Growth Study of 1922 to 1935." *New England Journal of Medicine* 327, no. 19 (1992): 1350-55.

National Association of State Boards of Education. "Healthy Schools: Fit, Healthy, and Ready to Learn. A school health policy guide." Web page [accessed 16 January 2004]. Available at http://www.nasbe.org.

National Research Council. *Recommended Dietary Allowances,* 10th ed. Washington, DC: National Academy Press, 1989.

Nicklas, T. A. "Calcium Intake Trends and Health Consequences from Childhood Through Adulthood." *Journal of the American College of Nutrition* 22, no. 5 (2003): 340-56.

Nielsen, S. J., A. M. Siega-Riz, and B. M. Popkin. "Trends in Food Locations and Sources Among Adolescents and Young Adults." *Preventive Medicine* 35, no. 2 (2002): 107-13.

Nieto, F. J., M. Szklo, and G. W. Comstock. "Childhood Weight and Growth Rate as Predictors of Adult Mortality." *American Journal of Epidemiology* 136, no. 2 (1992): 201-13.

Novotny, R. "Higher Dairy Intake Is Associated with Lower Body Fat During Adolescence." *FASEB Journal* 17(4) (2003): A453.8. Abstract.

Ogden, C. L., K. M. Flegal, M. D. Carroll, and C. L. Johnson. "Prevalence and Trends in Overweight Among US Children and Adolescents, 1999-2000." *Journal of the American Medical Association* 288, no. 14 (2002): 1728-32.

Ogden, C. L., R. J. Kuczmarski, K. M. Flegal, Z. Mei, S. Guo, R. Wei, L. M. Grummer-Strawn, L. R. Curtin, A. F. Roche, and C. L. Johnson. "Centers for Disease Control and Prevention 2000 Growth Charts for the United States: Improvements to the 1977 National Center for Health Statistics Version ." *Pediatrics* 109, no. 1 (2002): 45-60.

Pereira, M. A., D. R. Jacobs Jr, L. Van Horn, M. L. Slattery, A. I. Kartashov, and D. S. Ludwig. "Dairy Consumption, Obesity, and the Insulin Resistance Syndrome in Young Adults: The CARDIA Study." *Journal of the American Medical Association* 287, no. 16 (2002): 2081-9.

Powers, S. I., S. T. Hauser, and L A. Kilner. "Adolescent Mental Health." *American Psychologist* 44 (1989): 200-208.

Reilly, J. J., A. Kelly, P. Ness, A. R. Dorosty, W. H. Wallace, B. E. Gibson, P. M. Emmett, and and the ALSPAC Study Team. "Premature Adiposity Rebound in Children Treated for Acute Lymphoblastic Leukemia (ALL)." *Journal of Clinical Endocrinology and Metabolism*

86 (2001): 2775-78.

Rocandio, A. M., L. Ansotegui, and M. Arroyo. "Comparison of Dietary Intake Among Overweight and Non-Overweight Schoolchildren." *International Journal of Obesity and Related Metabolic Disorders* 25, no. 11 (2001): 1651-5.

Roemmich, J. N., S. M. Wright, and L. H. Epstein . "Dietary Restraint and Stress-Induced Snacking in Youth." *Obesity Research* 10, no. 11 (2002): 1120-26.

Rogers, K. B. "Parenting Processes Related to Sexual Risk-Taking Behaviors of Adolescent Males and Females." *Journal of Marriage and the Family* 61 (1999): 99-109.

Rolls, B. J., L. Roe, J. Meengs, and D. Wall. "Increasing the Portion Size of a Sandwich Increases Energy Intake." *Journal of the American Dietetic Association* 104, no. 3 (2004): 367-72.

Rolls, B. J. "Sensory Specific Satiety." *Nutrition Reviews* 44 (1986): 93-101.

Rolls, B. J., J. A. Ello-Martin, and B. C. Tohill. "What Can Intervention Studies Tell Us About the Relationship Between Fruit and Vegetable Consumption and Weight Management?" *Nutrition Reviews* 62, no. 1 (2004): 1-17.

Rolls, B. J., D. Engell, and L. L. Birch. "Serving Portion Size Influences 5-Year-Old but Not 3-Year-Old Children's Food Intakes." *Journal of the American Dietetic Association* 100 (2000): 232-34.

Rose, H. E., and J. Mayer. "Activity, Calorie Intake, Fat Storage, and the Energy Balance of Infants." *Pediatrics* 41 (1968): 18-29.

Ryan, A. S., G. A. Martinez, and A. F. Roche. "An Evaluation of the Association Between Socioeconomic Status and the Growth of American Children: Data from the Hispanic Health and Nutrition Examination Survey-NHANES 1982-1984." *American Journal of Clinical Nutrition* 51 (1990): 944S-52S.

Saelens, B. E., J. F. Sallis, P. R. Nader, S. L. Broyles, C. C. Berry, and H. L. Taras. "Home Environmental Influences on Children's Television Watching from Early to Middle Childhood." *Journal of Developmental and Behavioral Pediatrics* 23, no. 3 (2002): 127-32.

Satter, E. M. "Appendix G: Dietary Fat and Heart Disease-It's Not as Bad as You Think ." *Secrets of Feeding a Healthy Family*, 211-13. Madison, WI: Kelcy Press , 1999.

Satter, E. M. "Appendix H: Children, Dietary Fat and Heart Disease-You Don't Have to Panic." *Secrets of Feeding a Healthy Family*, 214-16. Madison, WI: Kelcy Press , 1999.

Satter, E. M. "Childhood Eating Disorders." *Journal of the American*

Dietetic Association 86 (1986): 357-61.

Satter, E. M. "The Feeding Relationship." *Journal of the American Dietetic Association* 86 (1986): 352-56.

Satter, E. M. "The Feeding Relationship: Problems and Interventions ." *Journal of Pediatrics* 117 (1990): S181-S189.

Satter, E. M. "Internal Regulation and the Evolution of Normal Growth as the Basis for Prevention of Obesity in Childhood." *Journal of the American Dietetic Association* 96 (1996): 860-864.

Satter, E. M. "A Moderate View on Fat Restriction for Young Children." *Journal of the American Dietetic Association* , no. 100 (2000): 32-36.

Saunders, R. B., C. B. Friedman, and P. R. Stramoski. "Feeding Preterm Infants: Schedule or Demand?" *Journal of Obstetrics, Gynecological and Neonatal Nursing* 20 (1990): 212-18.

Schwimmer, J. B., T. M. Burwinkle, and J. W. Varni. "Health-Related Quality of Life of Severely Obese Children and Adolescents." *Journal of the American Medical Association* 289, no. 14 (2003): 1813-19.

Serdula, M. K., D. Ivery, R. J. Coates, D. S. Freedman, D. F. Williamson, and T. Byers. "Do Obese Children Become Obese Adults? A Review of the Literature." *Preventive Medicine* 22 (1993): 167-77.

Shedler, J., and J. Block. "Adolescent Drug Use and Psychological Health: A Longitudinal Inquiry." *American Psychologist* 45 (1990): 612-30.

Shunk, J. A., and L. L. Birch. "Girls at Risk for Overweight at Age 5 Are at Risk for Dietary Restraint, Disinhibited Overeating, Weight Concerns, and Greater Weight Gain from 5 to 9 Years." *Journal of the American Dietetic Association* 104, no. 7 (2004): 1120-6.

Sills, R. H. "Failure to Thrive: The Role of Clinical and Laboratory Evaluation." *American Journal of Diseases of Children* 132 (1978): 967-69.

Simmons, R. G., F. Rosenberg, and M Rosenberg. "Disturbance in the Self-Image at Adolescence." *American Sociological Review* 38 (1973): 553-68.

Sinaiko, A. R., R. P. Donahue, D. R. Jacobs Jr., and R. J. Prineas. "Relation of Weight and Rate of Increase in Weight During Childhood and Adolescence to Body Size, Blood Pressure, Fasting Insulin, and Lipids in Young Adults: The Minneapolis Children's Blood Pressure Study." *Circulation* 99, no. 11 (1999): 1471-76.

Skinner, J., W. Bounds, B. Carruth, and P. Ziegler. "Longitudinal Calcium Intake Is Negatively Related to Children's Body Fat Indexes." *Journal of the American Dietetic Association* 103, no. 12

(2003): 1626-31.

Skinner, J. D., B. R. Carruth, K. Houck, J. Moran, A. Reed, F. Coletta, and D. Ott. "Mealtime Communication Patterns of Infants from 2 to 24 Months of Age." *Journal of Nutrition Education* 30 (1998): 8-16.

Stattin, H., and M. Kerr. "Parental Monitoring: A Reinterpretation." *Child Development* 71, no. 4 (2000): 1072-85.

Stayton, D. J., R. Hogan, and M. D. S. Ainsworth. "Infant Obedience and Maternal Behavior: The Origins of Socialization Reconsidered." *Child Development* 42 (1971): 1057-69.

Stice, E., R. P. Cameron, J. D. Killen, C. Hayward, and C. B. Taylor. "Naturalistic Weight-Reduction Efforts Prospectively Predict Growth in Relative Weight and Onset of Obesity Among Female Adolescents." *Journal of Consulting and Clinical Psychology* 67 (1999): 967-74.

Subar, A. F., S. M. Krebs-Smith, A. Cook, and L. L. Kahle. "Dietary Sources of Nutrients Among U.S. Adults, 1989 to 1991." *Journal of the American Dietetic Association* 98 (1998): 537-47.

Tanner, J. M., H. Goldstein, and R. H. Whitehouse. "Standards for Children's Height at Ages 2 to 9 Years Allowing for Height of Parents." *Archives of Disease in Childhood* 45 (1970): 755-62.

Taubes, G. "What If It's All Been a Big Fat Lie? " *New York Times Magazine*, 7 July 2002.

Taylor, R. W., I. E. Jones, S. M. Williams, and A. Goulding. "Body Fat Percentages Measured by Dual-Energy X-Ray Absorptiometry Corresponding to Recently Recommended Body Mass Index Cutoffs for Overweight and Obesity in Children and Adolescents Aged 3-18 y." *American Journal of Clinical Nutrition* 76, no. 6 (2002): 1416-21.

The Onion. "More U.S. Children Being Diagnosed with Youthful Tendency Disorder." 36, no. 34 (2000).

Toomey, K. A. "Caloric Intake of Toddlers Fed Structured Meals and Snacks Versus on Demand." *Verbal Communication* (1994).

Twenge, J. M. "The Age of Anxiety? Birth Cohort Change in Anxiety and Neuroticism, 1952-1993." *Journal of Personality and Social Psychology* 79 (2000): 1007-21.

Videon, T. M., and C. K. Manning. "Influences on Adolescent Eating Patterns: The Importance of Family Meals." *Journal of Adolescent Health* 32, no. 5 (2003): 365-73.

von Mutius, E., J. Schwartz, L. M. Neas, D. Dockery, and S. T. Weiss. "Relation of Body Mass Index to Asthma and Atopy in Children: The National Health and Nutrition Examination Study III." *Thorax*

56, no. 11 (2001): 835-38.

Wallace, J. R., T. F. Cunningham, and V DelMonte . "Change and Stablity in Self-Esteem Between Late Childhood and Early Adolescence." *Journal of Early Adolescence* 4 (1984): 253-57.

Wei, M., J. B. Kampert, C. E. Barlow, M. Z. Nichaman, L. W. Gibbons, R. S. Paffenbarger, and S. N. Blair. "Relationship Between Low Cardiorespiratory Fitness and Mortality in Normal-Weight, Overweight, and Obese Men." *Journal of the American Medical Association* 282 (1999): 1547-53.

Wolraich, M. L., D. B. Wilson, and J. W. White. "The Effect of Sugar on Behavior or Cognition in Children: A Meta-Analysis." *Journal of the American Medical Association* 274, no. 20 (1995): 1617-21.

Wright, C. M, L. Parker, D. Lamont, and A. W. Craft. "Implications of Childhood Obesity for Adult Health: Findings from Thousand Families Cohort Study." *British Medical Journal* 323, no. 7324 (2001): 1280-1284.

Wyshak, G. "Teenaged Girls, Carbonated Beverage Consumption, and Bone Fractures." *Archives of Pediatrics and Adolescent Medicine* 154 (2000): 610-613.

Zemel, M. B. "Mechanisms of Dairy Modulation of Adiposity." *Journal of Nutrition* 133, no. 1 (2003): 252S-6S.

Zlotkin, S., and A. McGowan. *Family Dynamics Correlates with Massive Obesity in Preschoolers.* Verbal communication, 1995.

INDEX

References to the major treatment of topics are printed in bold.

SECRETS OF FEEDING A HEALTHY FAMILY

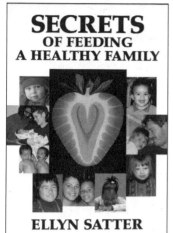

SECRETS
OF FEEDING
A HEALTHY FAMILY

ELLYN SATTER

A MUST-HAVE FOR GETTING A MEAL ON THE TABLE. The perfect companion to *Your Child's Weight*, this kitchen primer tells adults how to feed themselves and their families joyfully, appealingly and wisely. Satter's expertise in child feeding informs her suggestions for involving children in the kitchen and adapting menus for them. Recipe, planning and shopping chapters as well as fast tips, night-before suggestions, why-to, how-to.

Purchased by: WIC, Head Start, CACFP, Extension, PTA, early childhood organizations, child care providers, preschools, primary schools and universities as a text for nutrition for non-majors.

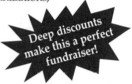

Deep discounts make this a perfect fundraiser!

1-9 books	$16.95 each
10-35 books (30% discount, no return)	$11.50 each
Carton of 34 books (60% discount, no return)	$230.00 carton

Kelcy Press, 1999, 240 pages, index, appendixes.

What Others Have Said

...a wonderful sense of bringing together a 'creative and explorative' spirit to meals and food preparation. The section on shopping, recipes and cooking is written so enthusiastically that it all seems new again.
　　　—*Journal of Nutrition Education*

I love this book! I just made another fabulous dinner for my family using the recipes from Secrets of Feeding a Healthy Family. *Ellyn tells you how to get started the night before, how to cook and even how to involve your child. Who knew cooking and eating a balanced dinner could be so fun!*
　　　—*Jennifer Hoots, parent*

I can't tell you how often I consult Secrets—*and how often I refer other people to it as my favorite all-around nutrition information book. Thanks so much for your great work!*
　　　—*Jon Robison, PhD, Health Educator, editor,* Health At Every Size *Journal*

CONTENTS

Chapters

1. The Secret in a Nutshell
2. You and Your Eating
3. The Feeding Relationship
4. Choosing Food For Your Family
5. How to Get (Started) Cooking
6. How to Continue Cooking
7. Enjoy Fruits and Vegetables
8. Planning to Get You Cooking
9. Shopping to Get You Cooking
10. Raising a Healthy Eater in Your Community

Appendixes - 10 in all, including:
- To diet or not to diet
- Children, dietary fat, and heart disease
- A primer on dietary fat

Samples and more information at **www.EllynSatter.com**

CHECK YOUR LOCAL BOOKSTORE OR ORDER DIRECTLY FROM US!

ORDER FORM

	Price Each	QTY	TTL

Your Child's Weight: Helping Without Harming
(10 or less) . . . . \$19.95 each   _____   \$ _____

Your Child's Weight: Helping Without Harming
(11 or more) (30% discount) . . . . \$13.97 each   _____   \$ _____

Your Child's Weight: Helping Without Harming
(carton) (60% discount) . . . . \$9.98 each   (call for details)

SUBTOTAL . . . . \$ _____

Wisconsin Residents
Add 5.5% tax or submit tax exempt number
(\$1.10 for a single copy) . . . . \$ _____

Shipping (\$5.00 first book, \$2.00 each additional book,
\$25.00 each case of books. International shipping rates may vary) \$ _____

BOOKS, TAX AND SHIPPING TOTAL (\$26.05 for a single copy) \$ _____

PAYMENT INFORMATION

Prepayment required on orders of less than \$50.

☐ Check is enclosed

☐ Purchase order for \$50.00 or more is enclosed #

Please charge: ☐ M/C   ☐ Visa   ☐ Discover

Card # _____ Exp_____

Name as it appears on card_____

Signature _____

Billing Address (must be the same as address on the credit card statement)

☐ Billing address is same as shipping address below

Address _____

City_____ State _____ Zip_____

Make checks payable to Kelcy Press. Return order form and payment to:

Kelcy Press   Telephone: 877-844-0857
4226 Mandan Crescent, Ste 57   FAX: 866-724-1631
Madison, WI 53711-3062

SHIPPING INFORMATION

Last name_____ Firstname_____

Profession_____ Place of work_____

Address_____

Address (Cont.)_____

City_____ State_____ Zip_____

Telephone_____ E-Mail (we do not spam)_____